The Food Medic:

The Female Factor

The Food Medic:

The Female Factor

Making women's health count – and what it means for you

Dr Hazel Wallace

Photography by Lizzie Mayson

This book is
dedicated to all
the women I have
had the pleasure of
providing care to.

Contents

Introduction

Welcome to *The Female Factor*. A lot has changed in the last few years, and you'll notice it in the content you'll find here in my third book. I've grown as a person and my mission with The Food Medic has evolved. So, to those of you who have read my first two books, and to those of you who are new here, in the words of Jay-Z, allow me to reintroduce myself:

The Food Medic was born out of a passion project of mine back in 2012 while at medical school. After losing my father suddenly to a stroke in my teens, I became fascinated by how nutrition and lifestyle can influence our health and genetic predisposition to disease. However, in lectures, only lip service was paid to non-medical interventions like diet, physical activity, sleep and stress management, so I set out to learn more about how our lifestyle shapes our health and started to blog about my findings in accessible, easy-to-follow articles and social media captions as 'The Food Medic'.

I wrote and published my first book – *The Food Medic* – in 2017, while working full-time as a first-year doctor in London, and released my second book – *The Food Medic for Life* – in 2018. Over this time, my passion for nutrition and public health continued to grow, which brought me back to university the following year to complete my master's in clinical nutrition and public health at University College London (UCL), allowing me to become dual-registered as a doctor and a nutritionist.

Nutrition will always be my biggest passion, but as a woman, and as a doctor to many women, I wanted to expand the work I do, especially when I discovered there was an unmet need within medicine and healthcare. I realised that our current model of male-centric medicine meant that women were understudied, underdiagnosed, misdiagnosed and undertreated. In most of the research I studied, it appeared that medicine sees our reproductive organs and hormones as our greatest source of difference to men and holds the assumption that pretty much everything else works in the same way, so can be fixed in the same way. But, in the words of Dr Stacy Sims, 'women are not small men'.

The more I shared female-focused research (albeit limited) and content online, the more women responded. My direct messages on Instagram would be filled with women who had similar experiences and felt like they weren't being listened to. Every post I curated that examined health topics under a female lens turned into an engaged and empowered discussion among my followers – among many of you. It made me want to learn more, to share more, to empower more. I knew there was an unmet need here and wanted to find some answers.

And so, for the past three years (in between COVID shifts at the hospital), I've dedicated most of my time to researching how to help *women* live healthier, happier lives.

And *The Female Factor* was born.

How Science Sees Women

The male body has always been the default body in biomedical research, and female subjects have been historically excluded. Here's the thing, we have so much incredible medical research available to us now, but most of it is based on male cells, male mice and male bodies, then simply applied to women.

I'll say that again for the people in the back: Most clinical research ignores the female sex and is centred around cis (a person whose sense of personal identity and gender corresponds with their birth sex.), endosex (a person born with sex characteristics that are considered typically male or female) men. It is also worth highlighting that transgender women are similarly excluded from medical research, even if their healthcare needs are not the focus of this particular book.

Even when it comes to research based on animals, there is a significant male bias in eight out of ten areas of biology.[1] For example, in studies of drug treatments, there is a five-to-one male-to-female ratio.[2] That's quite concerning considering women typically respond to drug treatments differently and experience adverse drug reactions nearly twice as often as men.[3] An analysis of prescription drugs withdrawn in the US market from 1997 to 2001 found that eight out of ten posed 'greater health risks for women'.[4] This is not simply because women are 'smaller men' (though on average we are smaller humans), but we also have smaller organs, more body fat (which can trap certain drugs), slower gut motility (affects drug absorption) and excrete drugs slower via the kidneys – all of which increase the risk of overmedication and adverse reactions, if not accounted for.[5]

Historically, researchers have argued that the female body is too complex to be included in studies due to fluctuating hormones and the risk of pregnancy, or that women are too difficult to recruit because of their caregiving responsibilities and the inflexibility of research trials. The latter being an argument that is simply infuriating and underpins the complex relationship between our sex (biology) and gender stereotypes (and the social norms that come with it), and how they both influence our health and the healthcare we receive.

Research into unique reproductive or gynaecological health problems that affect women and people assigned female biologically at birth isn't any better. For example, only 2.5 per cent of publicly funded research is dedicated to reproductive health, despite the fact that one in three women in the UK will suffer from a reproductive or gynaecological health problem in their life.[6]

Indeed, inequalities in health and research for women is also compounded by race and class. While it takes on average an already unacceptable eight years for a woman to be diagnosed with endometriosis, in the UK black women are shockingly half as likely as white women to be diagnosed.[7]

Our deeply embedded beliefs and unconscious biases that we hold about women and their health experiences are causing unnecessary – and preventable – suffering.

From research to healthcare, as well as the media narrative, it is all biased towards men, and the aim of this book is to dismantle and change that narrative.

Here's the thing: our fluctuating hormones may be considered a 'nuisance' for researchers, but actually they provide us with additional insight into the inner workings of our bodies. Sex hormones are not only orchestrating our reproductive health, but affecting our metabolism, as well as our bone, heart, gut and brain health . . . and even the way we sleep.

Similarly, across the lifespan, women experience important hormonal milestones – puberty, perinatally and after the menopause – which alter how our bodies function and can be windows of vulnerability for certain health conditions such as depression, anxiety and insomnia.

Although healthcare professionals strive for equal treatment of all patients, sex and gender bias exists throughout the healthcare system, from the interactions between patients and doctors to the medical research and policies that govern it. Indeed, this bias does not only affect one gender, but it disproportionately affects women and can have a serious impact on their health and healthcare. For example, women are diagnosed later for heart disease, not only because it is still largely considered a 'man's disease', but also because our understanding and diagnostic tests are male-biased. I wasn't aware of this at medical school – I hope that future medics will be.

Fortunately, in recent years there has been a big drive to improve the sex/gender gap in research, but there is still a long way to go and women are still being medically treated with outdated guidelines based on male subjects and a male-centric narrative.

Changing the Narrative

While you may not sit around reading research papers for fun (just me, right?), this gendered information is reaching you through the media, whether that be published or social. News headlines read 'Heart Attacks Kill Men', when in fact they're the biggest killer of both sexes.[8] Meanwhile, social media posts tell women to #Tone, #Sculpt and #Fast, instead of #Build, #Bulk and #Fuel.

Even from an early age, we are being sold the message that females are inferior – ask young children to draw a scientist and they are more than *twice as likely* to draw a man than a woman.[9] Unsurprisingly, children's science books contain pictures of males three times more often than females, reinforcing the stereotype that science is a man's pursuit and also influencing girls' perceptions of what they are (or aren't) capable of.[10] You might think that picture books aren't important, but they mimic what the advertising industry is doing every time we open a magazine, scroll through a social media app or watch TV. It's this glass ceiling that prevents women from achieving their full potential – but you are not weaker, you are not less smart, you are not less capable . . . and science backs this up!

Knowledge is power

My intention with this book is to empower women, not shout about all the ways in which we have been hard done by. This is also not a 'f*&k you' to men – I love men, but I dislike the repression and underrepresentation of women.

So, with this book, I am expanding the definition of 'women's health' from conditions that only affect our reproductive organs, to the study of all aspects of health and disease, with the recognition that presentation, diagnosis, treatment and prevention may be different between the sexes.

There are some things we can't change – like our genes – but by understanding our unique female physiology we can harness this information to improve our health and reduce our risk of illness. This book provides you with a method to do just that, helping you to make your body work with you, not against you.

I have written *The Female Factor* in four sections: Nutrition, Movement, Mood and Sleep. Each topic has been examined through the female lens, for a female audience. However, I believe this information is important for everyone. Knowledge is power, in my view, so I hope that the more you read about your unique physiology, the more empowered you will feel about supporting it. Each chapter guides you through the hormonal milestones most women experience: I explore how nutrition plays a role across our menstrual cycle; how our fitness is shaped by our physical make-up; how our hormones affect our mental health across our lifespan; and how sleep can save your sanity, no matter the day of the month. If I've done my job, by the time you've finished reading this book, you will feel empowered by your body, you will feel ready to support yourself in ways you never have before and you will share everything you've learned with every woman in your life.

What about food?

Of course, me being The Food Medic, there are recipes in *The Female Factor* too, but, if you've read my previous books or listened to my podcasts, you know that I don't sign up to the reductionist notion of using food as medicine. So, I'm afraid I'm not going to tell you to 'eat this' to 'cure that', but throughout the book I will make nutrition-based recommendations and suggest practical ways in which you can implement these into your diet, while signposting some recipes along the way.

A note on sex and gender

Sex and gender are terms that are often used interchangeably but are in fact two very different things.

Sex refers to the biological and physiological differences between males and females; that is genetics (XX and XY chromosomes), reproductive organs and hormones. While sex is normally assigned at birth, people can also change their sex through sex reassignment surgery and by taking hormones (biomedical gender transition). Also, conditions exist by which a person may be born with external genitalia that are ambiguous or do not match their chromosomal sex (intersex).

Gender, on the other hand, is a social, psychological and cultural construct and relates to the behaviours and attributes expected by different societies and cultures based on their understanding of what it is to be 'masculine' or 'feminine'. People may identify as a man, a woman, having no gender (agender) or as non-binary. A person's gender may correspond to their sex assigned at birth (cisgender) or they may identify with a gender that is not consistent with their sex assigned at birth (transgender).

Throughout this book I refer to both sex and gender and do my best to use them appropriately. However, even in the world of scientific research, sex and gender are often (incorrectly) used interchangeably and, as you will see throughout each chapter, both our sex and our gender influence our health and access to healthcare, but it can be difficult to disentangle and quantify the exact contributions of each.

Unfortunately, there is very little research that is inclusive of transgender people[11-13], which of course also has an impact on health outcomes for this group. While I acknowledge this in itself is problematic, it goes beyond the scope of this particular book. I have chosen to focus on the health of women and people assigned female at birth, and so when I use the words 'woman' or 'female' in this book, I am referring to people with female reproductive anatomy who identify as women, unless otherwise stated, and I recognise this may not speak to everyone who identifies as a woman. Also, I am a cisgender, white female and my experiences shared in this book may not be representative of other women.

Our Hormonal Lifespan

Just so that we're all on the same page, I want to begin with the basics. The female hormonal lifespan has three potential milestones: puberty, pregnancy and menopause. From our first bleed, menstruation shapes our lives, so it's important to know what a 'typical' cycle looks like, so we can know where we fit in and/or if something changes, what to do about it.

I want to stress that there are many variations to the norm when it comes to what is 'healthy' and, as we age, this may also change. What's important is knowing what is normal for you and looking out for any red flags, such as very erratic, irregular or absent periods, very painful periods, very heavy periods or bleeding in between periods, after sex or after the menopause.

The average menstrual cycle is said to be 28 days long, although most are not textbook and anything between 21 and 40 days is considered normal. Menstruation, or the period, occurs on day 1 and usually ends on day 5 or 6. The cycle is split into two main phases: the follicular phase (think follicular first) and the luteal phase (and luteal last), with ovulation sandwiched in between on day 14. All of this is orchestrated by the ebb and flow of four hormones in particular: oestrogen, progesterone, follicle-stimulating hormone (FSH) and luteinising hormone (LH).

In the first part of the follicular phase, oestrogen and progesterone levels are low and the lining of the womb (endometrium) sheds – this is the period. In the late follicular phase, oestrogen rises, peaking just before ovulation and, together with a surge in LH, ovulation is triggered. As the egg is released, oestrogen levels dip. Moving into the luteal phase now, progesterone levels rise and surpass oestrogen, preparing the lining of the womb for pregnancy. Oestrogen is also high during this time. If pregnancy does not occur, progesterone and oestrogen levels fall in the late luteal phase and a period occurs, starting the cycle once more (see charts overleaf).

Hormone levels in a menstrual cycle

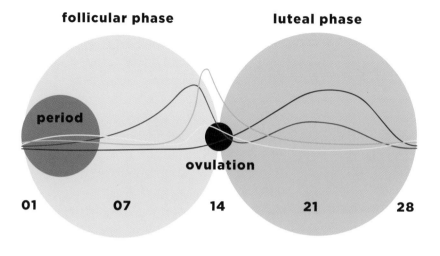

follicular phase　　　　**luteal phase**

period

ovulation

01　　　07　　　14　　　21　　　28

——— progesterone
——— oestrogen
——— luteinising hormone (LH)
——— follicule-stimulating hormone (FSH)

Follicular phase		Ovulation	Luteal phase
Menstruation: Oestrogen and progesterone levels are low and the lining of endometrium sheds. FSH levels gradually rise, causing stimulation of a few ovarian follicles.	Oestrogen rises, peaking just before ovulation. LH peaks ('LH surge') and triggers ovulation.	Egg is released. Oestrogen levels dip.	After ovulation and before the start of menstruation, progesterone levels rise and surpass oestrogen – preparing the lining of the womb for pregnancy. Oestrogen is also high during this time. If pregnancy does not occur, progesterone and oestrogen levels fall, and a period occurs.

When our reproductive years begin to pass us, we move into another phase of our hormonal lifespan: the menopause. It's funny how we learn about our first period at school, but we rarely talk about our last and what comes next – but, for many women, they will live a third of their life in the post-menopause phase. The menopause may signify the end of your reproductive life, but it does not signal the end of living. There are tools in this book that can help you to transition through this phase with as much ease as possible, but before we get into that, here are a few definitions so that you can understand what is happening to you, as you age:

- The menopause is a point in time 12 months after the final menstrual period. In the UK, the average age is 51 years, although this can vary between different ethnic groups. Post-menopause refers to the period after this in a woman's life.

- Perimenopause refers to the time during which your body makes the natural transition to menopause. It starts with irregular periods and ends 12 months after the last menstrual period. It typically lasts four years, but for some it's only a few months and for others it may be ten years.

- Early menopause occurs between 40 and 45 years of age, while a woman is said to have entered 'premature menopause' if it has occurred before 40 years of age.

- Premature ovarian insufficiency (POI) is the temporary or permanent loss of ovarian function before the age of 40 and is characterised by irregular or absent periods.

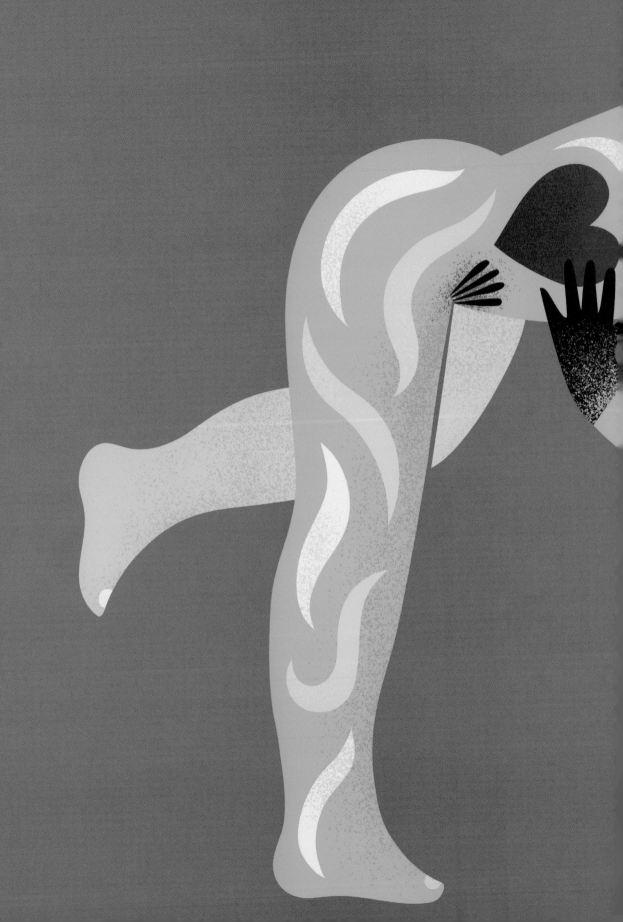

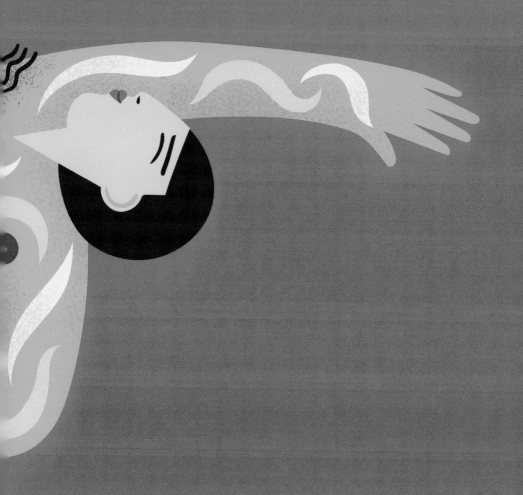

Nutrition

Nutrition

When I started writing this book, this was the chapter I was most excited about. As a qualified nutritionist and doctor, this topic is my bread and butter, but my enthusiasm and excitement were quickly diminished by the fact that there is little research, very few publications and minimal media focus on the specific nutritional needs of women beyond the usual calorie requirements, what foods to avoid when pregnant or breastfeeding and which nutrients best support fertility.

Of course, nutrition is extremely important during those critical periods and we will cover them in detail in this chapter, but a woman's nutrition should matter not (only) because of her pregnancy status or wish for children, but in order to be healthy and to thrive.

Here's the thing: yes, females (on average) require fewer calories overall than men (due to body size and muscle mass), but there are certain vitamin and mineral requirements that are of particular importance for women at certain points of their lives, such as iron after puberty, folic acid during pregnancy and calcium and vitamin D for bone health after the menopause.

Across the menstrual cycle, women have different calorie and nutrient needs too, due to fluctuations in sex hormones. Women also suffer from unique gynae issues, such as premenstrual syndrome (PMS), endometriosis and polycystic ovary syndrome (PCOS), all of which can be influenced by nutrition. Reproductive organs aside, women are also more likely to experience common nutrition-related gut issues such as irritable bowel syndrome (IBS), coeliac disease, constipation, haemorrhoids and anal fissures – oh, the joy!

Nutrition in females is a complex topic, not least because we have unique nutritional needs across the lifespan, but we also tend to have more food-related issues than men, such as extreme dieting behaviours and body dissatisfaction. Very few of us will escape our teenage years and twenties with a completely healthy relationship with food and will often (consciously or subconsciously) have ingrained food rules that we likely picked up from a tabloid magazine some years ago; for example, asking for salad dressing on the side, drinking water when we're hungry, never eating white carbs – or never eating carbs full stop.

Growing up, we are massively influenced by the people around us and absorb what we read in magazines and see on TV. Little things – like my older relatives praising me for turning down a biscuit or a piece of cake (but encouraging the boys in the family to eat up) or my mum cutting out bread in the weeks leading up to our summer holidays – make subtle but long-lasting changes to how we view food.

I'm not immune to diet culture and, as a teen, I had my own complex relationship with food and my body, and my diet-du-jour was usually mimicked from the 'what I eat in a day' feature of popular (very slim) celebs in magazines – I can't say I ever enjoyed the steamed fish and boiled veg for dinner or felt quite full after the afternoon snack of approximately three-and-a-half almonds. I also gave a juice cleanse a go after a neighbour commented on the fact that I was filling out. Looking back now, these practices seem pretty outrageous to me, but they felt totally normal and acceptable at the time.

Of course, boys and men are not immune to these stigmatised images of the 'ideal body' type and many men experience disordered eating and relationships with their bodies, but for women, it goes beyond this and is deeply entrenched in our cultural and societal beliefs of what it means to be 'a lady' or 'feminine' – from portion control to table etiquette.

Well, I am here to tell you that you deserve to eat regardless of your sex or gender, even if you haven't exercised, even if you're trying to lose weight, even if you ate more than usual yesterday, even if you're not having a 'good body day'.

In this chapter, we are going to explore how to eat for your unique female physiology and how to fuel it so that you can function at your best at every stage of life. I want to reframe food as fuel – not something you need to fear.

The Basics of a Healthy Diet

The majority of my readers know (vaguely anyway) what a healthy diet looks like, but the concept of 'balanced eating' or 'eating healthily' can still feel quite overwhelming and confusing. This is made worse by the *ton* of misinformation out there. To keep things really simple, a balanced meal can be built around the following rough guidance:

- Lots of colourful fruit and non-starchy vegetables ($1/3$–$1/2$ plate).

- About a fistful ($1/3$–$1/4$ plate) of grains or starchy vegetables such as potatoes, bread and cereals, ideally including some whole grains for additional fibre.

- A palm-sized portion ($1/3$–$1/4$ plate) of lean protein such as meat, fish, dairy or plant proteins, such as pulses and tofu.

- A thumb-sized portion (or sprinkle/drizzle) of fats, including some sources of unsaturated fats such as nuts and nut butter, seeds, avocado or plant-based oils.

- Occasional (optional) extras such as sweets and savoury snacks because, while sugar and salt are not hard to come by in a typical Western diet (and many of us could do with consuming a little less), having a little bit of what you fancy still fits into a balanced diet and makes it more realistic that you will eat well most of the time (rather than having an 'all-or-nothing' mindset). Allowing yourself to enjoy these foods is also an important part of a healthy relationship with food.

The above can be applied to most dietary types, but if you exclude certain foods altogether, such as dairy or animal products, you will need to take particular care to include fortified alternatives and, in some cases, supplementation. Check out my DIY Protein Poke Bowl on page 210 for a good example of a balanced meal.

Do Women Have Specific Nutrient Needs Across the Menstrual Cycle?

Let's start at the beginning. Your first period and the onset of puberty is where nutritional differences between males and females become apparent.

Over the course of the menstrual cycle, women have different calorie and nutrient requirements due to fluctuations in sex hormones, namely progesterone and oestrogen. These hormones not only influence our monthly cycle but also our body temperature, metabolism, hunger and food cravings.

The fact that we have a monthly bleed also puts us at higher risk for iron deficiency and iron deficiency anaemia. Between 15 and 18 per cent of women of childbearing age worldwide are iron deficient and, during pregnancy, one in four women in the UK will become anaemic, increasing to one in two women in low-income countries.[1]

What we eat and how much we eat can also impact our menstrual cycle, and eating too few calories can lead to very light, irregular or absent periods. Before we go any further, it might be helpful to return to page 11 for a quick recap of a 'typical', healthy menstrual cycle. Of course, there are many variations to the norm and what's important is knowing what is normal for you and looking out for any red flags (see page 12).

Why we crave chocolate before our period

During the luteal phase, when progesterone and oestrogen are high, there is an increase in resting metabolic rate.[2] This means that, at rest, we burn more calories in the second half of our cycle after ovulation – up to 300 calories more. The extent of this increase varies from day to day and woman to woman, along with other factors such as age, body composition, genetics, illness, physical activity levels, pregnancy and breastfeeding.

The human body is very clever at adjusting for changes in metabolic rate and so during this time we also often see a natural increase in food intake, in addition to increased hunger.[3] In particular, cravings for foods high in carbohydrate and fat are very common.[4]

Interestingly (as a bit of a side note), when it comes to food cravings, in general, women appear to crave chocolate more than men and it also appears to be the most frequently craved food among women.[5] I can personally absolutely vouch for that, but I'm pretty consistent across my cycle when it comes to my chocolate cravings and daily consumption!

Progesterone is thought to increase appetite, whereas oestrogen may suppress it, which is why we might observe these changes during the luteal phase.[6] Insulin sensitivity may also be lower in the luteal phase, meaning the body cells are less responsive to insulin and therefore we may require higher amounts of it to bring down blood sugar levels.[7] This may contribute to symptoms of PMS and increase food cravings during this time.

Cravings accross the menstrual cycle [8,9]

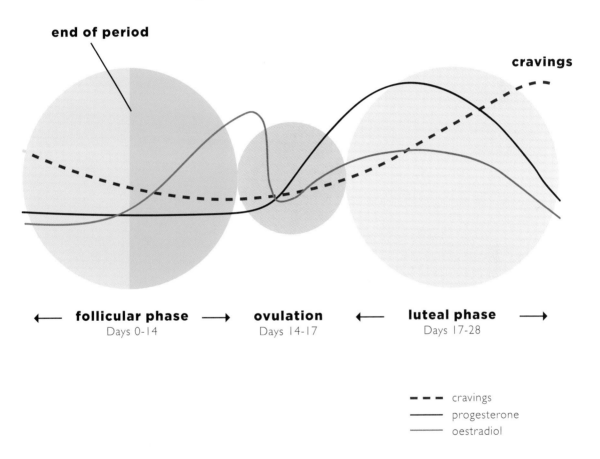

end of period

cravings

← **follicular phase** →	**ovulation** ←	**luteal phase** →
Days 0-14	Days 14-17	Days 17-28

- - - cravings
——— progesterone
——— oestradiol

Does the pill cause weight gain?

There are many different types and formulations of oral contraceptives, for example combined (oestrogen and progesterone) and progesterone only, which interfere with the natural fluctuations in hormones and will likely have differing effects on metabolism. A small number of studies have looked at the effects of oral contraceptives on calorie and nutrient intake, with some reporting higher intakes of calories and fat, and others showing no difference between pill users and non-users.[10] In terms of changes in resting metabolic rate, results have been conflicting over whether there is an increase, no difference or decrease in metabolic rate compared to non-pill users.[11] So yeah, basically anything could happen.

In terms of weight gain, which is often something women are concerned about when it comes to birth control, a review of 49 studies looking at the effect of pills or patches, using oestrogen and progesterone, found that most showed no large weight difference.[12] Overall, there is no real conclusive evidence to support that combined contraceptive methods cause major weight gain. Some women may find they retain some additional water and, as mentioned already, may find increases in appetite, but not every woman will experience this.

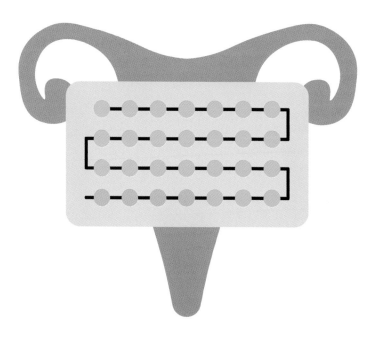

Beware 'Miracle Cure' Diets for Period Problems

A few years back, after months of irregular periods, I visited my GP to investigate what was going on. I had originally put it down to stress, and after my blood tests came back normal, my GP put it down to that too. He advised me to 'stress less' – easier said than done, was my response.

I incorporated meditation into my day, added yoga to my weekly routine, cut back on very intense exercise sessions and waited . . . but still nothing. So after a further three months, I went back to the GP and we agreed to arrange an ultrasound scan to have a look at my ovaries and womb. This scan was followed up by an appointment with a gynaecologist who decided to re-scan me before confirming that I had polycystic ovary syndrome, or PCOS.

The diagnosis offered me some relief but, despite my medical knowledge of the condition, I still had a lot of questions. My first (without much thought – or filter) was, 'Oh sh*t, can I have babies?' to which the gynaecologist replied yes, although having PCOS can make getting pregnant a bit more difficult. My next question was, 'Do I need treatment?' He explained that as I had a mild form of PCOS, no medication was necessary for now and to come back when I was planning for a baby. He didn't seem to want to discuss anything further and so I picked up my bag to leave. However, just as I was about to walk out the door, he did offer some 'lifestyle advice'. He suggested that as I was within a 'healthy BMI' range, I did not need to lose weight, but that I should 'just make sure to cut out the carbs'.

Oh, red flag!

First of all, not once did he ask me about my diet (I could have been on a low-carb diet already for all he knew) and, secondly, the role of diet in the management of PCOS is much more nuanced than simply avoiding carbohydrates. Luckily, I didn't take his advice on board, but it did leave me feeling a bit peeved – I mean, how many other women left that clinic fearing that bread was driving their condition?

This began my journey into researching the connection between food and PCOS (and later endometriosis, after a stint at a clinic that left me wishing I could help more in some way). It has been a long journey, but I have created a nutrition guide overleaf for any of you recently diagnosed with PCOS or endometriosis. They are relatively rare conditions, but that also means information on the best treatment is sparse on the ground too. So, check out Appendix 1 (page 246) for my advice on easing the symptoms.

Can food ease PMS symptoms?

If you have a menstrual cycle, it's likely you've experienced premenstrual symptoms at some point. The severity of symptoms occurs on a spectrum, and for some women they can be bad enough that they interfere with their daily lives, which then becomes premenstrual syndrome (PMS). We chat more about PMS, and the more severe version, premenstrual dysphoric disorder (PMDD), on page 95.

Unfortunately, you can't cure PMS, but there are some steps you can take to ease your symptoms, including nutrition and supplementation (discussed below), gentle exercise, limiting alcohol and stopping smoking.

Nutrition and supplementation

- **Carbohydrates:** Women are often advised to steer clear of carbohydrates, particularly sugars, to help improve PMS symptoms. However, there is no clear link between total, or type of, carbohydrate intake and the risk of PMS.[13] That said, opting for complex carbohydrates (whole grains, legumes, fruit and vegetables) more often than foods high in sugar (cakes, sweets, chocolate, ice cream) is certainly not a bad idea and may help control carbohydrate cravings and support mood and energy levels by stabilising your blood glucose levels.

- **Caffeine:** As this is a stimulant, it can impact our sleep, mood and gut function. So if you struggle with insomnia, anxiety or bloating before your period, it may be worth looking at your caffeine intake, and making sure to limit, if not avoid, caffeine later in the day.

- **Magnesium:** Magnesium supplementation has been shown to reduce PMS symptoms, mainly fluid retention (#periodbloat).[14] One study found that it works best in combination with vitamin B6 rather than taking it alone.[15] While these studies used supplements, magnesium can also be obtained through the diet in foods like pumpkin seeds, nuts, spinach and whole grains. So, if your symptoms are mild, including these foods in your diet may be a good place to start.

- **Iron:** One study found that women who consumed a high intake of non-haem iron had a 36 per cent reduced risk of PMS.[16] Non-haem iron is mainly found in plant-based foods such as fortified cereals, beans, pulses, soya products, nuts and seeds.

- **Salt:** If fluid retention is a PMS symptom issue for you, it may be wise to limit salt intake, as the sodium including salty foods like soya sauce, crisps, salted nuts, bacon and salami. This is because the body is constantly trying to maintain a balance of electrolytes so when you consume sodium, from salt, your body retains more water to maintain equilibrium.

- **Calcium and vitamin D:** Research shows that women with higher intakes of vitamin D and calcium in their diet had a lower risk of developing PMS compared to those with a low intake.[17] Studies where women received calcium supplementation, versus those who were given a dummy pill, also report fewer symptoms.[18]

- **B vitamins:** B vitamins are a family of vitamins involved in most processes in the body – from converting carbohydrates to energy, to supporting the brain and nervous system. Higher intakes of vitamin B1 (thiamine) and B2 (riboflavin) from food sources have been linked to lower rates of PMS from observational studies.[19] Pyridoxine (or vitamin B6) supplements are often still recommended, despite limited evidence. They're not something I recommend; however, some women find them useful in helping their PMS symptoms and I can't argue with that. Note: toxicity (including nerve damage) can occur with doses of vitamin B6 as low as 200mg/day so recommended doses are 25–100mg/day.[20] Head to Appendix 2 for a list of foods that contain B vitamins (see page 252).

- **Chasteberry (*vitex agnus-castus*):** The *vitex agnus-castus* fruit, also known as chasteberry, is produced by the chaste tree, and can be taken as a supplement in tablet or capsule form. It's often promoted as a dietary supplement for symptoms of PMS – particularly breast pain associated with PMS – infertility and other conditions. Surprisingly, a number of studies have shown a benefit when compared to a placebo.[21] While it may work (and it is generally considered safe), there are varying doses and formulations used in the different studies, so a standard recommendation is not available. The herb is believed to work through hormone modulation, and therefore it is not advised during pregnancy or while breastfeeding. It may also reduce the effectiveness of hormonal contraception.

- **Soya isoflavones:** A few small studies have found that consuming soya isoflavones from a supplement or in the diet (from soya-based foods such as tofu, tempeh and soya milk) may help to improve PMS symptoms, possibly due to the impact of high doses of soya on oestrogen.[22]

- **Omega-3 fatty acids:** Omega-3 supplementation has shown some promise in reducing mental and physical symptoms of PMS. However - we need more good-quality research to confirm this. In the meantime, adding omega-3 rich foods such as oily fish, walnuts and flaxseed is a good idea around this time.[23]

Let Nutrition Support Your Fertility Journey

There is a lot of misinformation out there when it comes to fertility and nutrition from superfoods to supplements, all claiming to boost your chances of conceiving. Here's the truth: nutrition does impact fertility and can support you and your partner with getting pregnant, but there's no single fertility diet or wonder food that exists.

Also, nutrition is only one piece of a very complex puzzle. Many couples struggle to conceive, and infertility impacts 8–12 per cent of couples worldwide (infertile = inability to become pregnant after 12 months of regular, unprotected sex).[24] There are many causes for this – and it can affect either partner, or both.

If you're planning to have children at some point – even if it's not any time soon – it's a good idea to be aware of some of the key nutrients that support fertility:

The Mediterranean diet

I know I said that a fertility diet doesn't exist, but based on the research, the best dietary pattern is the Mediterranean diet. That is one which is rich in colourful fruit and vegetables, whole grains, pulses, nuts and seeds, olives and olive oil, herbs and spices, and fish and seafood, with lower intakes of red meat, and sugary foods and drinks. This dietary pattern has been shown to improve both male and female fertility, as well as the chance of pregnancy after assisted conception (such as IVF).[25] This diet is also typically higher in omega-3 fatty acids (see below), which have been shown to support egg and sperm quality, and lower in trans fatty acids and saturated fat found mostly in confectionery and processed foods, which impair fertility in both men and women.[26]

Plant protein > animal protein

Opting for more plant-based sources of protein, and fewer animal sources, has been shown to improve fertility.[27] You do not need to forgo meat completely (and it also contains many nutrients such as iron and vitamin B12) but think more beans and pulses, soya-based products such as tofu and tempeh, nuts and seeds, and less red and processed meat.

Unsaturated fats

Women who consume diets higher in monounsaturated fat have higher fertility rates.[28] Omega-3 fatty acids (found in oily fish, chia seeds, flaxseeds and walnuts) can also support fertility including ovulation and egg quality.[29] Choose rapeseed oil, olive oil, nuts and seeds, and oily fish over foods high in saturated fat (found in butter, coconut oil, lard and meat).

Fats

Fats can be divided into saturated and unsaturated types. Unsaturated fats can be monounsaturated or polyunsaturated. Two essential fatty acids, omega-3 and omega-6, must be obtained through food as they cannot be synthesised by the body.

Antioxidants

Antioxidants are substances that can prevent or slow damage to cells caused by our body's reactions to environmental toxins, such as tobacco, drugs, alcohol, pollutants and other forms of stress. These reactions, known as free radicals, can impair both male and female fertility.[30] Fortunately, antioxidants can be found in abundance in the diet: fruits and vegetables, olive oil, nuts and seeds, and herbs and spices all contain antioxidants. The antioxidants zinc, selenium and vitamins C and E play a role in both male and female fertility.[31] Head to Appendix 2 (page 252) to read more about which foods contain these nutrients. Studies looking at fertility among women who take antioxidant supplements show a weak link at best, but they hold more promise for male fertility.[32] Supplementation with coenzyme Q10 (CoQ10) has also been shown to improve fertility in men and chances of pregnancy in women undergoing assisted conception, such as IVF.[33]

Rethink your cooking methods

Grilling, barbecuing, roasting, toasting and frying, while all delicious methods of cooking, have the potential to damage cells, including those needed for fertility. They increase the formation of compounds called advanced glycation end products (AGEs). These AGEs can cause oxidative stress in the body, leading to cell and tissue damage – including damage to developing eggs in the ovaries. Antioxidants can help prevent this from happening, but we can also reduce the amount of AGEs that are formed by using cooking methods such as steaming, poaching and microwaving, as opposed to those using dry heat.[34] Also using acidic marinades and dressings, such as lemon juice or vinegar, can reduce the formation of AGEs. Foods highest in AGEs are typically animal products, such as beef and eggs, and processed foods that are high in fat, such as cakes, pastries and pies.[35]

Iron

Iron, particularly non-haem iron (both from dietary supplements and from food), may help reduce the risk of infertility in women and increase the chance of pregnancy.[36] Non-haem iron is found mostly in plant foods, such as cereals, beans and lentils, but is slightly more difficult for the body to access and use. Plant-based sources of iron can also contain compounds, like tannins, polyphenols and phytates, which also affect absorption. To increase iron absorption it can help to:

- **add vitamin C to the meal** (such as strawberries, orange juice, kiwi, tomatoes, peppers or sweet potato)
- **avoid tea and coffee at mealtimes** (having them between meals instead)
- **soak grains and legumes before cooking**

If you're veggie or vegan, try to also include some iron-fortified foods: a medium (50g) bowl of fortified cereal contains roughly 70 per cent of the daily iron requirements for men and 40 per cent for women. See page 198 for my Tofu Katsu recipe, which uses a cornflake crumb! There is also some evidence that cooking food in cast-iron pots can help to reduce iron-deficiency anaemia by leaching iron into the food.[37]

Iodine

Iodine is crucial for the formation of thyroid hormones, which play an important role in metabolism and growth, and deficiency can lead to an underactive thyroid (hypothyroidism) and the development of a goitre (a swelling of the thyroid gland in the neck). Iodine is also essential for female fertility and becomes increasingly important during pregnancy and breastfeeding.

In the UK, from puberty onwards, women do not get sufficient iodine and this is thought to be partly due to the fact that more and more of us are opting to go veggie and vegan, which are diets typically lower in iodine.[38] Milk and dairy products, fish and shellfish are the main sources of iodine in the UK. It is possible to get iodine from a plant-based diet, but primarily through fortified foods, such as bread and certain plant milk alternatives (not all are fortified, so do check the label!).

Supplements

- **Folic acid (or methylfolate alternative):** Women who are trying to conceive should aim for a diet rich in folate (green leafy veg, legumes, avocados) in addition to taking a 400mcg folic acid (synthetic form of folate) supplement through preconception and up to 12 weeks of pregnancy to prevent neural tube defects. Some women who are considered high risk will be advised by their doctor to take up to 5mg per day. Folate is also important for male fertility as it is needed for the synthesis of DNA in sperm.[39]

- **Vitamin D:** Although vitamin D does not appear to offer much of a role in fertility in the absence of deficiency, adequate serum vitamin D levels are associated with more positive pregnancy tests, clinical pregnancies and live births in women undergoing artificial reproductive technology.[40] In the UK, it's advised to supplement with 10mcg per day, especially between October and March.

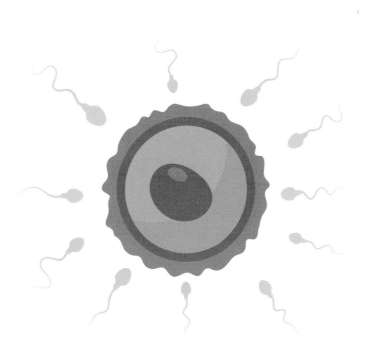

What You Eat During Pregnancy Matters

During pregnancy, good nutrition is so important, not only to support you through this period of growth, but for the health of your baby – now and in the future. We talk about the 'first 1,000 days', from conception to the child's second birthday, which is this incredibly unique, yet vulnerable, period when a child's brain begins to grow and develop and the foundations for their future health are built. So, the quality of a mother's diet during pregnancy also has a long-lasting impact on the health of her child. Your diet during pregnancy can also shape your child's food preferences later in life – which I find just fascinating – so feel free to start training those taste buds with a wide range of foods during your pregnancy!

Before you get too experimental, though, there are some foods which you should forgo, or limit, while pregnant. But first, let's look at what nutrients we need *more* of:

More of these please!

- **Energy:** It's a myth that pregnant women need to 'eat for two', but the body does need sufficient calories to not only account for the growing baby, but also for the mother's increased metabolism. In early pregnancy, energy needs are generally the same as non-pregnant women, but this increases as the pregnancy progresses. In the UK, the advice is that an extra 200 kcal of energy per day is required during the third trimester only.[41]

- **Protein:** Protein requirements increase during pregnancy to support foetal growth and development. In the UK, the guidance is to increase protein intake by an additional 6g per day.[42] For reference, one medium-sized egg or a handful of almonds provide about 6g of protein.

- **Omega-3 fatty acids:** DHA (docosahexaenoic acid), a type of omega-3, is of particular importance for the development of the brain and the retina. The European Food Safety Authority (EFSA) advises that pregnant women should consume an additional 100–200mg of DHA per day.[43] Oily fish is an excellent source of omega-3 fatty acids, although there are concerns of mercury contamination so advice in pregnancy (and for girls, women who are planning a pregnancy or may have a child some day, plus breastfeeding women) is to consume no more than two portions of oily fish per week.[44] Avoid taking cod liver oil supplements as they can contain high levels of vitamin A, which can be harmful to the baby.

- **Iodine:** We've already spoken about the importance of iodine (see page 26), but it is especially important when it comes to pregnancy. During pregnancy, women should consume 200mcg a day (50mcg higher than non-pregnant women).[45] Those who may be at risk of iodine deficiency, such as anyone who avoids fish and/or dairy products, may wish to consider taking an iodine supplement of no more than 150mcg.

- **Iron:** Iron needs are higher during pregnancy, as the amount of circulating blood volume increases by 20–30 per cent(!), which increases the demand for iron to make haemoglobin.[46] Iron is also extremely important in foetal brain development, and low levels during pregnancy can lead to anaemia which has been associated with preterm delivery and low birth weight.[47] Don't stress as iron levels are routinely measured at the first antenatal appointment and again at week 28. If iron levels are low, iron supplements may be recommended.

- **Supplements during pregnancy:** Even with the increased demand for the nutrients mentioned above, most women will be able to get everything they need from a healthy balanced diet. The exception, of course, is a folic acid supplement which should be continued until the twelfth week of pregnancy and, in the UK, pregnant women are also advised to take a 10-mcg vitamin D daily supplement. For convenience, some pregnant women may decide to take a specially formulated prenatal supplement, which usually contains optimal levels of vitamin D and folic acid, as well as some other vitamins and minerals. Those who follow a plant-based diet may need to take additional supplementation of iodine and omega-3 fatty acids.[48]

Less (or none) of these please!

And now for the less good news – foods that should be limited and/or avoided during pregnancy:

- **Avoid unpasteurised dairy and mould-ripened cheeses:** This is because these types of cheese can harbour listeria, a type of bacteria that is dangerous to an unborn baby. However, theses cheeses should be fine to eat if they have been well-cooked and are hot all the way through, so make sure to check with whoever is cooking your dish.

- **Avoid raw shellfish and certain forms of fish:** High-mercury fish, such as shark, marlin and swordfish, have the potential to harm foetal development and should be avoided. Tuna should also be limited to two tuna steaks, or four medium-sized tins, per week. Oily fish is fab (nutrient-wise) but can contain other pollutants, so should be limited to two 140-g portions per week. Sushi is safe to eat if it's been made with cooked fish or shellfish, or pre-frozen raw wild fish – make sure to check first or, if in doubt, avoid.

- **Avoid raw or partially-cooked eggs:** This is due to the risk of salmonella food poisoning. However, eggs with a British Lion stamp are considered safe to be consumed during pregnancy when raw or partially cooked.

- **Avoid raw or undercooked meat, and game:** Meat should be cooked until there is no trace of pink or blood left, and any cold, cured meats (like prosciutto, salami, pepperoni and chorizo) should also be cooked thoroughly. This reduces the risk of getting an infection called toxoplasmosis, which can increase the risk of miscarriage. Game meat, such as goose, partridge or pheasant, should also be avoided due to potentially high levels of lead.

- **Avoid a high intake of vitamin A:** This vitamin is still important for healthy development of the baby, but high levels can cause birth defects. Avoid any supplements that contain vitamin A, as well as liver and liver pâté. (It's also recommended to avoid all types of pâté due to the risk of bacterial contamination.) Pregnant women (and those trying to conceive) are advised to avoid prescription acne drugs (such as isotretinoin) and topical retinols as a precautionary measure.

- **Avoid liquorice root:** Liquorice root may not be top of your list anyway, but this is advised as a precaution based on a study that found that liquorice consumption may negatively impact foetal development.[49]

- **Avoid alcohol and caffeine:** Despite the discussion around safe limits of alcohol during pregnancy, I don't think the evidence is strong enough to exclude the risk of harm. To be safe, I would therefore advise avoiding alcohol during pregnancy. Caffeine should be limited to 200mg a day, as high amounts have been linked to low birth weight and risk of pregnancy loss.[50]

> Food hygiene is important for everyone, but it's particularly important to be careful how you prepare, handle, store and reheat food during pregnancy. This includes washing fruit and vegetables thoroughly, washing hands, equipment and work surfaces well after handling raw food and ensuring any reheated food is piping hot all the way through. This reduces the risk of food-borne infections.

Troubleshooting in pregnancy

During pregnancy, you may also have to make changes to your diet to help ease some of the common symptoms such as constipation, morning sickness and heartburn.

Constipation

Hormones during pregnancy can slow down the transit of stool through the gut and this slo-mo process also allows more water to be absorbed from the poop, which makes it harder to pass. Later in pregnancy, pressure from the growing baby also adds to the problem. Constipation combined with straining can also lead to haemorrhoids. Fun times!

Tips to soften that stool (this advice applies to non-pregnant women too!) include:

- Drink plenty of fluids.

- Increase your intake of fibre by eating more fruits, vegetables, whole grains, beans and pulses – and prunes too!

- Try adding some flaxseed to the diet, gradually building up to 1 tablespoon per day.

- Aim to do some form of regular physical activity (this basically massages the gut and helps with the movement of the stool).

- If you need to poo, don't put it off! This can worsen symptoms.

- When you are ready to go, it can help to place a footstool under your feet, so your knees are higher than your hips. Lean forwards, resting your elbows on your knees – and relax.

- Certain prenatal vitamins, especially iron supplements, can contribute to constipation. Speak to your doctor or midwife if you think this might be the case.

Note: Laxatives are usually safe for pregnant women to take because most of them are not absorbed by the digestive system. This means that your baby will not be affected. Speak to your GP or midwife about what laxatives are most suitable for you.

Morning sickness

Around eight out of every ten pregnant women feel sick or vomit during the first few weeks of pregnancy.[51] I'm sure many women who have been pregnant will back me up here – despite the name, this does not just happen in the morning, and it can linger on past the first trimester. We don't really know the exact reason why some women are affected and others are not, but it's thought to be due to the increases in hormones that occur during pregnancy. Women who are having twins or multiples are at higher risk of experiencing nausea and vomiting.[52]

Unfortunately, there is no quick fix, but here are some tips that may help:

- **Graze:** Try to eat smaller, more frequent meals across the day.
- **Stay hydrated:** Sip water regularly throughout the day as vomiting can cause dehydration. If you are vomiting a lot,* a sports drink that contains some sugar, salt and electrolytes will help replace what your body has lost and provide some energy.
- **Ginger:** Although it is not conclusive, there is evidence to suggest that consuming ginger can help with nausea during pregnancy.[53]
- **Bland foods:** Stick with plain foods and avoid those with strong aromas or flavours.
- **Eat what you can:** Something is always better than nothing, so eat what you can, when you can.

If the vomiting is severe to the point where you are losing weight, or you are unable to keep down food for over 24 hours, this could be more than morning sickness and a condition known as hyperemesis gravidarum (HG). Contact your midwife or doctor as soon as possible.

Heartburn

Indigestion, or heartburn, affects as many as half of all pregnant women.[54] During pregnancy, the muscle between the oesophagus and stomach relaxes due to hormonal changes (allowing the contents of the stomach to move upwards) and, at the same time, the growing baby puts upwards pressure on the stomach – the perfect cocktail for heartburn. Unfortunately, women who experienced heartburn before are more likely to experience it during pregnancy.

Try these tips if you're struggling:

- **Eat little and often** and avoid eating too close to bedtime.
- **Avoid spicy and fatty foods** (some people report other food triggers like citrus fruits and onion). Caffeine can also contribute – even more reason to cut down.

- **Sleeping with the head of the bed slightly elevated** (for example, using an extra pillow) may help.

- **Most standard over-the-counter heartburn treatments are safe during pregnancy**; however you should consult your pharmacist or GP to see what is appropriate for you.

Note: If you experience severe pain in the upper right side of your abdomen under your ribs, you should speak to your doctor as it could be a sign of something else, such as pre-eclampsia or gallstones.

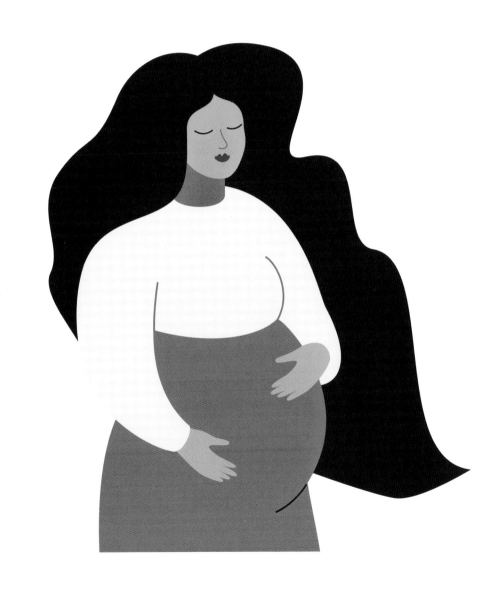

Good Nutrition Doesn't Stop When You Give Birth

During pregnancy, many women pay close attention to what they're eating in order to give their baby all the nutrients they need to grow and develop, which is amazing, and absolutely the right thing to do. However, nutrition matters even after the baby is born. I know that, practically speaking, when in the throes of motherhood and taking care of a newborn, looking after your own nutrition may not exactly be at the top of your list of priorities, but your health matters too. I say this without any judgement, but with your best interests in mind. This goes for mammas who are breastfeeding and those who are not.

Unfortunately, there are no official guidelines for postnatal nutrition for mothers who are not breastfeeding, but your body goes through a lot during pregnancy and birth, and still needs sufficient nutrition to recover and heal. Additionally, nutrition also plays a role in mood and risk of postnatal depression, which I discuss in Chapter 3 (see page 82). The best advice is to follow general healthy eating recommendations. These, of course, will need to be adapted to work with your new routine (and time constraints). It may be that you end up having lots of smaller meals in between feeds and sleeps – and that's OK.

My sister always had a water bottle next to her in those first few weeks of new parenthood and lived off a lot of bananas, peanut butter and toast. Parents of newborns also might find having the occasional sweet and savoury snack to be a convenient energy boost, and that's fine, but choosing complex carbohydrates (like wholegrain bread and cereals) with protein (such as eggs, peanut butter or yogurt) may sustain that energy a little longer. Note to friends and family of new parents: the best gift right now is food.

In addition to general healthy eating guidance (see page 17), if you choose to breastfeed, there are a few things you need a little extra of:

- **Fluids:** Breastfeeding women have higher fluid requirements – about 700ml extra.[55] All drinks count towards fluid intake so this can be water but also milk, diluted juices and herbal teas. Tea and coffee should be limited, however, as caffeine is excreted in breast milk and may keep a baby awake – something most parents want to avoid!

- **Calories:** If you're breastfeeding exclusively for the first six months, you may need up to an extra 500 calories per day.[56] If you're giving some formula feeds this will be less.

Extra nutrients:

- **Protein:** An extra 11g of protein per day is needed for the first six months of breastfeeding; this decreases to an extra 8g per day after six months.

- **Calcium:** Requirements increase by 550mg per day.

- **Omega-3:** Daily DHA requirements remain 100–200mg higher during breastfeeding as compared with pre-pregnancy.

- **Iodine:** Requirements remain at 200mcg, which is higher than pre-pregnancy.

- **Vitamin D:** Breastfeeding women in the UK are also advised to consider supplementing with 10mcg vitamin D supplement.

Unfortunately, if you're breastfeeding, there are still some foods you're advised to limit or avoid, even after birth, as they can affect the baby:

- Limit caffeine to less than 200mg per day – the same as during pregnancy.

- Keep oily fish to a maximum of two portions per week, and shark, swordfish or marlin to once a week.

- It's recommended not to drink any alcohol for the first three months when breastfeeding and no more than two units (one standard glass of wine or a pint of lower-strength beer) of alcohol once or twice a week after that.[57] The odd drink is unlikely to cause any harm to your baby, but it's advisable that you leave a few hours between drinking alcohol and breastfeeding as alcohol can pass to the baby in breast milk. You could always plan ahead and express some milk beforehand.

Eat to Ease Your Menopausal Transition

The menopause is a universal experience for all women at some point in their life (see page 11 for more detail on the hormonal lifespan). However, while it may signal the end of our fertility, women spend a third of their lives in the post-menopausal phase so there is so much life yet to be lived! We should be supporting women to thrive and be as healthy as possible during the menopausal transition.

Unfortunately, the drop in oestrogen that occurs during this time not only puts a stop to periods, but impacts bone health, heart health and brain health – not to mention marking the start of menopausal symptoms of hot flushes, headaches, difficulty sleeping, low libido, irritability and low mood.

That said, not all women experience these symptoms and some sail through the menopause just fine. However, the risk of certain health problems, such as heart disease and osteoporosis, still exists so it's important that we are proactive when it comes to looking after ourselves through this transition. Lucky for you, you're in the right place.

Keep an eye on your heart

Up to the menopause, women are relatively protected against heart disease, compared to men of the same age. This is believed to be due in part to the protective effect of oestrogen, which helps keep the blood vessels flexible, meaning they can relax and expand to accommodate blood flow. After the menopause, the blood vessels become increasingly stiff and narrow, bumping up the risk of heart disease. Around this time, traditional risk factors for heart disease tend to go in the wrong direction for women:

- Weight gain of 2–2.5kg (over three years) is typical during the menopausal transition, in part due to reduced activity levels and other lifestyle factors such as changes to eating habits, but also due to a reduced metabolism that occurs with age.[58]

- Body fat distribution shifts from the hips and bum to the abdomen. These are often referred to as 'pear' and 'apple' shapes respectively – and the latter increases the risk of type 2 diabetes and heart disease.[59]

- Blood pressure rises more steeply in post-menopausal women compared with men. Oestrogen has a positive effect on blood vessels, which allows them to dilate and for blood to flow more easily. This is lost somewhat after the menopause.

- The cholesterol profile changes after the menopause with an increase in total cholesterol and low-density lipoprotein (LDL) – sometimes called 'bad' cholesterol – and a decrease in high-density lipoprotein (HDL) – the 'good' cholesterol.[60] High levels of LDL cholesterol raise your risk for heart disease and stroke.

- Type 2 diabetes, although likely due to age, becomes more common in women after the menopause.[61]

Because these changes that occur at menopause lead to an increased risk of heart disease, it's even more important now than ever that we focus on the factors that we can control. In fact, certain risk factors for heart disease – such as smoking, diabetes and high blood pressure – increase the risk of a heart attack more in women than in men.[62] This means women may need to be more vigilant when it comes to managing their lifestyle factors (diet, exercise, sleep and smoking cessation) at a younger age to prevent heart disease later in life.

I also urge women in their midlife to have a discussion with their doctor about their individual cardiovascular risk and have regular blood pressure, cholesterol and blood glucose checks. In the UK, you will be invited for a free NHS health check every five years from the age of 40 to 74 years to check whether you're at higher risk of heart disease, stroke, diabetes and kidney disease.

While the risk is increased at menopause, there are nutritional changes you can make to support your heart health:

- **Replace foods high in saturated fat and trans fatty acids** (found in butter, lards, coconut oil, pastries and fried food) for foods high in monounsaturated and polyunsaturated fats (found in olive oil and other plant oils, avocados, nuts and seeds).

- **Reduce red and processed meat intake**, and aim to include at least one portion of oily fish per week, such as salmon, mackerel, herring, trout, sardines and kippers.

- **Increase your intake of whole grains.** Whole grains (such as wholemeal bread, wholegrain cereals, oats, barley, brown rice, spelt and rye) can reduce risk of cardiovascular disease, with the greatest benefits at three or more 30g servings per day (think breakfast, lunch and dinner!).[63] You can also make little changes elsewhere, like swapping some white flour for wholewheat or spelt flour when baking (or do half and half) – check out my Quinoa + Chia Loaf on page 238.

- **Up your fibre intake.** As well as keeping your gut healthy, eating more fibre has been linked with a lower risk of heart disease.[64] Dietary fibre can be found in all plant-based foods so make sure to include a good variety from fruit and veggies, pulses, grains and cereals, and nuts and seeds. Beta glucan, a soluble dietary fibre in oats and barley, appears to have a particularly positive effect on total and LDL cholesterol levels.[65] Perhaps try an oat-based meal for breakfast such as porridge, muesli or homemade granola (I have a few options for you to try in the recipes section from page 134).

- **Aim to get your five-a-day** from a range of different coloured fruits and vegetables every day – *all* types count (fresh, frozen, tinned, dried or juiced). Fruit and vegetables provide vitamins, minerals, fibre and other plant nutrients such as antioxidants that help protect your heart. You could add a handful of antioxidant-rich berries to a smoothie or your morning porridge.

- **Introduce some soya into your diet.** Soya-based foods (such as tofu, soya mince, edamame beans and soya-based milks/yogurts) have the potential to reduce blood cholesterol by 3–4 per cent – and therefore to reduce the risk of heart disease.[66] This is based on a 25g per-day intake of soya protein, which is not based on the total weight of a soya-based product, but the amount of soya protein within the food. For example, in 100g of firm tofu, there is about 8g of soya protein; in 250ml of soya milk there is 8.5g; and 10g in an 80g serving of fresh or frozen edamame beans.

- **Go nuts (within reason).** A 30g portion of nuts (roughly a small handful) has beneficial effects on heart health by reducing total cholesterol, LDL cholesterol and triglycerides (another type of fat found in the blood).[67] These can be consumed as snacks or sprinkled on top of salads, soups or breakfast bowls.

- **Watch your salt intake.** A high intake of salt can increase blood pressure which can, in turn, increase the risk of heart disease and stroke.[68] Cut down on your intake by getting into the habit of not adding salt to meals, checking food labels (low salt = less than 0.3g of salt per 100g) and cutting down on foods typically high in salt such as savoury snacks, ready meals, smoked and cured meats.

- **Look out for foods with added sterols and stanols.** Sterols and stanols are plant chemicals that are a similar size and shape to cholesterol. They are absorbed from the gut into the bloodstream and prevent some cholesterol from being absorbed and lowering the cholesterol in your blood.[69] We get a small number of sterols from plant-based foods but not enough to reduce cholesterol. Food products now exist on the market with added sterols and stanols, such as yogurt drinks, spreads, milk and yogurts: 1.5–3g per day is recommended to reduce cholesterol.[70] (PS There is no real benefit if you don't have high cholesterol.)

- **Try to limit alcohol** to no more than 2–3 units per day and consume no more than 14 units of alcohol per week, with some alcohol-free days in between.

Make bone health a priority

Bone health is important for everyone through every stage of life, but women are at risk of osteoporosis, particularly after the menopause when levels of oestrogen decline. Muscle loss and strength are also accelerated after the menopause, which also contributes to the risk of fractures and falls – both of which have a huge impact on other aspects of health, independence and quality of life.

There are a number of key nutrients that work together for strong and healthy bones – in particular calcium, vitamin D, protein, magnesium, phosphorus and vitamin K.

Sufficient calories are important for not only directly helping to maintain and build healthy bones, but also indirectly as inadequate calorie intake often comes hand in hand with lower intakes of important nutrients involved in bone health, such as calcium. This is important for women at *all* stages of life.

Calcium and vitamin D

Calcium is essential for building and maintaining strong bones at all stages of life, but our requirements are slightly higher at certain periods, including after the menopause.[71] Those who have certain health conditions, such as osteoporosis, coeliac disease and inflammatory bowel disease (IBD), also have higher recommended daily needs (1000mg/day).[72] The richest sources of calcium in the UK diet are dairy products (milk, cheese and yogurt), but calcium can also be found in tinned fish with bones. Calcium can be found in plant-based foods such as fortified plant milk alternatives, calcium-fortified cereals and orange juice, nuts and seeds, and tofu (if set with calcium chloride or calcium sulphate), and in smaller amounts in leafy green vegetables such as kale. In the UK, white and brown flour must be fortified with calcium.

Top tip: Make sure to shake your carton of plant-based milk alternative before pouring as fortified nutrients like calcium can sink to the bottom.

Supplements are generally not needed on top of a healthy, balanced diet, but for individuals who are struggling to get enough calcium every day, they can be helpful. Just like too little calcium can impair health, so can too much, so speak to your doctor before starting anything new.

It's worth noting that calcium alone does not equal healthy bones. Vitamin D helps to absorb calcium from food, and can be found in foods such as eggs (in the yolk), oily fish, liver, mushrooms grown under UV light and certain fortified foods like breakfast cereals, margarine and plant-based drinks – and supplementation.

Protein

Better known for its role in muscle-building, protein actually makes up 50 per cent of bone volume and a third of its mass. It produces hormones and growth factors that are involved in bone formation. After the menopause, women may need even higher intakes than younger adults to maintain and build muscle (approximately 1–1.2g/kg bodyweight and at least 20–25g protein at each main meal).[73] Instead of worrying about weighing your food, I would suggest simply aiming to have a source of protein at each meal and opting for high-protein snacks such as Greek yogurt, cottage cheese and oatcakes, edamame beans and mixed nuts.

Other key nutrients for bone health

- **Magnesium:** Magnesium is another important mineral that is involved in bone formation and vitamin D regulation. Good food sources of magnesium include nuts (almonds, cashews, Brazil nuts), seeds (pumpkin, sunflower, chia), spinach, soya beans, black beans, potatoes and whole grains – dark chocolate is also a source! You should be able to get all the magnesium you need from a healthy balanced diet without the need for supplementation.

- **Vitamin K:** Vitamin K switches on a protein known as osteocalcin, which is necessary for bone-building and bone-healing.[74] Good sources include green leafy vegetables (chard, kale, spinach), turnip, broccoli and soya beans (especially nattō – a traditional Japanese food made from fermented soya beans). Most healthy people should be able to reach their recommended daily intake through diet. Those taking warfarin should not take vitamin K supplements.

- **Phosphorus:** Phosphorus combines with calcium to form the structural basis and rigidity of bones and teeth. Too much or too little phosphorus can both negatively impact bone health. Phosphorus deficiency is rare as it is found in a variety of sources, such as dairy, meat and poultry, fish, nuts, beans and whole grains.

- **Potassium:** Potassium is involved in maintaining the acid–base balance in the body, preventing bone loss and calcium excretion in the urine.[75] Sources include bananas, broccoli, Brussels sprouts, nuts and seeds, pulses, fish and shellfish, and meat and poultry.

Take the heat out of hot flushes

One of the most common complaints about menopause is hot flushes (or hot flashes), which usually start in the perimenopause, affecting up to 85 per cent of menopausal women.[76] The reason this is thought to happen is due to the effect of reduced oestrogen levels on the body's internal thermostat (the hypothalamus of the brain), making it more sensitive to slight changes in body temperature.[77]

If you've not experienced one before, it's described as a sudden feeling of intense heat, usually spreading through the chest, face and neck. They're not only annoying and interfere with daily activities, but they also disrupt sleep which can, over time, lead to worse mood and poor health.

Simple changes you can try at home include reducing room temperature, using fans, dressing in loose-fitting clothing and avoiding triggers, including certain foods (see below) and stress. However, if you are experiencing pretty significant symptoms, there are other options to help, so please don't suffer in silence. Treatment options include hormone replacement therapy (HRT), psychological support and lifestyle changes.

- **Caffeine and alcohol:** Caffeine and alcohol can make the severity of hot flushes worse in some women.[78] Another factor to consider is that caffeine and alcohol are also known to disrupt sleep (more on this on page 127) and many women going through menopause have trouble sleeping. Perhaps keep a diary and opt for more decaf drinks throughout the day and reduce alcohol intake to a minimum.

- **Spicy food:** Avoiding spicy foods is a common recommendation for women experiencing hot flushes, but evidence to support this is limited.[79] I recommend relying on your personal experience here and, if you see a pattern with the severity or frequency of your symptoms and spicy foods, then it makes sense to reduce them in your diet.

- **Phytoestrogens:** Phytoestrogens are oestrogen-like compounds that are found naturally in many plants. For some women, these effects could be sufficient to help relieve mild menopausal symptoms, particularly hot flushes.[80] Foods that naturally contain phytoestrogens include soya beans and soya-based products, chickpeas, peanuts, flaxseeds, barley, grapes, berries, plums and green and black tea (try my Banana, Flax + Walnut Bread on page 236).

Making a decision on HRT

HRT replaces hormones that naturally fall to lower levels during the transition through and after the menopause. There are a few different types, regimes and ways of taking HRT (such as tablet, patch or gel). The specific regime you are given will always contain oestrogen, but the progesterone component is only needed if you still have a womb as this decreases the risk of endometrial cancer. Testosterone can also be given.

What most women want to know is whether HRT is safe. For most women, yes it is, but it depends and, as with any medical intervention, we always have to weigh up the risks versus the benefits, which are summarised in the table opposite. For women under the age of 60, the benefits generally outweigh the risks, but this balance starts to tip in the other direction after 60 years of age. For women under the age of 50 who go through the menopause the risks of HRT do not apply as you are simply replacing the hormones you would normally have at this age.

Potential risks versus potential benefits of HRT

The next question I get asked is, whether you should take it. Although there have been concerns raised about HRT, it still remains the most effective solution for the relief of menopausal symptoms and also carries some other benefits. However, it's not completely risk-free and it is not suitable for everyone. I know it is deeply annoying when people sit on the fence about things like this, but this is something where there is simply no one-size-fits-all approach.

If you're under the age of 60, have no medical reasons not to take HRT and are struggling with debilitating menopausal symptoms that are affecting your quality of life, then I would absolutely consider it. Also, to reiterate, for women under 50 years of age who have gone through the menopause, the benefits are significant, even without symptoms.

Ultimately, you need to discuss with your doctor whether HRT is a suitable option for you and to ensure you have no medical reasons that prevent you from safely taking it (for example, a recent clot in your leg or lung, or a diagnosis of breast cancer, now or in the past). They can help work out the best option for you which can offset some of the risks mentioned. There are also several alternatives to HRT if it is not suitable for you including complementary and alternative treatments, non-hormonal medications and lifestyle measures.

* * * *

The role of nutrition in women's health is poorly understood (and under-researched). I hope this chapter has helped you to understand how to eat for your unique female body and how to fuel it so that you can function at your best at every stage of life.

Potential risks and benefits of HRT

Potential risks	Potential benefits	Inconclusive
• Small increased risk of breast cancer with combined HRT (little to no increased risk with oestrogen-only HRT).[81] • Increased risk of endometrial cancer with oestrogen-only HRT – in women with a womb.[82] (This is why oestrogen is always given with progesterone in women who still have a womb to protect the endometrial lining.) • Combined or oestrogen-only HRT taken orally slightly increases your risk of stroke.[83] This also depends on dose and route, so there is no increased risk with transdermal oestrogen, for example. • Increased risk of blood clots (venous thromboembolisms) in the legs or lungs with oral HRT, but not patches or gels.[84]	• Reduction in menopausal symptoms including hot flushes, sleep disturbances, joint aches and pains, mood changes and vaginal and urinary symptoms.[85] This has a knock-on benefit of improving overall quality of life and relationships. • Protection against osteoporosis and risk of fracture.[86] • Many offer cosmetic benefits on skin ageing.[87] • May improve muscle mass and strength.[88] • Decrease in cardiovascular risk if started within 10 years of the menopause or under the age of 60.[89]	• Possible increase in ovarian cancer, but results conflicting.[90] • Research into dementia risk and HRT is mixed and inconclusive, and so HRT is not currently recommended for the prevention of dementia.[91] • Possible risk reduction in colorectal cancer.[92]

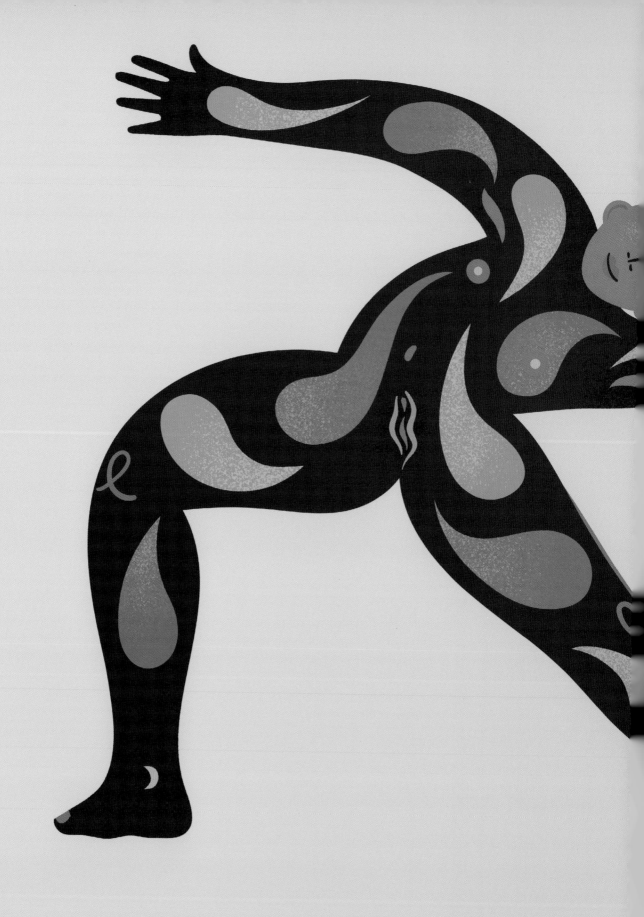

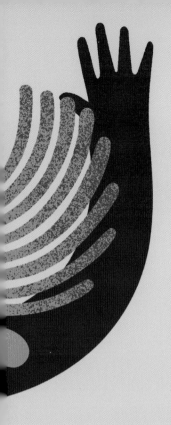

Movement

Movement

When several women reportedly collapsed after the 800-metre race at the 1928 Amsterdam Olympics, the International Olympic Committee (IOC) banned women from running any race longer than 200 metres.[1] However, it transpired that this was, in fact, poor journalism and though some women lay down beside the track after crossing the finish line, none of them dropped out or collapsed from exhaustion.[2] I don't know about you, but I would be pretty spent after that too. Unfortunately, this falsified version of events prevented women from competing in the women's 800 metres until 1960. This reinforced a commonly held belief that women were somehow not physiologically capable of endurance activity; that it would damage their reproductive health and femininity. Some warned that a woman's womb might fall right out (!) should she attempt to run such distances.

In 1967, Kathrine Switzer was the first woman to run the Boston Marathon (even as an official tried to physically stop her and wrestle her to the ground) and it wasn't until 1972 that women were officially 'allowed' to run the New York City Marathon (on the condition they started ten minutes before the men).[3]

Thank goodness times have changed and recent efforts to get more of us active and involved in sport are paying off. For example, at the elite level, the number of women taking part in the Olympic Games increased from 10.5 per cent in 1952 to 49 per cent in the Tokyo 2020 Olympics – making it the most gender-equal Olympics since the Olympics started.[4]

Despite all this, society is still treating women as smaller, weaker versions of men. This narrative is outdated and incorrect. Women have their own strengths, and we must start paying closer attention to the unique needs of our bodies to level the playing field.

Unfortunately, it's not easy to optimise and support women's health and performance when we don't study them! As it stands, women are massively underrepresented within sport and exercise science research. In fact, we only make up 34 per cent of participants in this field, and only 6 per cent of this is carried out on females only.[5]

We also see this inequality in how women are portrayed in the media when it comes to sport and exercise, placing more emphasis on how we look rather than how we perform. The Norwegian beach handball team offered the perfect example of this when they recently made headlines while competing in the European Beach Handball Championships prior to the Olympics. The news stories were not focused on their performance, but on what they were wearing, after they were fined because their shorts were *too long*. Yes, you read that correctly. After decades of being told to cover up, these women were fined for not showing enough skin.

From feminised gym classes to sexist sporting kits, we don't care about how fit, strong or healthy women are, as long as they look good, right? With a narrative like this, it's no surprise that women choose to exercise for weight loss and toning more than men, while men report doing it for enjoyment more than women.[6]

On top of that, the terms 'physical activity' and 'exercise' are often used interchangeably in the media, in research and by healthcare professionals. While exercise is a form of physical activity, it is not the *only* form. Physical activity represents any form of movement produced by the body's muscles and requires energy to be used. This could be everyday activities, such as walking the dog, cycling to the shops, gardening or playing with the kids, but could also include exercise and sporting activities.

Exercise, on the other hand, is a structured form of physical activity that is planned and repetitive, with the intention of improving or maintaining physical fitness or body condition (for example, attending an exercise class such as Pilates or yoga; or doing a strength-training programme).

The difference is key because pushing an exercise-only message makes it less achievable and inclusive for all women, of all abilities. So I really want to emphasise that all activity counts and that some amount of physical activity is better than no activity at all.

We have different athletic expectations of women: that we can't lift those heavy weights, or run that distance, or exercise during pregnancy or after the menopause. But you can, we can, #ThisGirlCan. It's time to rewrite the story and rewire old ways of thinking.

I want you to come away from this chapter understanding the major key health considerations that you need to know in order to be the fittest, healthiest and strongest version of yourself now and in the future, no matter which physical activities you choose to enjoy.

Before You Pull On Your Trainers . . .

Everyone needs a certain amount of energy (in the form of calories) to simply stay alive, even if all we do is lie in bed. Reading this sentence requires energy. It's no surprise then that exercise requires additional energy in the form of calories. Diet culture has taught us women that calories are things to be avoided or 'burned off', but calories are units of energy and allow us to thrive and survive. When we reframe them in this way, it doesn't make much sense to restrict them; am I right?

I want you to visualise an 'energy pool' that contains all the energy that we take in from food. This energy pool must meet specific demands: allowing your body to function as normal and meeting your activity demands. As the day goes on, this energy pool shrinks in size, as we use up our reserves.

When we remove the energy needed to cover the demands of exercise from the pool, the residual energy is known as energy availability (EA) and, if this falls below the minimal level required for a person to function optimally, the body goes into a state of low EA. This may happen if someone is not eating enough calories to meet daily energy requirements (*not enough energy going in*) or if there is an increase in energy used (such as through exercise) without an increase in calorie intake to meet that need (*too much energy going out*).

Low EA is like the energy-saving mode on your smartphone; the light is dimmed, the device slows down and background refreshing of apps is turned off. That is essentially what happens to the body here. This means that certain bodily functions that are not immediately life-sustaining (such as regular menstruation and the ability to conceive) get sidelined until more energy becomes available.

So, before you tie up those trainers, I want you to consider how you're fuelling your body to make sure it stays as healthy as possible. Activity and exercise are great for our health, but only when we're using all the tools we can – including the energy we consume – to set ourselves up to thrive.

Energy availability

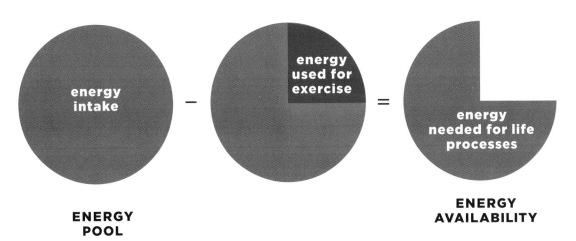

ENERGY POOL

ENERGY AVAILABILITY

Fuel Your Fitness

You can work out all you like, take all the supplements in the world and try out the latest recovery technique, from cryotherapy to saunas, but if your nutrition is not quite right, then you're unlikely to make progress and you're ultimately setting yourself up for failure. We need calories and the right nutrients to grow, repair and recover. However, what we are starting to realise is that, compared to men, women have different needs when it comes to fuelling sport and physical activity.

Here's the thing: carbohydrates and fat are the key energy sources used during exercise. As exercise intensity increases, carbohydrate contributes the most energy, whereas fat is a more important fuel at lower-intensity exercise. This holds true for both sexes. However, compared to men, women tend to burn *more fat for fuel at the same relative intensity of activity*. In other words, women rely on carbohydrates *less* and burn *more* fat for fuel than men do at a higher intensity.

Theoretically, this might prevent women 'hitting the wall' early and make them more suitable for endurance sports, *but* in practice men still outperform women in endurance sports and events (but the gap is as low as 4 per cent in ultramarathons and even less in ultra-cycling events). Women also tend to outperform men in long-distance open-water swimming. The reason for this is also down to differences in muscle fibres and fatigability, lower energy requirements and the amount and distribution of body fat.

Across the menstrual cycle, our reliance on carbohydrates versus fat for fuel also changes. Research shows that, during moderate-intensity endurance exercise, women rely less on carbohydrates for fuel in the luteal phase (second half of the cycle) compared to the follicular phase (first half).[7] In addition to this, there is also increased use and breakdown of protein, which comes with higher metabolism at this time.[8] As we spoke about earlier, women often report hunger, cravings and food intake during this time too, especially in the late luteal phase (see page 19).[9]

That said, most studies have only seen minor differences, with others having found none, so right now we don't have enough evidence to start making blanket recommendations for nutrition across the menstrual cycle. However, for women who really want to squeeze out that extra 1 per cent from their training and in races, during the luteal phase keep the following things in mind:

- **It may be beneficial to increase dietary fats in this phase.** Include plenty of healthy fat sources in the diet such as avocado, nut butter, nuts and seeds, and at least one portion of oily fish per week.

- **It may also be more beneficial to think about protein intake here.** Protein is also satiating and can help with increased hunger and cravings.

- **Carbs are still important!** Opting for complex carbohydrates (whole grains, legumes, fruit and vegetables) over foods high in sugar (cakes, sweets, chocolate and ice cream) may help control carbohydrate cravings and support mood and energy levels by stabilising your blood glucose levels.

- **Hydration** is especially important in the mid-luteal phase due to rising progesterone increasing body temperature.

Let's talk about fat

Females naturally have more fat than males. While the word 'fat' often makes women (and men) squirm, I cannot emphasise enough how vital it is – having enough body fat is actually essential for life and making new life. Body fat stores in females, especially in the lower body, are believed to be an evolutionary adaptation for times of increased demand (such as pregnancy and breastfeeding) and also as an energy supply for times of food shortage and malnutrition.[10]

Fat is not just used as an energy store; it also forms part of cell membranes, brain tissue, nerve coverings and as protection around important organs (such as the heart and kidneys). We call this 'essential fat', and women have more of it than men for reproductive and hormonal functions. The second component of fat is storage fat, which can be found under the skin (subcutaneous) and around the organs (visceral).

An adequate amount of body fat is absolutely essential for a regular menstrual cycle, which is why women who have a very low body fat percentage often suffer with menstrual cycle disturbances (see page 66).[11] The good news is that this is recoverable – when sufficient body fat is achieved and enough energy (calories) is available.

Where females store fat is also different to males. We tend to store it in the lower part of our bodies (hips, thighs and bum) compared to males who store their fat centrally (around their stomach). Interestingly, this pattern of fat distribution in females is actually favourable when it comes to cardiovascular risk, as although we may have more subcutaneous fat (the fat under your skin) we also have less visceral fat (the fat around your organs) which carries the greatest risk with respect to metabolic disorders such as heart disease and type 2 diabetes. This degree of protection lasts until a woman goes through menopause, when fat distribution becomes more 'male-like', which unfortunately pushes up the chances of heart disease and related diseases.[12] Read more on supporting your heart health during menopause on page 36.

Cheat sheet: What to eat before, during and after your workout

Before

If you're under-fuelling going into a session, you may be making the workout harder on yourself. You can get away with exercising fasted if the workout is less than an hour and at low intensity, but anything more than that and I would recommend getting some fuel in the tank. Women also tend not to tolerate fasting very well and often report changes to their menstrual cycle as a result, which is one of the reasons I am very cautious to recommend this in females.

Aim to have your pre-workout meal (three to four hours before) or snack (one to two hours before) before you work out – ideally you want to avoid eating large meals too close to exercise to avoid any digestive issues. Your pre-workout meal should be based around carbohydrates and protein, with a smaller amount of fat.

Pre-workout meal and snack ideas

- porridge made with milk (or plant alternative*) and a spoonful of nut butter (try my Coconut, Quinoa + Oat Porridge on page 149)
- stuffed sweet potato with tuna and sweetcorn or veggie chilli
- pasta with tomato sauce and cheese
- peanut butter and banana sandwich on wholemeal bread
- granola or fruit and nut bar (check out my On-the-Run Fruit + Nut Bar on page 224)
- 1–2 bananas

fortified soya-based dairy alternatives tend to have the most similar nutritional profile to cow's milk products.

During

If you're exercising for fewer than 60 minutes, water is generally all you need during your workout – this will apply to most gym-goers. However, if your workout lasts longer than 60–90 minutes (such as a long run or cycle), you will need to top up your energy stores by taking on some extra carbs. In this case, start fuelling 45–60 minutes into your workout with 30–60g of carbohydrates per hour for exercise lasting up to 1–2.5 hours. Ideally, it should be high in carbohydrate, low in fibre, easy to digest – and familiar to you to avoid gut upset. Personally, I like taking malt loaf on my long runs, but some other ideas can be found opposite.

For endurance exercise greater than 2.5 hours, this can be increased up to 90g/hour in the form of a mixed carbohydrate (glucose and fructose) source. This can be in the form of energy drinks (with a 2:1 or 1:1 ratio of glucose to fructose) or dried fruit.

Snack ideas for during your workout

- malt loaf
- handful of dried fruit
- bananas
- jam and/or peanut butter sandwich
- fruit and nut bar or flapjack (check out my On-the-Run Fruit + Nut Bar on page 224)
- sports energy gels
- 500ml sports drink
- jelly babies

After

Your post-workout meal or snack should include protein (to repair and build muscle) and carbohydrate (to replenish energy stores) – and, of course, don't forget fluid (or electrolyte) replacement. There is no major urgency to eat straight away (unless training twice per day), but it is generally advisable to get some fuel in whenever you can and continue to fuel throughout the day beyond the 'post-workout window'. Some ideas for good post-workout meals and snacks are in the box below.

Post-workout meal and snack ideas

- a smoothie made with milk (or plant alternative), yogurt (or protein powder), banana and berries (check out my PB + Jelly Smoothie on page 141)
- a pot of yogurt with fruit and granola (try my Chunky Granola Clusters recipe on page 142)
- oatcakes with peanut butter and strawberries, or hummus
- overnight oats made with porridge oats, milk, yogurt and fruit (check out my Good-For-Your-Gut Overnight Oats on page 146)
- veggie chilli made with kidney beans and quinoa, served with brown rice (or served as a burrito)
- keep it simple with chicken or fish, rice and your choice of veggies

Finding the Right Sports Bra

When it comes to exercise and physical activity, our breasts bounce with us, so it makes sense that we protect them with a supportive sports bra. Did you know that the very first sports bra was made out of two jock straps sewn together? And do you know who came up with the idea? A woman. Fed up with breast pain while running and the discomfort that her regular bra caused, Lisa Lindahl created the first sports bra in 1977 called the 'Jogbra'.

Lindahl paved the way for women in sport and exercise, and despite the progress we have made with sports bra development, the industry still largely holds a 'one-size-fits-all' approach, and really very few sports bras are scientifically informed to create the best support. To add to that, most women don't know what they're looking for in a sports bra or can't find one that gives them what they need.

When I set about designing my own sports bra, I reached out on social media and asked *you* what makes finding the right sports bra so hard. Most of you were in resounding agreement that there are lots of very pretty-looking bras on the market, but they aren't fit for purpose and don't provide enough support – with many women resorting to wearing *two*!

Similarly, those that are supportive don't tend to be very flattering or attractive. In terms of sizing, most sports bras are categorised as small, medium or large and not by cup size, which can be challenging for women with larger breasts and smaller ribcages, or vice versa. So, you might have to shop around to find the right sports bra that fits your body type and, to do so, there are a few things you need to know – which is where I come in.

Why is it important?

The wrong sports bra, or the right sports bra that is poorly fit, can lead to breast pain, breast ptosis (breast sag) and embarrassment, and it can negatively affect performance and act as a barrier to exercise. The prevalence of exercise-induced breast pain has been reported in a whopping 72 per cent of exercising females.[13] Over a third of female runners surveyed at the 2012 London Marathon reported breast pain, with 17 per cent reporting it affecting their participation.[14]

While the source of exercise-induced breast pain is surprisingly not yet clear, studies have linked it to the displacement of the breasts – not just up and down, but also side to side and forwards and backwards. From the research, unsupported breasts move by up to 4cm in walking, up to 15cm during running and almost 19cm during a jumping jack.[15]

If left unsupported, this repetitive motion can strain and stretch the Cooper's ligaments – the fibrous, relatively weak connective tissue that helps to hold up the breast. The amount of movement and breast pain increases with the type of exercise (for example, low- versus high-intensity exercise) and also the size of the breast. In fact, women with large breasts are more likely to take part in less vigorous exercise, report increased pressure and pain from shoulder straps (which can also cause arm tingling and numbness due to nerve compression), more frictional injuries from sports bras and greater difficulty finding the correct bra fit than smaller-breasted women.[16]

What to look for in a sports bra

1. Type

Largely speaking, there are three types of sports bras:

1. **Compression (crop tops):** This type of sports bra is usually made of thick elastic material with the aim of reducing breast movement by compressing the breast tissue to the chest, and is more suitable for smaller-breasted women of size D or less.

2. **Encapsulation:** This type of sports bra contains two moulded cups formed by seams, panels or underwire. The aim of this bra is to limit movement by individually lifting each breast and holding them in place. Research promotes use of this style for larger-breasted (larger than a D cup) women to reduce movement and discomfort.[17]

3. **Combination:** This type of sports bra incorporates both encapsulation and compression elements with two separate cups that elevate and support each breast independently, covered by an external layer that compresses the breasts against the chest wall. This type of bra may reduce exercise-induced breast pain by minimising 'breast slap'.[18]

2. Underband

Most of the support should actually come from the underband with only a small amount coming from the straps to reduce pressure on the shoulders. An adjustable underband is advised for greatest comfort and reduction in breast movement. When checking the fit of the underband, it should feel secure without pinching the skin. For a quick test, raise your arms when you're trying it on and check that it does not ride upwards.

3. Shoulder straps

In terms of comfort, a wide, padded vertical strap appears to be preferable for women with larger breasts. Non-vertical straps (cross-over or racerback) can help to prevent the straps slipping off the shoulders, but strap orientation is largely a personal preference.[19] When adjusting your straps, you might find that each may be a different length as most of the female population have asymmetrical breasts, with the left often larger than the right![20]

4. Cups

Cups with padding can protect the breasts in sport and also provide additional support.[21] The breast should not bulge over the cup or neckline (a sign the bra is too small), nor should there be wrinkles or gaping (a sign it's too big). The gore (the bit between the cups) should sit flat on the breastbone (not on your breast tissue); if this is floating away from your chest, either the cups may be too small or the underband too big.

5. Neckline

In general, the higher the neckline, the more supportive the bra – for every 1cm increase, bounce reduction increases by 0.75 per cent.[22] We must remember that the breast tissue extends all the way up to the collarbones and also up into the armpit, so it's important that the sports bra is as supportive as possible.

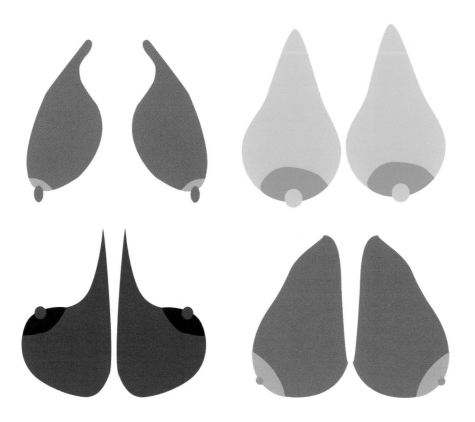

Taking Care of Your Breasts

Breast health goes far deeper than choosing the right sports bra and, like everything, 'knowledge is power'. Your first port of call should be getting to know your breasts, by look and feel, so you can notice any changes immediately.

During a Sunday binge of my latest favourite Netflix series, I was lying on the sofa when I noticed a small – but discrete – firm lump in my right breast. I rolled it under my fingertips and began to quickly examine myself. It was firm, smooth, rubbery, about the size of a grape, and it moved under the skin.

As someone who has worked as a doctor in breast surgery during one of my surgical rotations, I was used to treating patients of all ages (many younger than me) with breast cancer and so I knew not to dismiss this new breast lump. I arranged a consultation with my GP the next morning and he referred me to the 'One Stop' breast clinic at my local hospital. This is a fast-track diagnostic clinic where you are seen by a breast consultant or senior registrar, and often involves having some investigations or tests to speed up the diagnosis.

The breast surgeon who examined me wasn't quite sure what the lump was and so sent me for an ultrasound scan of my breast. As I lay on the examination bed while a radiologist ran a probe over my breast, I stared at the ceiling and fell into a black hole of all the potential outcomes of this scan. It didn't help that the radiologist remained deathly silent throughout the examination.

The suspense was killing me so I chipped in with, 'Sorry to disturb you, but can you talk me through what you're looking at? I'm also a doctor.' He cleared his throat, shifting slightly on his stool, and said, 'Oh, sorry! Well, I've found what you're feeling, and I don't think you have anything to worry about.' He pointed to what he was looking at on the screen and explained that it was essentially a dense collection of fibrous tissue (aka lumpy breast tissue) and that a biopsy wasn't needed. Relief!

A part of me felt a little silly for losing sleep over a little lumpy bit of tissue, but I quickly reminded myself of what I tell my patients and the women in my life: **knowing your boobs and what is normal for you could save your life.**

What is your normal?

Breast cancer is now the most common cancer in the UK and is by far the most common cancer in women, with one in seven women in the UK developing it during their lifetime.[23] While it is more common as we age, breast cancer is the second most commonly diagnosed cancer in women under the age of 30 in the UK. We all have breast tissue and people of all genders and sexes can get breast cancer. Being breast aware, knowing what is normal for you and noticing any new changes is the first step in detecting breast cancer in the early stages.

How to check your breasts

Look

Stand in front of the mirror bare-breasted and scan your breasts for any changes (if you have large breasts, lift them up and look underneath). Repeat this standing to each side, with your hands raised above your head, and finally with your hands on your hips pushing inwards so that you tense your chest muscles.

Things you're looking for include:

- changes in skin colour
- obvious lumps
- changes in texture, such as puckering or dimpling (like the skin of an orange)
- redness or a rash on the skin and/or around the nipple
- changes to the nipple (inversion or change in direction)
- nipple discharge

Feel

Feel each breast. This ideally should be done lying down, but can be done standing up if you have small breasts. As doctors we are trained to examine breasts with patients lying down at 30–45 degrees which you can replicate at home with two or three pillows under your head. Examine one breast at a time, using the opposite hand to feel the opposite breast and placing your free arm behind your head.

Using the flat underside of your fingers (not pressing down with your fingertips) gently push the breast tissue against your ribcage. Check the entire breast using a systematic approach – in quadrants or in a clockwise fashion, for example. Don't forget to feel all the way up to the collarbones and into the armpits.

Breasts are naturally a bit lumpy – they are not typically smooth, hard and round like 'melons', but soft, squishy and dense. If one breast feels lumpy, check the other side and it's likely it will feel the same. The majority of breast lumps are not cancerous and may in fact be caused by normal breast changes or a benign (not cancerous) breast condition such as cysts or fibrous tissue. But, if a lump appears and doesn't go, it's really important to get it checked out.

You might also notice that at certain points in your menstrual cycle your breasts will feel lumpier than usual, so keep a track of when in your cycle you check.

Things to feel for include:

- unusual change in size or shape of the breast

- any lumps in the breast, armpit or around the collarbone

- thickening of the skin

- discomfort or pain in one breast*

*Breast pain is a rare symptom of breast cancer, but new-onset pain should be assessed.

If you find a lump or notice a change, or even if you're not quite sure, pop along to your GP as they are the best person to check for you and also refer you for any scans or further tests as needed.

If you're aged 50–70 in the UK you will also be invited for routine breast screening.

How Do We Compare to Men?

With your breast health covered, it's good to think about the ways in which your body may differ from men's in terms of strength and physical activity, so you know where you can excel.

Run like a girl

In studies using MRI (magnetic resonance imaging) machines, men have 30–40 per cent more muscle mass than women, and this is greatest in the upper body.[24] In addition to having *more* muscle, the type of muscle fibres also differ. In females, type I or 'slow-twitch' muscle fibres (used for endurance activities, such as long-distance running) tend to be larger than the type II or 'fast-twitch' muscle fibres (used for quick, powerful movements such as sprinting or weightlifting), whereas the reverse is true for males.[25]

Another reason why women may have an edge on men when it comes to running marathons is that women are generally more resistant to muscle fatigue and are better at using fat for fuel during endurance activity, which prevents them hitting the wall and slowing down.[26] So while women may not out-lift men, it seems we can keep going – for longer.

Is it harder for women to build muscle?

While men do have – and can build – more muscle, women can build it just as fast. Hear me out. This is because the rate at which males and females build muscle, in response to resistance training, is essentially the same.[27] That said, we can pump all the iron we like, but physiologically, females cannot develop as large muscles as males. The bodybuilding community is a good example of this: one study found that the biceps of competitive male bodybuilders were twice as large as their female bodybuilders, after years of equivalent training.[28] Additionally, the male bodybuilders had a larger number of muscle fibres, meaning more muscle-building potential to begin with.

So, while men gain more than twice the *total amount* of muscle mass from lifting weights, we need to remember that women have much less muscle mass to begin with. For example, if you take a 90-kg man and a 60-kg woman, if they both increase their muscle mass by 10 per cent, the man will have gained more (9kg versus 6kg) muscle tissue. But, compared to their starting point, females gain similar amounts of muscle as males.

Size aside, are men stronger than women? In absolute terms – yes. On average, women are 52 per cent as strong as men in the upper body and 66 per cent as strong as men in the lower body.[29] This is because males are generally larger but leaner humans, with longer and thicker bones and bigger muscles that are better equipped for strength (type II muscle fibres ensure men have a greater power output).[30] So while we may be closing the gap on endurance sport, women are not going to out-squat men anytime soon.

All in all, men will always outperform women when it comes to strength and power, but it's important to understand that women benefit just as much as men in terms of relative improvements in strength from their baseline.

#GirlsWhoLift

Although sex and hormones are crucial factors when it comes to building muscle, biology is not the only thing preventing women from making gains in the gym. Not only do gender-specific workout guides and classes still exist, but there is still this ingrained belief that women should avoid building too much muscle as it is not considered a 'feminine' trait.

Despite the #StrongNotSkinny era, research has found that many female lifters report holding back when lifting weights, in order to avoid gaining too much muscle. This phenomenon is known as the 'glass ceiling' of female masculinity, in which women describe an upper limit on the quest for muscular strength and muscle gains; women strive to build muscle – just not *too* much.[31] As such, women in fitness may find that their bodily agency and empowerment are not limited by their biology (they have the capacity to build more muscle and gain strength) but instead by ideologies of emphasised femininity. In response, we have developed a feminised language to talk about muscularity – 'tone', 'sculpt' and 'firm' are girl code for gaining muscle and losing fat. Let's reframe that.

Women are strong. Women have muscles. Women are athletes.

Cardio is hardio

Males also have an advantage in that they're leaner (good for speed), they have a bigger set of heart and lungs (a bigger engine) and they have slightly higher levels of haemoglobin (so more oxygen gets to the muscles and organs). Because of these differences, men typically have a higher 'VO2 max' (a measure of how much oxygen is used during exercise). This value is regarded by most exercise scientists as the best test of a person's cardiorespiratory fitness and endurance capacity. That said, this gap can be narrowed with the right training, and many elite female athletes have significantly higher values than untrained men and women – some even higher than elite male athletes![32]

Down to the Bone

In terms of our bones and skeleton, males and females differ there too. Males typically have longer and thicker bones, which assist with power output and also mean they are better at withstanding injury.

We acquire most of our bone mass by the time we are 18 (earlier in females), but peak bone mass isn't achieved until about the age of 25–30 and, after that, bone loss occurs faster than bone formation. This process happens faster still and at a younger age, in females.[33] This can result in osteoporosis, a condition characterised by very low bone mineral density (BMD), where bones are more fragile and prone to fractures. Osteoporosis is known as a 'silent disease' as you typically won't have symptoms and it is not often diagnosed unless it is screened for or until a fracture occurs.

Oestrogen plays an essential role in the development and maintenance of bone mass. This is why, after the menopause, women lose bone density at a rate several-fold faster than that in men of the same age or premenopausal women.[34] In fact, women over the age of 50 have a four times higher rate of osteoporosis and twice the rate of osteopenia (lower than normal bone density), and they tend to have fractures five to ten years earlier compared with men.[35]

This can also happen in younger women who have suppressed oestrogen levels, for example, those who have had their ovaries surgically removed or have gone through an early menopause for other reasons, or in young women who are not having regular periods due to anorexia nervosa or functional hypothalamic amenorrhoea (FHA) – see page 67.

All of that said, females are not destined to have brittle bones and there are things that we can do instead that will help protect bone health in the future. There are a number of factors that determine our bone health and peak bone mass, some of which we can't change, such as our genes, sex or age, and some of which we can, including our diet, staying physically active and not smoking. In fact, lifestyle factors influence up to 20–40 per cent of adult peak bone mass, so optimising them today can help reduce your risk of osteoporosis later in life.[36] See page 39 for advice on what to eat for bone health and page 80 for the best exercises to strengthen your bones.

Bone mass across the lifespan[37]

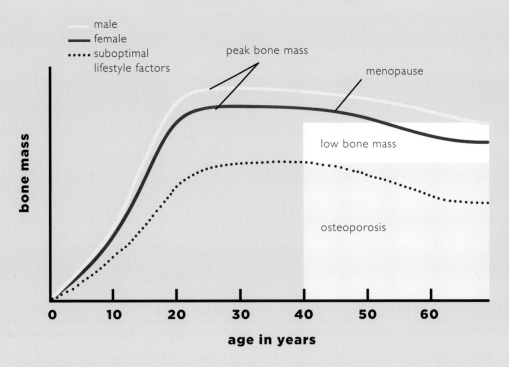

- male
- female
- •••• suboptimal lifestyle factors

peak bone mass

menopause

low bone mass

osteoporosis

bone mass

age in years

0   10   20   30   40   50   60

Factors influencing peak bone mass

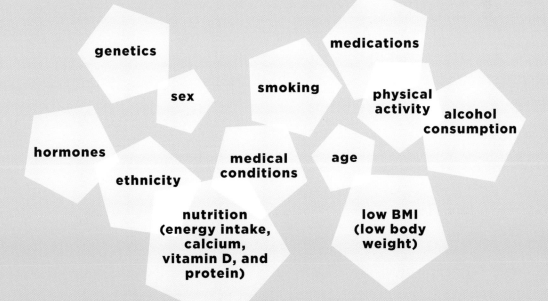

genetics

medications

sex

smoking

physical activity

alcohol consumption

hormones

ethnicity

medical conditions

age

nutrition (energy intake, calcium, vitamin D, and protein)

low BMI (low body weight)

Can I Exercise on My Period?

British athlete Jessica Judd says the effects of her menstrual cycle can be 'the difference between finishing first and last', but not all women are affected in the same way.[38] Paula Radcliffe allegedly started her period the morning of the 2002 Chicago Marathon and went on to break the world record.[39]

Historically, women have been advised not to exercise during their period with the fear that it may impair fertility. Over the last few decades, we have accumulated a modest amount of research exploring the effects of exercise on the menstrual cycle and vice versa – the effects of the menstrual cycle on performance in exercise.

We now know that women can safely and confidently exercise – even at high intensities – without it impacting their cycle or fertility. The caveat, however, is that EA (energy expended exercising versus energy taken in from food) must be balanced, as we discovered earlier on in the chapter (see page 48). First, let's take a look at how our menstrual cycle affects performance in exercise and sport, and then we'll go on to discuss whether exercise can affect your period.

Can my period affect performance?

Across the menstrual cycle, some women will experience changes in their strength, performance and recovery when it comes to sport and exercise, but for others, this difference may be so subtle that they notice no changes at all.

These changes are down to the fluctuations in oestrogen and progesterone that occur across the menstrual cycle and are not necessarily positive or negative, but by understanding them, we have the potential to make the most of our training and recovery.

Early follicular

From the research, there seems to be a slight dip in performance (both strength and endurance) during your period when compared with other phases in the menstrual cycle.[40] That said, if you do feel up for moving your body, it is totally safe to do so and may help to ease menstrual symptoms – and boost your mood at the same time.[41]

Late follicular

After your period, as oestrogen rises and progesterone remains low, this might be a good time to make some gains in the gym. Oestrogen helps to boost energy levels, promotes muscle-building and enhances recovery, including reducing next-day muscle soreness and swelling (often referred to as DOMS – delayed-onset muscle soreness).[42] Now is a good time for higher intensity and strength training.

Ovulation

Strength and performance remain strong around ovulation, with the added help of testosterone, but be careful before tearing up the pitch as knee injury (particularly ACL – anterior cruciate ligament) is particularly common in women during this time.[43] The research is still inconclusive here, but perhaps take caution with exercises that require a rapid change of direction or impact and make sure you're sufficiently warmed up beforehand.

Early/mid-luteal

Oestrogen levels (which initially dropped off at ovulation) start to rise again and may enhance aerobic performance during this time. However, progesterone also rises and peaks mid-cycle, which is thought to inhibit some of the beneficial effects of oestrogen, as well as increasing body temperature, fluid retention and bloating. So while endurance training may be a good idea, emphasise recovery and hydration.

Late luteal

During this part of your cycle both oestrogen and progesterone begin to decline, and you may experience premenstrual symptoms, but light to moderate exercise may help with that. Sleep is likely to be disrupted around now, which could affect your concentration and alertness, so it may not be the best time for highly skilled or precision training. Typically, now is a good time to take some extra rest days and focus on active recovery like walking and yoga.

Across the menstrual cycle you may feel stronger, more motivated and more energetic during certain phases, *but* research in this field is limited and conflicting and every woman experiences her cycle differently. The table below should be used as a guide – not a rule.

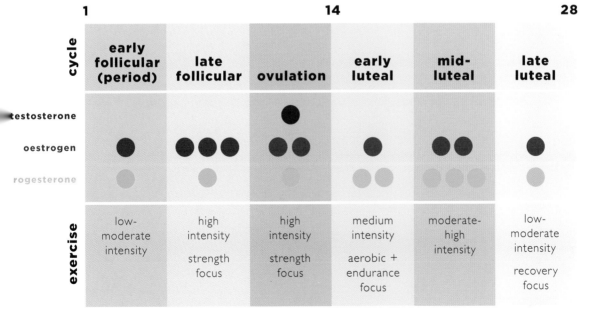

	1		14			28
cycle	early follicular (period)	late follicular	ovulation	early luteal	mid-luteal	late luteal
testosterone			●			
oestrogen	●	● ● ●	● ●	●	● ●	●
progesterone	●	●	●	● ●	● ● ●	●
exercise	low-moderate intensity	high intensity strength focus	high intensity strength focus	medium intensity aerobic + endurance focus	moderate-high intensity	low-moderate intensity recovery focus

How does the pill affect exercise?

To date, most of the research has not shown a change in strength or high-intensity performance between pill-users and non-users, or between pill-taking and pill-free days.[44] A recent review found that pill-users might have slightly reduced exercise (both strength and endurance) performance when compared to non-users, but no changes between pill-taking and pill-free days.[45]

It's likely that some women may find the pill affects their performance, strength or recovery, while others do not. At the end of the day, only you know your body.

Can exercise affect my period?

One of the most common complaints I hear from women who are avid gym-goers, runners or triathletes is that their period is either out of whack or has totally disappeared.

This is more common than some may think. A study of women who exercised regularly found that half had menstrual disturbances and over a third had no period at all.[46] Anecdotally, one of the most common reasons women contact me directly is because they've lost their period, and while there are many reasons why someone may be experiencing amenorrhoea (the absence of menstruation), one of the most common causes in active females is functional hypothalamic amenorrhea (FHA).

What is the hypothalamus?

The hypothalamus is a small part of your brain with many roles – it is essentially the master regulator of all the endocrine (hormone) glands in the body, including your ovaries. The hormonal connection between the brain and ovaries is known as the 'hypothalamic-pituitary-ovarian' axis, or the HPO axis. Hormones released from these key areas in the brain travel through the bloodstream and stimulate the ovaries to ovulate and produce oestrogen and progesterone.

Functional hypothalamic amenorrhea (FHA)

FHA is thought to be responsible for 20–35 per cent of cases of secondary amenorrhoea (previously had a period, now it's gone versus never having had a period) with rates higher in athletic women.[47] This is caused by low calorie/nutrient intake, excessive exercise, weight loss, stress or a combination of these factors.

Firstly, FHA is a diagnosis of exclusion, which means that all other medical conditions that could be potentially causing amenorrhoea first must be ruled out by your doctor.

Secondly, regardless of what you're training for or how fit you think you are, *it is not normal or healthy to not have a period*. It is a sign that your body is undergoing significant stress, so please don't ignore it. The menstrual cycle is much more than just a period. In fact, many clinicians are now calling for the menstrual cycle to be recorded as a fifth vital sign when assessing overall health status; just as we would take your blood pressure, temperature, heart rate and breathing rate.[48]

You might be thinking, well it's just my period and I'm not thinking about having children at the moment (or at all), but not having a regular cycle can have far-reaching effects in the body beyond reproduction, including bone density, other hormonal disturbances (such as thyroid hormones) and impaired immunity, and it can affect your mental health too.

Before you make any self-diagnoses, you first need to be reviewed by a medical doctor to do a full work-up and rule out other causes for your symptoms. Recovery should ideally occur with the support of a doctor and a registered dietitian, but ultimately when it comes to getting your period back, addressing the root cause is key. This often involves increasing your daily calorie intake and/or reducing the amount or intensity of exercise – likely both. In addition to consuming enough calories, you also want to ensure you're eating sufficient amounts of protein, carbohydrates and fats. Often, this will mean restoring lost weight or gaining some additional weight. Optimising sleep and aiming to reduce as much external stress as possible are also really important for recovery (see Chapter 4 for lots more about sleep).

> **Regardless of what you're training for or how fit you think you are, it is not normal or healthy to not have a period. It is a sign that your body is undergoing significant stress, so please don't ignore it.**

Can I Stay Active While Pregnant?

'Can you be an athlete? You pregnant? You a mother? That depends. What is an athlete? Someone who moves? Sounds like you.'[49]

This is how one of Nike's maternity ads titled 'The Toughest Athletes' begins, featuring women engaging in various forms of activity while pregnant and in the postpartum period. While the advert features famous athletes such as Serena Williams and Alex Morgan, the underlying message aims to be inclusive and redefine who and what an athlete is and looks like, stating that 'no matter what you do or how you do it, you are the toughest athlete'. And they're not wrong – research has shown that in terms of energy expended, pregnancy is basically like running a 40-week marathon and is one of the most energy-demanding challenges the human body can sustain.[50]

Pregnancy was previously considered a time of rest, but we now know that staying active during pregnancy not only offers the usual benefits of regular physical activity, such as improved sleep and mood, but also a reduced risk of pregnancy complications such as gestational diabetes, blood pressure disorders and the risk of postpartum depression.[51]

Benefits of physical activity in pregnancy[52]

- fewer newborn complications
- reduced risk of diabetes in pregnancy
- reduced risk of excessive gestational weight gain (see opposite)
- reduced risk of blood pressure disorders (such as pre-eclampsia)
- may reduce risk of Caesarean and instrumental delivery
- improved mood and reduced risk of postpartum depression
- reduction in severity of lower-back and pelvic girdle pain
- reduced risk of urinary incontinence (with pelvic floor training)
- usual benefits of physical activity, including improved sleep and fitness

Despite the benefits for mum and baby, it is estimated that only 3–15 per cent of pregnant women are meeting the physical activity guidelines compared with 24–26 per cent of non-pregnant women.[53] There are a number of reasons why this may be, but let's start with the fact that learning to move in a pregnant body is naturally going to feel very different than when not pregnant. Not to mention symptoms commonly experienced by pregnant women, such as morning sickness, tiredness, backache and pelvic pain, which are likely to act as a barrier to activity.[54]

A note on weight gain in pregnancy

Weight gain is a positive sign of a healthy pregnancy. This additional weight is mostly due to the weight of a growing baby, the amniotic fluid that surrounds the baby, increased blood volume circulating in your body, and also increased body fat stores, which are needed to provide energy for breast milk production. Weight gain during pregnancy varies considerably from woman to woman and also between pregnancies. Gaining too little weight or too much can both carry health risks for mother and baby. However, in the UK there are no official guidelines on how much weight a woman should gain during pregnancy. Weight loss or restrictive dieting is not recommended during pregnancy as it can be harmful to the health of the growing baby. If you're concerned about your weight or any other aspect of your health while pregnant, ask your midwife or GP for advice.

Of course, there are situations, such as certain health conditions or pregnancy complications, where physical activity may be advised against or specialist input may be required (see table below). If you do fall into one of these categories, please speak to your consultant or midwife.

Conditions and pregnancy complications where exercise may be contraindicated[55]

Absolute contraindications	Relative contraindications
• severe respiratory diseases (such as chronic obstructive pulmonary disease (COPD), restrictive lung disease, cystic fibrosis and so on) • severe acquired or congenital heart disease with exercise intolerance • uncontrolled or severe arrhythmia • placental abruption • vasa praevia • uncontrolled type 1 diabetes • intrauterine growth restriction (IUGR) • active preterm labour (regular and painful uterine contractions before 37 weeks of pregnancy) • severe pre-eclampsia • cervical insufficiency	• mild respiratory disorders, such as well-controlled asthma • mild congenital or acquired heart disease • well-controlled type 1 diabetes • mild pre-eclampsia • preterm premature rupture of membranes (PPROMs) – waters breaking • placenta praevia after 28 weeks • untreated thyroid disease • symptomatic, severe eating disorders • multiple nutrient deficiencies and/or chronic undernutrition • heavy smoking (>20 cigarettes per day) in the presence of comorbidities

Staying fit and safe

Most forms of physical activity are safe during uncomplicated pregnancies, whether that be walking your dog or heading to the gym. However, some carry significant risk and should be avoided.

Activities to avoid:[56]

- activities with higher risk of falling or high-impact injuries, such as skiing, gymnastics, off-road cycling and horse riding

- contact sports, such as rugby, soccer, boxing, basketball and martial arts

- scuba diving (due to the possibility of decompression sickness and gas embolism)

- skydiving or vigorous exercise above 6,000 feet (due to potential lowering of uterine blood flow)

- activity in excessive heat, especially with high humidity

After first trimester:

- sports where there is a risk of being hit in the abdomen by equipment, such as tennis or squash

- exercise involving lying flat on the back, due to venous compression and hypotension (note that pregnancy-specific yoga or Pilates classes should not include these exercises and are safe)

Top tips for staying active safely in pregnancy:

- stay cool, comfortable and hydrated. Try to avoid sessions longer than an hour in duration, especially on warmer days

- due to an increase in the hormone relaxin, joints become more lax as pregnancy progresses. Shoes that support the ankles and arches can help prevent injuries

- due to progressive weight gain, a shift in the centre of gravity and increase in the hormone relaxin, postural balance can be affected, which increases the risk of falls and injury. Therefore, try to avoid bumpy terrain and stick to flat surfaces – plan your activity in advance

- don't bump the bump

Safety guidelines are there to guide you, but it's so important to listen to your body and adapt accordingly. If it feels pleasant, keep going; if it's uncomfortable, stop and seek advice.

If you experience any of the following red flags, stop and seek medical advice:

- vaginal bleeding

- abdominal pain

- regular and painful contractions

- amniotic fluid leakage

- shortness of breath before exertion

- persistent excessive shortness of breath that does not resolve with rest

- persistent dizziness or faintness that does not resolve with rest

- headache

- chest pain

- muscle weakness affecting balance

- calf pain or swelling

Finally, you might be surprised to hear that the recommended amount of activity is actually not dissimilar to the advice for all adults, that is 150 minutes of moderate-intensity physical activity per week and muscle-strengthening activities twice per week.[57] A simple measure of moderate intensity is the talk test; if you're doing moderate-intensity activity, you can talk but not sing during the activity. This might include brisk walking, water aerobics or swimming – even gardening. It may sound like a lot of minutes, but activity should be accumulated across the week, and no one is expecting you to count these minutes (unless, of course, you want to!). So while 150 minutes is the official recommendation, every little counts.

How Soon Can I Move Postpartum?

Remaining active in the postnatal period is so important for your mental and physical well-being. In addition to the usual benefits of improving fitness, sleep and strength, physical activity can help improve mood and emotional well-being, and reduces the risk of postnatal depression.[58]

The act of taking time out for you each day to do some type of movement is essentially a form of self-care for your mind and body. You may wish to include your baby in this, or you may want 10 minutes to yourself. It can also be a good opportunity to connect with new mums or catch up with friends. The period following birth can be quite isolating, so building and maintaining strong social connections is equally important for your health.

While the guidelines for physical activity following childbirth do not differ to those for pregnant women, postpartum women should aim to gradually build back up to 150 minutes of moderate-intensity physical activity across the week and to doing muscle-strengthening activities twice a week.[59] It is also advisable to break up long periods of sitting time with light forms of activity.

It's generally safe to start gentle activity as soon as you feel up to it, but it's different for all new mums. For Caesarean sections or more complicated vaginal births, recovery times may be longer, so check with your doctor if you're unsure. Remember, physical activity does not need to be intense or a structured form of exercise in order to provide benefits.

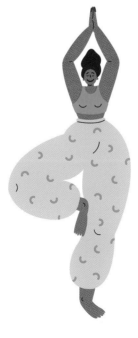

Why Is the Pelvic Floor So Important?

The female pelvic floor is made of muscles and connective tissue that form a 'sling' or 'hammock' across the base of the pelvis. Its role is not only to keep all the pelvic organs (your bladder, uterus/womb and rectum) in place, but to also ensure urinary and faecal continence, support increases in intrapelvic/abdominal pressure (for example, during activities such as coughing or lifting heavy objects) and also help to stabilise the spine and bony pelvis. The pelvic floor muscles also provide additional support during childbirth. In fact, antenatal pelvic floor muscle training (PFMT) can reduce the need for operative delivery and Caesarean section.[60]

Finally – but crucially – a strong pelvic floor can also improve your sex life. Come again? (No pun intended.) Research shows that women with better pelvic muscle strength have more desire, excitement, lubrication and orgasm than women with weak pelvic floor muscles.[61] Pelvic floor muscles appear to improve sexual function through increased blood flow to the pelvis, enhanced clitoral sensitivity and attainment of orgasm.[62]

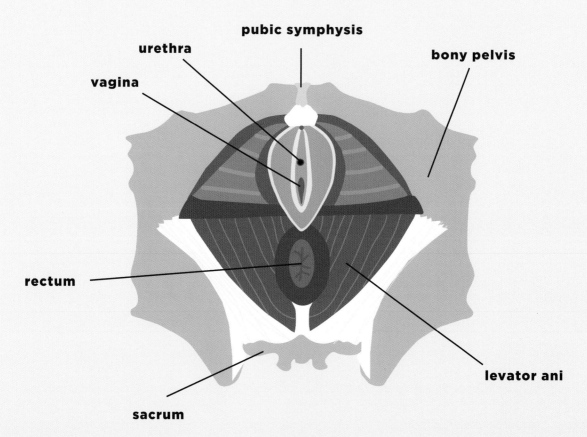

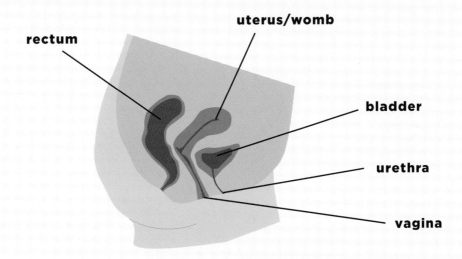

rectum

uterus/womb

bladder

urethra

vagina

Signs of a weakness

If your pelvic floor muscles are not working optimally, you may have pelvic floor dysfunction (PFD), which could present with one or a few of the following symptoms:[63]

• urinary incontinence (leakage), sudden urgency to wee and increased frequency of having to go to the toilet

• bowel incontinence, sudden urgency to have a bowel motion, leakage of wind and/or stool

• obstructive defecation

• pelvic organ prolapse (often described as a feeling of something coming down, or a 'heaviness' or bulge in your vagina)

• painful sex or reduced sexual arousal

• pelvic pain

Note: pregnancy and childbirth are not the only risk factors for PFD. Constipation and straining, breath-holding when lifting or exercising, a high BMI, smoking and a persistent cough can also increase the risk.

Vaginal flatulence (also known as 'queefing' or fanny farts) may also be a sign of PFD. However, it is normal to queef when you're doing certain exercises (such as yoga) or during penetrative sex – due to air becoming trapped inside the vagina and then escaping again. Fanny farts (what a terrible name!) are not actual farts and do not smell because it's literally just air. It's nothing to be ashamed or embarrassed about, and a very common thing that most women experience (easier said than done, you're thinking).

However, in some rare cases, vaginal flatulence can be a sign of a more serious medical condition or issue. If you find yourself queefing more than usual, or it's accompanied by one or more of the symptoms listed above, speak to your GP.

How do I find my pelvic floor?

One method of locating your pelvic floor is stopping the flow of wee when you're on the toilet – that's your pelvic floor working. This is an effective method for locating your pelvic floor muscles, but you shouldn't use it as a way of exercising your pelvic floor (also known as Kegel exercises).

How do I train my pelvic floor?

1. Make sure you are comfortably lying, sitting or standing.

2. Inhale through your nose and, as you exhale through your mouth, squeeze your anus as if you're trying to stop yourself from passing wind. As you do this, you should feel your perineum (the bit between the anus and vaginal opening) contract and lift.

3. Try to hold this squeeze for a few seconds and then let go and relax. As you're holding this position, try to breathe normally (just as you would when holding a plank).

4. After relaxing, repeat the exercise ten times, aiming to hold for ten seconds each time (it may take some weeks to build up to this).

5. After your longer holds, follow with ten short squeezes. Make sure that you slowly release and relax between each squeeze.

Train your pelvic floor every day, at least once a day, and up to two to three times a day if you have PFD symptoms such as incontinence.

Check out the NHS app 'Squeezy' for pelvic floor exercise regimes and daily reminders – plus a directory for pelvic health physiotherapists.

Staying Active After Menopause

The perimenopause and the menopause are periods in every woman's life that are rarely discussed (unless within the four walls of a doctor's surgery) and almost never celebrated.

Unlike sex education at school for puberty, there's no adult version for the menopause, and though we support and celebrate women who are pregnant with 'baby on board' badges and bespoke exercise classes, we still refer to the menopause as 'the change' or the 'M word' as if it is this big dirty secret that we shouldn't talk about.

So I'm sure that it comes as no surprise when I tell you that there is little guidance for women when it comes to staying active after the menopause. Unsurprisingly, 30 per cent of women report becoming less active after the menopause and 38 per cent of women aged 45–54 do not meet the government guidelines for physical activity.[64]

An independent survey found that social stigma and lack of social support, menopausal symptoms and lack of self-confidence and knowledge when it comes to physical activity were major barriers to staying active after the menopause.[65] Women of this 'sandwich generation' are often taking care of elderly parents and their own children and grandchildren (financially, emotionally and physically), which zaps them of their time and energy.

There is now robust evidence to show that physical activity after menopause not only adds years to life, but also adds life to years by improving quality of life, independence and mood. Physical activity can also offset the risk of health conditions that are more common after the menopause, such as heart disease, osteoporosis and incontinence.

Unfortunately, there are no menopause-specific physical activity guidelines out there, so the same generic guidelines for adults apply (see overleaf).

Benefits of physical activity after the menopause

- improves bone health and reduces risk of osteoporosis[66]

- reduces midlife weight gain[67]

- improves balance and risk of falls[68]

- improves heart health and associated risks (such as high blood pressure and type 2 diabetes)[69]

- improves cognition and reduces the risk of dementia[70]

- improves sleep quality[71]

- improves mental health, including symptoms of depression and anxiety[72]

- improves some menopausal symptoms (see below)

- reduces risk of certain cancers including breast, endometrial and colon[73]

Can exercise reduce menopausal hot flushes and night sweats?

Unfortunately, the evidence is conflicting on this one and, overall, it seems we don't have enough good evidence to say yes. That said, there are a few studies that have found positive effects, and many women report that increasing their physical activity has positive effects on their menopausal symptoms.[74]

Getting Started

It's never too late to start being active – and any amount of exercise is better than no exercise at all. For all adults, including those over 65 (who are generally fit and have no health conditions), the advice is to do at least 150 minutes of moderate-intensity activity a week or 75 minutes of vigorous-intensity activity, or a combination of both.[75] If you're unable to meet this goal due to health conditions, you should aim to be as physically active as your abilities and conditions allow. There is also emphasis for adults to include activities that improve strength on at least two days of a week, and for those over 65 to include activities that improve strength, balance and flexibility.

Aerobic exercise

When it comes to heart health, aerobic exercise (sometimes called 'cardio'), such as cycling, walking, jogging/running, swimming and dancing, is considered the best. This form of exercise has been shown to strengthen the heart muscle and the health of the blood vessels, while also improving blood cholesterol levels, blood glucose and blood pressure. (Note: if you have high blood pressure or a heart condition, it is important to check with your doctor or cardiac team before starting any new exercise programme.)

Moderate intensity (You can talk, but not sing)	Vigorous intensity (You can't talk in full sentences without pausing for a breath)
• brisk walking • water aerobics • riding a bike • dancing • doubles tennis • pushing a lawn mower • hiking • rollerblading	• running • swimming • riding a bike fast or on hills • walking up the stairs • sports, like football, rugby, netball and hockey • skipping • aerobics • gymnastics • martial arts • spinning • interval training: circuits, sprints, weightlifting

Weight-bearing activities

Weight-bearing activities that provide some form of impact appear to be the most effective at strengthening bones and maintaining bone health. But what do we mean by 'weight-bearing'? This is essentially any activity where you are standing on one or both feet. So that includes walking, jogging, hiking, jumping, dancing and most types of team or racquet sports. Generally, higher-impact activities (such as running) that involve dynamic movements have a greater effect on bone density than lower-impact activities (like walking). Muscle-strengthening exercises are also bone-strengthening exercises. This is because the muscles essentially apply a stress to the bones which respond by renewing themselves and strengthening – more on this next!

Lower impact	Moderate impact	High-impact
• walking • marching • stair climbing • stamping • gentle heel drops	• Highland dancing • jogging or running • team and racquet sports • skipping and hopping • low-level jumps • vigorous heel drops and stamping	• basketball • volleyball • track events • star jumps • tuck jumps • high-level jumps[77]

Muscle-strengthening exercises

Muscle-strengthening exercises, often called strength-/weight-/resistance training, offer multiple benefits beyond building and strengthening muscles. Ideally, you should aim to do muscle-strengthening exercises on at least two days of the week, working your major muscle groups (legs, arms, back and core). This can involve weights, resistance bands and bodyweight exercises (such as lunges, squats or push-ups). Other activities such as heavy gardening, yoga and Pilates also count.

Move More, Sit Less

Finally, in addition to moving more, we also need to spend less time sitting. This is because being sedentary (spending time sitting or lying) is an independent risk factor to physical inactivity, for heart and circulatory disease and general poor health. This means that, even if you meet your physical activity recommendations per week but spend the majority of your day sitting down (yep, we can all raise our hands here), then you are still at increased risk.

Unfortunately, sitting has become the norm in modern society. In fact, the average UK adult spends almost 30 hours a week watching TV – this is equivalent to 64 days a year![78] Make sure to break up your sitting time with regular breaks, standing while taking the bus or train, going for a short walk on coffee and lunch breaks, walking while taking phone calls or during meetings, or perhaps setting a reminder to stand up and do a few squats every 90 minutes.

This advice applies to us all, whatever stage of life we're currently living through, so keep the motto of 'move more, sit less' under your belt, and it should hold you in good stead.

* * * *

I hope you end this chapter feeling strong and empowered, knowing that you are capable of great physical achievements and a strong and healthy body. As women, we have a unique physiology that impacts how fast we move or how strong we are, but instead of viewing it as a disadvantage, view it as a difference. By understanding your unique needs and tuning into your body, you're able to maximise on your strengths and achieve great things. Women are not small – nor *weak* – men.

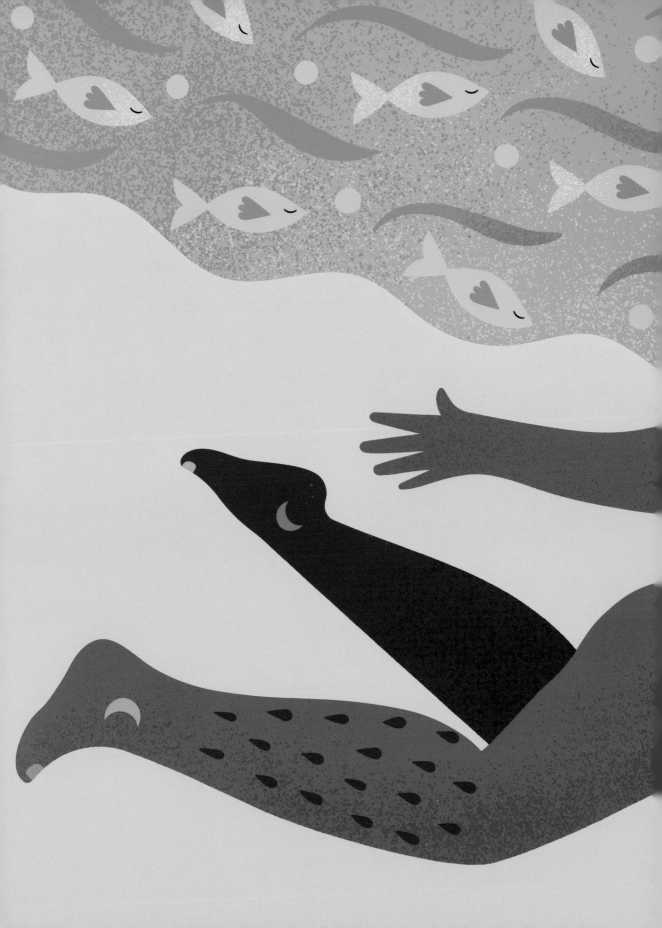

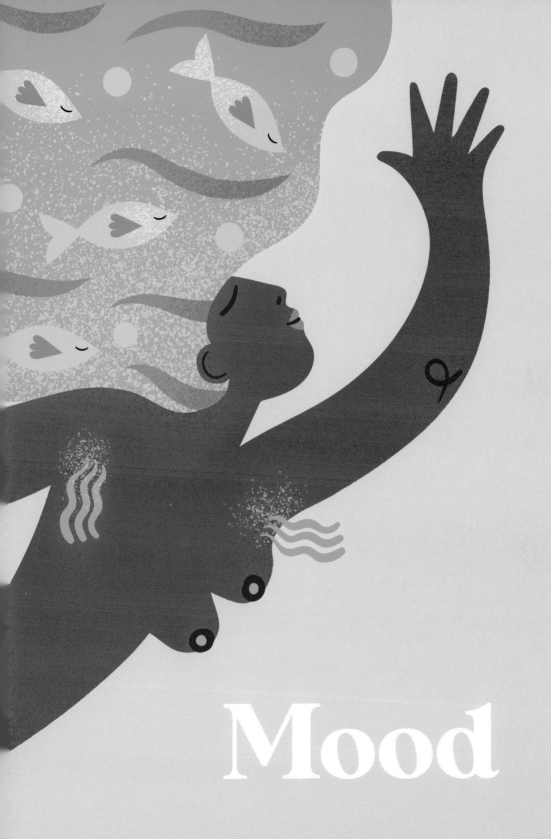

Mood

Mood

Throughout my teenage years, I suffered with low mood, anxiety and panic attacks. This was exacerbated by the grief of losing my dad when I was 14 years of age, but the signs and symptoms had been bubbling under the surface for a few months before that.

I didn't label it – and neither did my family. I guess the assumption was that it was all part and parcel of teenage angst or 'puberty blues'. Now, don't get me wrong, I am not suggesting my family or teachers ignored or dismissed the signs – on the outside I was still a very highly functioning, relatively happy teenager. This is the thing with anxiety though; it can be insidious and inconspicuous, masking as other things and manifesting in weird and wonderful ways.

For me, it started as insomnia and sleep paralysis, to the point where I started to fear going to sleep. I would ruminate and catastrophise every scenario, which resulted in me over-working and becoming a top-level student (out of fear of failure, not through motivation for success). I started to withdraw into myself and avoid social events, despite my friends' best efforts to pull me in closer. The cloud lifted somewhat when I went to university, but it wasn't until I was an adult that I sought help and was given a formal diagnosis of anxiety, along with the tools to help me recognise and manage my symptoms.

Writing this book, and diving deeper into the research, made me realise a few things.

The first realisation for me was that anxiety (along with other mental health conditions) remains taboo and this prevents people from getting the help they need. When I tell people I have anxiety and see a therapist, they almost recoil out of fear, but if I disclose that I have PCOS and see a specialist doctor for that, they don't bat an eyelid.

The reality is that one in five women in the UK reports symptoms of common mental disorders (CMD) such as anxiety and depression compared to one in ten women who experience PCOS.[1] I'm not saying one is more or less important than the other, but it just puts into perspective how common mental health conditions are. Despite the overwhelming evidence that many more of us are presenting with CMD symptoms, I think people would much rather assume it's just a bad day or that they are going through a phase. That sometimes may be the case, but when it's a series of bad days or your life is a constant haze, it's time to get help.

My second realisation was a question: why, when it comes to women and their emotions and mood, are we so quick to blame hormones? There's still this pervasive belief that when a woman presents with physical symptoms that they are either related to hormones or psychosomatic. How many times have you heard 'it's all in your head'?

This medical gaslighting of women needs to stop. As we will learn in this chapter, there are periods of vulnerability throughout a woman's lifespan where mental health disorders are more common – and this is closely aligned with major hormonal shifts. That said, it's also closely aligned with other life changes and lifestyle factors – like how supported we feel! So while hormones are sometimes the loudest voice in the crowd, they are not the only voice.

Do Women Respond to Stress Differently?

Everyone 'knows' that stress is bad for you – the media tells us it can make you ill and even make you die younger. While there are elements of truth to that messaging, it's the *dose* and the *duration* of stress that make the poison.

There is no single definition of stress, but essentially, we feel 'stressed' when real or imagined pressures (stressors) exceed our perceived ability to cope. So, what may cause a feeling of 'stress' in one person, may not cause stress to another. Even events that may seem positive – like the arrival of a new baby or a wedding (or writing a book!) – can induce a feeling of stress. Our perception depends on our genetics, early life experiences, personality and other social circumstances.

When we perceive something as a threat (the stressor), this triggers a physiological response in our bodies, through the activation of our sympathetic nervous system (SNS) and hypothalamic-pituitary-adrenal (HPA) axis. The SNS acts first, causing the adrenal glands to release adrenaline (epinephrine) and noradrenaline (norepinephrine), which travel around the body causing our hearts to beat faster, our breathing rate to increase, our pupils to dilate, an increase in blood glucose and the redirecting of blood to the muscles. It's essentially preparing us to fight, flee or freeze. Activation of this system also makes us more alert, increases arousal and attention and even acts as a pain reliever (analgesic).[2]

As the body continues to perceive the stressor as a threat, the brain activates the HPA axis. The HPA axis is a hormone system that chemically connects the hypothalamus and the pituitary gland in the brain to the adrenal glands, causing the release of the 'stress hormone' cortisol. Cortisol allows the body to continue to stay on high alert; it also increases blood glucose levels, suppresses insulin levels, dampens the immune response, reduces wound healing and alters appetite and mood.[3]

From an evolutionary perspective, the stress response is nature's fundamental survival mechanism. It kicks our butt into gear when we need to run from a grizzly bear or oncoming traffic, or when we are approaching a deadline or about to present to a room full of people.

The Yerkes-Dodson law describes how we perform better (mentally or physically) when we experience stress, but only up to a certain point.[4] If we surpass this tipping point, and levels of stress become too high, performance impaired (see chart overleaf).

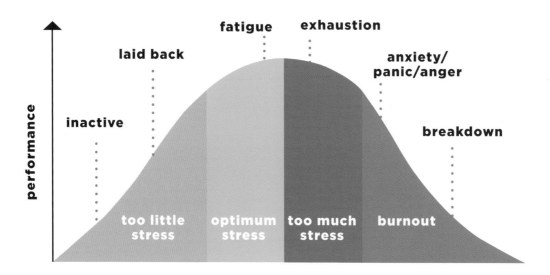

The stress curve [5]

fatigue exhaustion

laid back

anxiety/
panic/anger

inactive

breakdown

performance

too little
stress

optimum
stress

too much
stress

burnout

So stress is not inherently a bad thing, but if we perceive a stressor as intense or we are exposed to it over a long period of time (chronic stress), the response becomes maladaptive and leads to worse performance and poor health, including depression, anxiety and heart disease – and in females, it can also lead to menstrual disturbances, including irregular, infrequent or absent periods.[6]

While most people can handle the day-to-day stresses of life, how we cope and respond to stress matters, and this can either reduce or intensify its effects. Research shows that men and women respond to, and cope with, stress differently.[7] This is, in part, believed to be one of the reasons why women are more likely to experience stress-related conditions, such as anxiety, depression and post-traumatic stress disorder (PTSD), than men.

Women also experience their own unique mental health conditions that manifest during periods of major hormonal transition: premenstrual dysphoric disorder (PMDD), postpartum depression (PND), postpartum anxiety disorders and perimenopausal depression. However, our unique female physiology and hormone profiles are certainly not the only culprits here.

Our psychology, behaviours and gender stereotypes also seem to be driving this divergence in mental health conditions between men and women. For example, women are more likely to be informal caregivers to family, friends, parents and neighbours, and are more likely to put the needs of others first.[8] Women also tend to have lower self-esteem and greater emotional dependency than men which massively influences mental health.[9]

This chapter is going to dive deep into anxiety and depression, which are the most common mental health disorders and disproportionately affect women. This is not an inevitable fate or part and parcel of being a woman, but I'm going to be straight with you: there are particular periods across the lifespan when we are most vulnerable and at higher risk of poor health. However, information is power, and we will explore ways in which you can proactively take steps to protect and improve your mental health.

Is It Anxiety or Something Else?

Anxiety is a word that gets thrown around a lot, and it means different things to different people. The same goes for depression. People claim to be 'depressed' because the weather messed up their plans or having 'anxiety' before a driving test. Feeling a bit p*ssed off with the weather or nervous before a test is a very normal reaction. However, living with depression or an anxiety disorder is much more than a natural fluctuation in mood or a short-lived feeling. It occurs when, for a consistent period of time, we experience extreme shifts in our mood that we can't shake, affecting our sleep, draining us of energy, causing us to over- or undereat and interfering with our ability to function in everyday life.

Anecdotally, I see a lot more women with anxiety written in their medical notes than I do men, and this matches up with what the statistics say. Women are indeed twice as likely as men to be diagnosed with anxiety.[10] This is true of all the anxiety disorders, including panic disorder, agoraphobia, social anxiety disorder, specific phobias and generalised anxiety disorder (GAD), although the extent of the sex difference varies for each.[11]

Male: Female ratio common behavioral disorders [12]

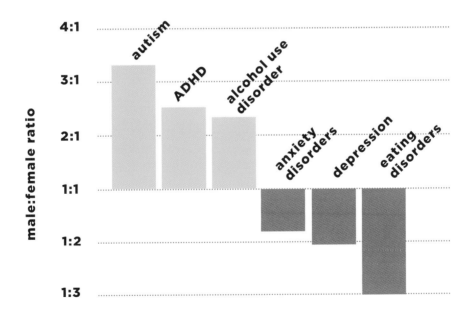

Additionally, women tend to have higher rates of drug prescriptions for anti-anxiety meds and antidepressants, which, interestingly, can't be explained by differences in mental health status or how often they visit the doctor.[13]

Medical professionals have manuals and guidelines with specific criteria to help us to diagnose mental health conditions, such as anxiety disorders and depression, but my inkling is that a lot of people are given this label or diagnosis perhaps inappropriately, before meeting sufficient criteria. There is also some evidence that the overdiagnosis of depression in women is more frequent than underdiagnosis in men.[14]

I don't want to trivialise the fact that a huge number of women do indeed suffer with these mental health disorders – and I say this not only as someone who has treated people with depression and anxiety, but as someone who has a diagnosis of GAD myself. So trust me when I say that I understand the gravity of these diagnoses and the toll it can take on your mental and physical health.

However, in the words of Dr Alyson McGregor, author of *Sex Matters*, 'Anxiety should be the diagnosis of exclusion, not the diagnosis of default' in women.[15] Historically, women have been considered weak and emotional, and therefore predisposed to mental health disorders, but also often blamed and shamed for not having mental wellness.

Let's not forget 'hysteria', a (fake) diagnosis unique to any owner of a womb, which can be traced back to ancient Egyptian and Greek medical texts.[16] The term hysteria derives from the Greek word for uterus, *hystera*, and served as a catch-all for a variety of miscellaneous symptoms and behaviours that were believed to arise from the uterus. Symptoms included everything from fainting, seizures, nervousness, increased (or decreased) sexual desire and a 'tendency to cause trouble for others'. In the nineteenth century it became a psychiatric diagnosis and was only removed from classification in the *Diagnostic and Statistical Manual of Mental Disorders (DSM) III* in 1980.[17] Yes, 1980 – shocking, isn't it?

Hysteria may be a diagnosis of the past, but gendered stereotypes, where women are considered irrational, emotional or sick if they're not well-tempered (and submissive), are hugely problematic and can lead to worse health outcomes in women.

When it comes to medical appointments, it's almost as if men present with symptoms, while women present with feelings, and I believe it is because of this that the diagnoses and care differ. I suspect this is more than just linguistics, but highlights a gendered bias, which echoes the messaging of the age of hysteria.

Compared to men, women are more likely to be given a psychiatric diagnosis than a physical one for a number of health conditions and, unfortunately, having anxiety on your medical record can sometimes act as a red herring and distract from the underlying issue.[18] Indeed, anxiety can manifest with physical symptoms including heart palpitations, nausea, diarrhoea, sweating, headaches and insomnia (and this is not an exhaustive list), and therefore mimic other illnesses. Similarly, the symptoms of many physical conditions, such as thyroid disease and heart disease, can mimic those of anxiety. So yes, it's often on our list of differentials, but it shouldn't be our go-to diagnosis in women.

For example, one study found that male doctors were more likely to offer an X-ray to male patients presenting with symptoms suggestive of irritable bowel syndrome (IBS), whereas female patients presenting with the same symptoms were provided lifestyle advice and anti-anxiety medication.[19] (Just as a little medical side note: we can't diagnose IBS on an X-ray, but they are often ordered when someone turns up to A&E with abdominal pain to rule out other more serious conditions.)

Similarly, in comparison to men, women who are having a heart attack are more likely to assume their symptoms are stress or anxiety (21 per cent versus 12 per cent) and women who experience an abnormally fast heart rhythm (known as paroxysmal supraventricular tachycardia) are far more likely to be misdiagnosed with anxiety, depression or stress, compared to men.[20] This ultimately leads to women being referred for treatment later, which can lead to devastating consequences.

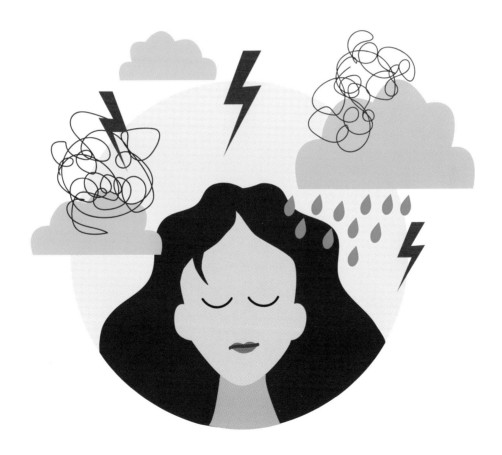

Myth: Heart disease is a man's disease

Truth: if I had a penny for every woman I have met who has been having a heart attack, while trying to convince both herself and me that it's just a panic attack or a touch of indigestion, I would be a rich woman. I have yet to meet a man in the same situation who has downplayed his symptoms or tried to assure me it was something else.

I can vividly recall one female patient who came into the acute medical unit with chest pain, referred by her GP who wanted to rule out that it wasn't heart-related. It was a busy shift, the waiting room was full and I had one more patient to see before this woman. While rushing back to the clinic room to see my next patient, I overheard her ask the receptionist how long it would take, highlighting how busy her day was and how her grandchildren needed to be picked up in a few hours. My mind was already ticking over what the cause of her chest pain might be – perhaps stress-induced heartburn.

In the meantime, the nurse did an ECG (electrocardiogram or trace of the heart) and took her vital signs. The ECG didn't look like a typical heart attack, but her heart rate was a bit fast and her blood pressure was high. I called her into the room and began to ask her some questions. She was in her early fifties with a high body weight. She looked flustered, flushed and had beads of sweat on her forehead. From her history, she explained the chest pain was heavy in nature and located in the centre of her chest; it came on while she was cleaning the house and did not go away after she sat down. She also felt nauseous and assumed it was her reflux, which had been bothering her lately, though her antacids hadn't been helping. The pain had now subsided, but red flags began to wave in my mind.

I explained to her that she could have had a heart attack, but we needed to wait for her blood results to come back and take it from there. Her response? 'I don't have time to have a heart attack, Doc, so can you please speed this up?' To cut a long story short, behold, her blood results came back and shifted the diagnosis towards a heart attack. She was admitted under the cardiology team for further investigations and treatment (after much persuasion).

With that story in mind, it might not surprise you to hear that coronary heart disease (CHD) is the single biggest killer of women (so not just men) worldwide, and in the UK, CHD kills more than twice as many women as breast cancer every year.[21] Research shows that at every stage – presentation, diagnosis, treatment and aftercare – women who have heart attacks receive

inferior care than men. In one study over ten years in England and Wales, women were twice as likely as men to die in the month after heart attack.[22]
Why? In part, it's down to biology, but it's also down to bias:

- **Arrival time:** Women tend to arrive at hospital later than men when having a heart attack.[23] Reported reasons for why this may happen include lack of awareness of risk, attributing symptoms to something else (such as a panic attack), waiting at home until symptoms worsen, attempting to self-medicate and conflicting work or family responsibilities.[24] If you suspect you're having a heart attack, call 999 and ask for an ambulance. A heart attack is a medical emergency.

- **Presentation:** It's been suggested that men experience 'typical' and women experience 'atypical' symptoms while having a heart attack. While research shows that women are more likely to present with pain between the shoulder blades, nausea or vomiting, and shortness of breath, it's not wholly accurate to say that there are distinct sets of 'male' and 'female' symptoms, as there is huge overlap, and – regardless of sex – chest pain is the most common presenting symptom.[25]

- **Diagnosis:** A woman is one-and-a-half times more likely than a man to receive the wrong initial diagnosis for a heart attack.[26] This is not just an inconvenience, but leads to delays in time-dependent treatment which are associated with increased risk of death.[27]

- **Treatment:** Following the diagnosis of a heart attack, urgent, time-dependent treatment is needed to get blood flowing into the heart muscle again, yet research shows that women are less likely to receive a number of potentially life-saving treatments in a timely manner.[28] This is also compounded by the fact that women are more likely to have a diagnosis of anxiety and depression, and evidence shows that those with a mental health diagnosis receive less screening and lower-quality treatment for heart disease.[29]

- **Discharge:** Following a heart attack, women are less likely to be prescribed risk-lowering medications, such as statins and beta blockers, to help prevent a second attack.[30]

- **Rehabilitation:** In the UK, women are less likely than men to be recruited for and access important cardiac rehabilitation following a heart attack (29 per cent versus 71 per cent), and even when they do attend, they do not seem to gain the same benefit as men in terms of outcomes.[31]

- **Risk factors:** Well-established risk factors for heart disease, including smoking, type 2 diabetes and high blood pressure, may put women at an 'excess risk' of a heart attack compared to men.[32]

So, when it comes to heart attacks, from symptom onset to discharge, the odds are stacked against us. I don't believe that this is the fault of any individual or organisation, but largely due to the deeply embedded unconscious biases that we hold about women and heart disease. From research to healthcare, as well as the media narrative, it is all biased towards men.

We All Have Bias

I should be clear that I am not implying that doctors intentionally do not take women seriously or dismiss their symptoms, but rather that we all hold unconscious biases – doctors, patients, you and me – and this can harm any gender.

For example, women are more likely to report when feeling anxious, whereas men, typically, are more stoic, suck it up and lean on things like alcohol instead.[33] These behavioural norms attributed to men and women can be traced right back to when we were kids and our parents and teachers (subconsciously) reinforced 'appropriate' behaviours based on our gender. We raise boys to be brave, assertive and independent, and praise girls for being caring and empathetic.[34] This idea that 'big boys don't cry' may be why men are (typically) less likely to speak up and ask for help when experiencing symptoms of anxiety or low mood.[35] This can lead to devastating consequences such as suicide, with male rates more than three times higher than female.[36]

While the evidence is not completely conclusive, it seems that men are more physiologically reactive to stress compared to women, who appear to have a somewhat blunted stress response.[37] This response also varies across the female lifespan and during the menstrual cycle, suggesting sex hormones are involved. For example, research has found that during the second half (luteal phase) of the menstrual cycle, women have a similar cortisol response as men, while in the first half (follicular phase) of the menstrual cycle, menopause and when taking oral contraceptives, the cortisol response is lower.[38]

These differences may also, in part, explain behavioural differences that have been observed between men and women when it comes to stress. So, while men are more likely to 'fight or flee' in response to an acute threat, women are more likely to 'tend and befriend'. This theory suggests that women are less likely to put themselves first in the face of danger, have the desire to protect their offspring (*tend*) and seek out support from others to promote survival (*befriend*).[39] This may, in part, buffer the stress response.[40]

Of course, not *all* females and not *all* males respond in this way. However, one thing it does highlight is how important social connection and support are for a woman, especially during times of stress. One hormone in particular that may be at play here is oxytocin. Many know it better by its nickname as the 'love hormone' due to its role in social bonding, reproduction and childbirth. Oxytocin is believed to downregulate the stress response, particularly in women, and, coupled with other sex hormones, may encourage maternal and affiliative behaviour in response to a threat or stress.[41]

There are also psychosocial influences at play. For example, women (again *on average*) tend to ruminate (worry and overthink) more than men, report lower self-esteem and are more likely to meet the needs of others, at the expense of their own – all of which can increase the risk of anxiety.[42] Trauma and abuse are big risk factors for anxiety and poor mental health and, while both men and women can be victims, women are more likely to experience repeated and severe forms of abuse, including domestic and sexual violence. They are also more likely to have experienced sustained physical, psychological or emotional abuse.[43]

So I guess you could say, sex/gender differences when it comes to anxiety are complicated and emphasise how both our biological sex and the gender we identify as, play a huge role in our health and our experience of the healthcare system.

How Hormones Affect Our Mood

Isn't it funny (read: not funny at all) how we automatically assume changes in a woman's mood or behaviour are down to hormones or TOTM? (Side note: can we ditch 'time of the month', as if a woman's period is that taboo? It's almost equivalent to 'he-who-must-not-be-named' from Harry Potter.)

Many of us would be insulted if a man turned around to ask us if we are on our period simply because we got upset or angry over something, and yet we often do it to ourselves. Think back to the last time you cried out of the blue or found yourself getting highly irritated by your work colleague. I'm sure you blamed it on hormones or questioned, either to yourself or out loud, if your period was due.

Let me just say that you don't need a biological excuse for feeling the feels. Life has its ups and downs, which can have an effect on how we feel on any given day. That said, our hormones and our menstrual cycle can indeed influence our mood, no matter what we're living through at the time.

On (almost) a monthly basis, many women report changes in mood, including anger, irritability and tearfulness, in the days leading up to their period and, as if that wasn't enough, can also experience a worsening of pre-existing mental health conditions, such as anxiety and obsessive compulsive disorder (OCD).[44] On top of this, our sex hormones fluctuate enough to further influence our mood and mental health around puberty, pregnancy and perimenopause. So, I want you to be compassionate with yourself and stock up on ways to cope through these shifts.

Where it all begins

The first big challenge is puberty, which brings enormous hormonal changes into a young person's life. In childhood, the rates of depression and anxiety are similar in girls and boys, but from puberty onwards this shifts where girls are twice as likely to be affected as boys, and this continues through to adulthood.[45]

However, while these differences coincide with a surge in sex hormones, there is actually no firm evidence to say hormones directly cause 'puberty blues' – but they do play a role.[46] Thinking more widely, back to your own puberty, perhaps, it's not just a time of internal change. Your body physically changes (as does your relationship with it), but this often coincides with the transition from primary to secondary school (which is stressful in itself), increased pressure to perform academically or otherwise, and changes in relationship dynamics, whether they be with friends, parents, siblings or romantic interests. All of these changes come with their own storm of confusing emotions and thoughts. So, while, yes, puberty is a time of hormonal change, it typically reflects other life changes, which can be extremely destabilising for a teen.

I'm not a parent (yet), but I've experienced puberty as a girl, and I would like to publicly apologise to my parents for my emotional outbursts. I also get that it's not always easy to distinguish between the typical mood swings of puberty and mental health conditions, but signs it might be something else include persistent changes in mood, significant changes in behaviour and signs that it's affecting other areas of life like school, friendships and sport.

Mood across the menstrual cycle

Bloated tummy, tender boobs and a blubbering mess – sound familiar? If you have a menstrual cycle, it's likely you've experienced premenstrual symptoms at some point. In fact, it is estimated that 80–90 per cent of women experience some premenstrual symptoms (there are over 150 of them!) including bloating, breast tenderness, headache, acne, constipation and mood changes.[47] A recent study of 40,000 Dutch women found that abdominal pain (or cramping) was the most common experienced premenstrually.[48] The second-most common symptom was psychological complaints, such as low mood or irritability, experienced by over 77 per cent of women.

Premenstrual symptoms occur on a spectrum and, for most women, they are relatively mild and do not disrupt day-to-day activities. However, some women have symptoms so severe that they stop them from getting on with their daily lives, which is diagnostic of premenstrual syndrome (PMS). This collection of physical and emotional symptoms can occur in the two weeks before you have your period, usually gets better once your period starts and often disappears by the end of it.

A smaller number (3–8 per cent) of women get an even more intense form of PMS known as premenstrual dysphoric disorder (PMDD).[49] The symptoms of PMDD are similar to those of PMS, but are more severe and often have more psychological than physical symptoms, including feelings of hopelessness, depression, extreme anger, anxiety and irritability. If you are getting severe symptoms (physical, mental or emotional) in the days leading up to your period and it is interfering with your day-to-day life, do speak to your doctor.

However, like PMS, symptoms should resolve when the period starts – if not, there could be something else causing them, such as depression (which can be exacerbated premenstrually) or another cyclical mental health condition, such as bipolar disorder.

As with many things related to female health, due to a lack of scientific research, we don't know exactly what causes PMS or PMDD, and why some women are affected and others are not. Based on the research we do have, we think it's largely due to the rise and fall of oestrogen and progesterone, which influence mood-enhancing neurotransmitters in the brain, such as serotonin (often dubbed 'the feel-good hormone'). Compared to women who don't suffer from intense PMS, those who do have similar levels of oestrogen and progesterone but appear to be *more sensitive* to these hormonal fluctuations. Interestingly, global rates of PMS reporting vary quite drastically by country, which begs the question: can it be *purely* down to hormones if it varies so much by social environment?[50]

I was surprised to read that a review from 2012 (inclusive of 47 studies) measuring links between mood and women's menstrual cycles found that only 15 per cent of studies provided evidence of a link between the premenstrual phase and negative mood.[51] This was followed up by a study of women (aged 18–49) exploring the extent to which women's daily moods are influenced by their menstrual cycles. The participants were asked daily questions about their mood over six months via a smartphone questionnaire, but were not told that this had anything to do with mood and the menstrual cycle, which helped to reduce bias.[52] They were also asked about other things such as physical health, perceived stress and days of their menstrual cycle. What the study found was that only 1 in 20 showed any clear variation in mood based on where they were at in their cycle, and actually, physical health, perceived stress and social support were much stronger predictors of mood.

So does this mean that our mood isn't influenced by our menstrual cycles and it's all a myth? I don't think so, and I think that suggesting PMS is 'all in your head' minimises the lived experiences of many women who are sensitive to these hormonal changes. However, I do think – again – that we shouldn't be so quick to always assume it's our hormones and, when it comes to changes in mood, considering that other factors in our life – such as our relationships, the stress we are under and our overall well-being – are just as, if not more, important. I'm a big advocate of tracking your mood, in addition to physical symptoms, when tracking your menstrual cycle. This will give you a useful insight into the patterns that you experience and allows you to better understand your body and needs.

What about hormonal contraception?

I'm sure most people reading this will know at least one or two women who have said their contraception has affected their mood, making them more irritable, emotional or tearful.

Several studies have explored this link between hormonal contraception and changes, and the results have been conflicting. One large study, that is often quoted in the press, was published in 2016 and included over 1 million women (aged 15–34 years) in Denmark.[53] The researchers accessed 14 years of health data from medical records and found that hormonal contraception users were more likely to be diagnosed with or treated for depression, for the first time, than those who were non-users.[54] The strongest link was seen in teenage girls. Understandably, this caused a lot of widespread panic.

Looking deeper into the data, what the study found was that women who used combined oral contraceptives had a 23 per cent increased risk of requiring antidepressants for the first time, which jumped to 80 per cent for adolescents. Shockingly high, right? I thought so too. Well, this is the *relative* risk and not the *absolute* risk – the latter tells us more about our individual risk. In this study, the absolute risk increase is four to five women per 1,000 per year for users of oral hormonal contraceptives. This, I imagine, changes the situation for many women who are weighing up the risks and benefits of hormonal contraception.

Other studies looking at depression and hormonal contraception have found conflicting results – with some even reporting *lower* levels of depression in women using hormonal contraception and others reporting links between the use of hormonal contraception and the likelihood of being prescribed antidepressants.[55] The age at which women start using hormonal contraceptives seems to make a difference. In short, younger teens (aged 12–14) are far more likely to be prescribed antidepressants versus adult women (where it is virtually nil) when using hormonal contraceptives.[56]

Ultimately, we don't have enough evidence to say that hormonal contraception causes depression (or reduces the risk), but some women do report worsening mental health with certain forms of contraception – and we shouldn't ignore that. We really need more research here to better understand the link between hormonal contraception and depression. So unless you are noticing side effects from your current form of contraception, there is no evidence to suggest you should stop. Also, if you do decide to stop and are not intending on getting pregnant, please ensure you use another reliable form of non-hormonal contraception as unwanted pregnancy in and of itself is not without psychological risk.

How Long Do the Baby Blues Last?

It's normal to feel emotional, tearful or low during the first few days after giving birth. For most women, these feelings, often called the 'baby blues', go away within a week to ten days, without any intervention. However, if these feelings persist beyond two weeks and become worse, it may be a sign of postnatal depression (PND, also called postpartum depression).

Did you know? 10 to 15 in every 100 women who have a baby experience postnatal depression.

PND is not just feeling a little cranky or tearful – it's a serious mental health condition, and it's more common than you may think. In fact, it is *the* most common complication of pregnancy, affecting 10–15 per cent of women and, devastatingly, suicide accounts for up to 20 per cent of all postpartum deaths.[57] Anxiety is also common in the postpartum period, but receives considerably less attention, with an estimated 8.5 per cent of postpartum mothers experiencing one or more anxiety disorders, such as GAD and OCD.[58]

The symptoms of PND are similar to those in depression at other times and can be so severe that it makes caring for yourself and your baby very difficult. Symptoms usually occur within the first few weeks after giving birth, but can start any time in the first year after giving birth, and include:

- feeling low or tearful most of the time
- loss of interest or pleasure in things you normally enjoy
- exhaustion and lack of energy
- difficulty sleeping
- feeling anxious and irritable
- having negative and guilty thoughts
- avoiding people
- thoughts of self-harm or suicide

A small number of women with very severe depression develop psychotic symptoms, including hearing voices or holding unusual beliefs. If this happens, or if you're having thoughts about harming yourself, you should seek medical attention urgently.

Myth: Pregnancy protects women from depression

Truth: while most people recognise that in the postnatal period, baby blues and mood disorders are common, during pregnancy, there is this myth that women are protected from depression and anxiety and ought to be glowing and blissfully happy. But antenatal depression affects one in ten pregnant women, with even higher rates in low- and middle-income countries.[59] Yet, as few as 20 per cent of pregnant women with depression receive adequate treatment.[60] The underdiagnosis and undertreatment of depression, or any mental health disorder, in pregnancy does not only affect the health of the mother but also the health of the baby, including premature birth and low birth weight.[61]

During pregnancy, emphasis is often placed on physical health over mental health, which can make pregnant women less likely to offer up how they're feeling without being prompted. That said, even if mood is explored by a midwife or doctor, it can be tricky to diagnose antenatal anxiety, as symptoms may overlap with normal changes during pregnancy, such as increased (or decreased) appetite, low energy, poor concentration or insomnia, and also it's normal to have some level of anxiety over the pregnancy itself.[62] But if you experience persistent symptoms of depression and/or anxiety and it's affecting your day-to-day life, please do seek support as there is help available for you.

Hormone levels during pregnancy and after birth[63]

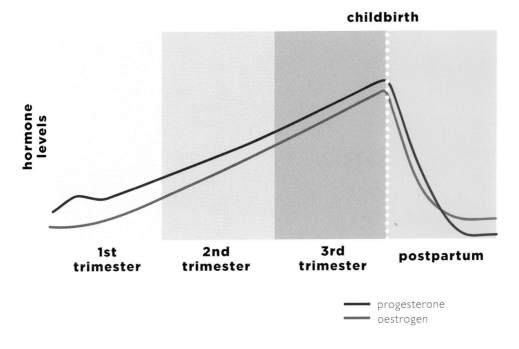

Research suggests that the sudden, dramatic, drop in sex hormones that occurs after delivery has a strong effect on mood and may be the driver behind low mood in the postnatal period.

During pregnancy, levels of oestrogen and progesterone are at an all-time high, but fall off a cliff after childbirth; not too dissimilar to what happens premenstrually, just far more significant. Levels of oestrogen and progesterone increase several fold during pregnancy, and there are also increases in other hormones such as oxytocin and prolactin – and a few others that are currently under investigation for their role in PND.

While most hormones return to pre-pregnancy levels within one to two weeks, in women who breastfeed, prolactin remains elevated, and bouts of breastfeeding actually trigger bursts of both prolactin and oxytocin.[64] These hormones are known to have mood-boosting effects and, additionally, there is some evidence to suggest that breastfeeding may protect against PND or assist with a speedier recovery.[65] Not all women can breastfeed, however, and those experiencing PND are also less likely to do so.[66]

Additionally, the drop in reproductive hormones isn't the only hormonal change that happens: levels of thyroid hormones may also drop after giving birth, which can also contribute to low mood.[67] Various other systems in the body are thought to be involved, including the immune system and the stress response (that HPA axis again – see page 85).[68]

It's also important to say that *all* women experience this drop-off after childbirth, and not everyone will experience PND. However, for those who do seem to be more sensitive to these hormonal shifts, it appears to be due to their own individual risk factors such as genetics, early life adversity or history of mental health conditions. Similar story to PMS and PMDD, hey? Women are also at increased risk if they have previously experienced (or have a family history of) depression or other mood disorders, if they've experienced recent stressful life events (such as a break-up or bereavement), if they've gone through domestic violence or abuse or if they're lacking support from friends and family.

While we have not yet been able to pinpoint the cause of PND, it's likely to involve many factors (not too dissimilar to those contributing to depression at other times of life) including biological, psychological, social and – now – baby-related. Indeed, new dads can also experience PND, as can non-biological and adoptive mothers.

After a woman gives birth, the newborn is not the only 'new thing' to deal with. In addition to changes in hormones, there are also physical changes to the body, and oftentimes pain related to delivery or perhaps breastfeeding. Nutrition is usually not great, not to mention sleep. Finding time or energy to do any form of physical activity is often difficult, as are other aspects of lifestyle, which may mean loss of that vital 'me time'. The birth of a baby can also have a huge impact on your relationships with your partner, family and friends. However, right now, social support is exactly what a new mother needs and is possibly the most important factor to protect against PND, plus it is a variable we can influence.

The transition into motherhood is a vulnerable period for mental health, but this does not mean that all women (or parents) will develop depression postnatally.

I think the media – particularly social media – can give a false impression and unrealistic expectations of what motherhood should look and feel like, which can put a lot of pressure on new mums (and dads!). I think this can make mothers feel like they're failing themselves or their baby if they ask for help when they are struggling – when that's simply not true. There are support and treatment options available, depending on how severe the PND is, including talk therapy or medication, or a combination of both. Your GP and health visitor can help you decide what kind of help you need. There are also many support groups, both online and in person, for new parents – and, as we have learned, our social support is so important to help buffer some of that stress.

The Highs and Lows of Menopausal Transition

So far, we have learned that women have higher rates of depression after puberty and throughout the reproductive years, compared to men, until after the menopause when rates become similar between the two. However, the transition into menopause, known as perimenopause, is where we next see an increased risk of low mood and rates of depression.[69]

A woman is said to have gone through the menopause after 12 months without a period (so by definition it is one day in a woman's life). After this, women are said to be post-menopausal. However, perimenopause occurs in the years before your periods stop – and can last anywhere from a few months to many years. Unlike the menopause, it's not always super obvious when a woman is going through the perimenopause and the symptoms are often attributed to something else or not recognised.

During perimenopause, sex hormones do not just gradually decline in a nice linear fashion giving us time to calibrate, but rather they erratically fluctuate as they decline, which means hormonal blood tests during this time are not reliable in aiding a diagnosis. These hormonal ups and downs contribute to the often unpredictable physical and psychological symptoms that women experience during this time – from hot flushes, irregular periods and insomnia, to mood swings, brain fog and changes in sexual arousal.

Hormone levels during the menopause transition[70]

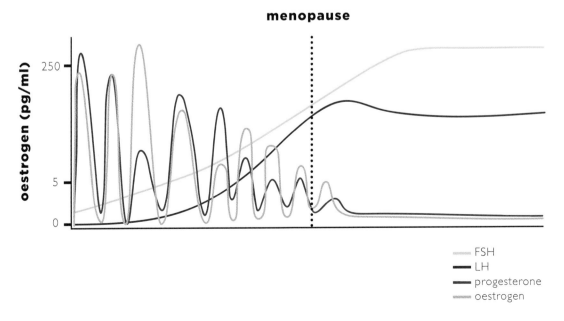

menopause

oestrogen (pg/ml)

250

5

0

FSH
LH
progesterone
oestrogen

Finding yourself in a brain fog

'Brain fog' isn't a clinical or scientific term; it's often used by people to describe when they're feeling forgetful, having difficulty concentrating and just feeling a bit mentally fuzzy.

We all forget things (like where we put our keys) and have brain farts (like 'Why did I come into this room again?'). However, women often report this more frequently and severely as they go through perimenopause – some refer to it as the 'menofog' or 'menobrain'. This isn't too dissimilar to the 'baby brain' that women often report during pregnancy and early motherhood. The fears many women have later in life, if this occurs, is whether what they're experiencing is just part and parcel of the menopausal transition or if it is, in fact, early warning signs of dementia.

The research does seem to back up anecdotal reports of women during the perimenopause experiencing some cognitive changes, such as mild memory loss and word-finding difficulties.[71] However, while this menopause-related brain fog may mimic some of the symptoms of dementia, for most women it is temporary and recovers to baseline after the transition.[72] We also need to remember that some normal age-related decline is to be expected, so that baseline may look a little different to where it was in the premenopause. These relapses in memory and concentration are also compounded by perimenopausal-related changes in sleep and mood, not to mention troubling symptoms like hot flushes. There is a 'but', though, and unfortunately, and for a small subset of women, brain fog may be the beginning of something like dementia. In fact, two-thirds of those with Alzheimer's, the most common form of dementia, are women.[73] As always, if you have concerns that the fog could be signs of something else, do speak to your GP about it.

As discussed earlier in the chapter, there are multiple biological, psychological, social and cultural factors that can influence our mood and development of depression. Similar to other periods of major hormonal transitions, this is, in part, thought to be due to fluctuations in sex hormones and their influence on neurotransmitters in the brain. For some women, these hormonal dips can set off a depressive episode, especially for those who have had a diagnosis of depression in the past, including PND or premenstrual mood disorders, suggesting that some have a genetic vulnerability to these periods of major hormonal shifts. Other risk factors for perimenopausal depression are also similar to other times, such as stressful life events and a history of trauma or abuse. Finally, other major life events are also often happening for a woman during this time – empty-nest syndrome with kids growing up and leaving home, career pressure, divorce, ageing parents – all of which can trigger depression.

Lifestyle factors also play a role in the timing of the menopause; in fact, cigarette smoking can almost double the risk of entering the menopause early compared to never-smokers.[75] Women in their mid-life (40–50 years of age) who report depressive symptoms are also less likely to meet physical activity guidelines.[76] So, moving more may offer some protection against mood disturbances during the menopause transition.

However, we not only need to move more, to sit less (that includes all of us, FYI – see page 81). One study reported that women aged 50–55 who sat for seven hours or more a day and did no physical activity were three times more likely to experience depressive symptoms than those who sat for fewer than four hours a day and met physical activity guidelines.[77] Need a movement refresher? Head to Chapter 2 (see page 44) to learn more about what exercise you should be prioritising during this time.

Finally, sleep disturbances are very common during the perimenopause, which in and of itself is a symptom of depression, but can also lead to more severe depressive symptoms – a bit of a chicken-and-egg scenario. However, improvement in sleep quality has been shown to improve symptoms of depression in women going through this menopause transition.[78] Check out Chapter 4 (see page 112) for more on this.

I want to be clear that the menopause does not *cause* depression, but it is a period of vulnerability. Further to that, experiencing low mood during the menopause does not necessarily mean that you have depression. There have been recent news reports of GPs pushing antidepressants on women inappropriately to treat symptoms of the menopause.

Antidepressants should not be given first-line for low mood associated with the menopause in women who do not have depression.[79] In these scenarios, you may be offered HRT, which can help with low mood associated with the menopause. Another option is cognitive behavioural therapy (CBT) for low mood or anxiety as a result of menopause.

However, if you are struggling with your mood, regardless of how mild or severe or what age you are at in life, I can't emphasise enough how important it is that you seek help from a medical professional. There are many treatment options available, depending on the severity of your symptoms and what is suitable for you. When it comes to treating mental health conditions, there is not really a one-size-fits-all model that works for everyone, and different people respond to different treatments.

What Can You Do to Help Yourself?

There are many lifestyle changes that have a big impact on our mood and risk of mood disorders.

Nutrition

Unfortunately, when it comes to food and our mood, it's not as easy as 'eat this, not that', but there is a pretty powerful link between what we eat and our risk of depression. Unsurprisingly, the diet that seems to come out on top, when it comes to reducing the risk and perhaps even the symptoms of depression, is a Mediterranean diet.[80] As we saw in Chapter 1 (see page 24), a Mediterranean diet is one that is rich in colourful fruit and vegetables, nuts and seeds, whole grains and legumes, olive oil, fish and seafood, moderate consumption of dairy, and lower intakes of red and processed meat and alcohol. This dietary pattern also places emphasis on cultural and lifestyle elements, such as cooking, physical activity, adequate rest, traditional and local produce, biodiversity and seasonality and socialising – the take-home message being: it's not only what we eat, but how we eat that matters.

Nutritionally speaking, what makes this diet so good for your brain?

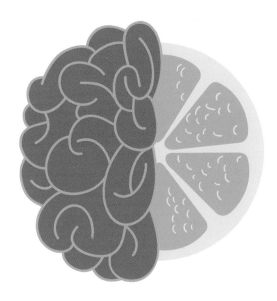

Omega-3 fatty acids

The reason nutritionists and dietitians love oily fish is because it is an incredibly rich source of the omega-3 fatty acids eicosapentaenoic acid (EPA) and docosahexaenoic acid (DHA). EPA and DHA are critical for normal brain function and development. They are both involved in the structure and function of cell membranes in the brain and also have anti-inflammatory effects.[81] As such, higher omega-3 intakes have been associated with lower rates of depression and, in fact, omega-3 supplementation has been shown to improve depressive symptoms during pregnancy and the postnatal period, in addition to depression at other stages of life.[82] EPA and DHA can be made through another omega-3 fatty acid called alpha-linolenic acid (ALA), found in plant-based foods such as walnuts, chia seeds, flaxseeds and soya beans – although the amount converted isn't great.[83] Check out my recipe for Walnut, Chia + Kidney Bean Meatballs on page 204 to stock up on your omega-3 fatty acids! I'm not big on supplementation (unless indicated) but if you have a plant-only diet, this is one supplement I would consider for the future health of your brain.

Antioxidants

There are many different nutrients and compounds that can act as antioxidants, which help to reduce oxidative stress caused by free radicals (see page 25), and, in turn, reduce neural damage. Vitamins C and E, zinc and selenium, for example, act as antioxidants, as do phytoestrogens (found in soya, pulses and flaxseed) and polyphenols (found in dried herbs, cocoa, nuts and seeds, dark berries, tea and coffee).[84] Olives, olive oil and green leafy vegetables, which are found in a Mediterranean diet, are also great sources of antioxidants. Instead of chasing down these individual foods, or using antioxidant supplements, focusing on plant diversity in your diet (research suggests we should aim for 30 different plant-based foods per week) will ensure you're getting a good dose of vitamins and antioxidants.[85]

B Vitamins

Did you know there are actually eight B vitamins? They all have different roles – from helping the body use carbohydrates as energy to supporting the brain and nervous system. Vitamin B12 is particularly important in long-term brain and nerve health. It helps to form the fatty sheath that covers nerves, which helps to speed up the transmission of signals from one nerve cell to another. Deficiency can lead to a number of symptoms, from fatigue, pins and needles and numbness to low mood and memory loss. Unfortunately, vitamin B12 must be obtained from animal products, so unless you consume meat, fish, eggs or dairy, then it is essential that you supplement. Certain fortified plant-based foods provide vitamin B12, but the safest and most reliable option is to supplement.

Folate (B9) is another key nutrient for our brain and nervous system, and deficiency three months prior to pregnancy and in the first trimester can lead to neural tube defects, which is why we strongly recommend supplementing when trying for a baby and continuing until week 12 of pregnancy (see page 27). But it's not just important for a growing baby – both B12 and folate deficiency are associated with a greater risk of depression in adulthood.[86]

Vitamin B6 is involved in making neurotransmitters for the brain, such as dopamine, serotonin and the hormone melatonin, which regulate mood and sleep.[87] Deficiency of this vitamin has also been associated with cognitive decline and dementia, although clinical trials testing the effects of vitamin B supplementation have generally shown a lack of benefit in terms of cognition.[88]

In general, when it comes to the brain, a lot of the research focuses on the three B vitamins I've just mentioned (folate, B6 and B12), but all B vitamins play a role in brain health on some level, often working in concert, so it's important we are getting a good dose of all the B vitamins.

Fibre

A healthy gut is essential for a healthy brain, and vice versa. This connection goes both ways via a long nerve from brain to belly called the vagus nerve, but also through chemical messengers and active metabolites produced by the trillions of microbes that live in the gut. These gut bugs feed on, and ferment, prebiotic fibre-rich foods (such as onions, artichokes, leeks, garlic, nuts, beans and legumes) and produce beneficial short-chain fatty acids (SCFA) such as butyrate, propionate and acetate. These SCFAs support gut health but also have far-reaching effects on other organs, including the brain and, as such, have been linked to a number of neuropsychological diseases, such as Alzheimer's and Parkinson's.[89] Research has largely been focused on animals, but it has been found that faecal SCFA concentrations are lower in women with depression, and transferring faeces from a depressed patient into mice has been shown to induce depression-like behaviour.[90]

In addition, just as gut bugs affect the brain, the brain can also have a profound impact on the gut microbiome, and stress can actually suppress levels of beneficial bacteria. In 2008, researchers found that, during exam week, university students' stool samples contained fewer lactobacilli than they had during the relatively untroubled first days of the semester.[91] Stress also increases gut motility and fluid excretion – which can lead to diarrhoea – which may sound familiar if you reflect on any high-pressure events in your past such as exams or presentations. Right now, we don't have direct evidence to prove an altered gut microbiome causes depression or vice versa, but maintaining a healthy gut is likely to contribute to better overall health in general – with the bonus of possibly improving mood. To support the hard work of these fibre-feeding bugs, aim to include a variety of plant-based foods in your diet, including fruit and vegetables, pulses and whole grains, and nuts and seeds. Check out my Good-For-Your-Gut Overnight Oats recipe on page 146.

What about probiotics?

There is emerging evidence to suggest that probiotics (live bacteria) could play an important role in mood and depression. A review from 2020 of the (albeit limited) research found that probiotics – either alone or in combination with prebiotics – may help reduce depressive symptoms.[92] No significant difference was found for anxiety. So it's interesting (and exciting!), but we need more research to learn more about which specific probiotics and strains should be used here as it's rarely one size fits all.

This is by no means an exhaustive list of nutrients that play a role in the health of our brain – some other key nutrients include:

- **Carbohydrate:** in the form of glucose, is virtually the only source of fuel for the brain (except in periods of starvation).

- **Protein:** which is needed for overall body function, and an amino acid called tryptophan is needed to make serotonin (aka the happy hormone). A balanced diet that provides enough protein also provides enough tryptophan, so there is no need to consume a high-tryptophan diet to support your mood.

- **Choline:** a nutrient needed to create an important chemical messenger in the brain called acetylcholine which is used by the nerves to control breathing, heart rate and muscle contraction. It is also important for parts of the brain involved in memory and mood – and is critical during foetal brain development in the womb. The human body can make some choline, but it can also be obtained through the diet (eggs, organ meats and legumes are the best sources) to top up our levels. Choline requirements are higher during pregnancy and breastfeeding, and also after the menopause and in men – thought to be due to oestrogen's ability to enhance synthesis of this nutrient.[93] Check out my Aubergine, Soft-boiled Egg + Hummus Pitta Pockets on page 162.

Other important vitamins and minerals include iron, magnesium, vitamin D and vitamin K.

Flick to Appendix 2 to find out where to find these brain-boosting nutrients (page 252).

Connection

It may surprise some people to learn that social connection was found to be the most important protective factor when it comes to depression.[94] The opposite of connection, social isolation, has a negative effect on health, both physically and mentally, and can increase depressive symptoms. This is not about having loads of friends or a huge family, but simply having people you trust who you can connect with and confide in. Of course, living in an abusive or toxic relationship (be that familial, romantic or a friendship) is likely to be more harmful than being alone.

Smoking

Smoking is often used by people to cope with stress, with some saying it helps them to relax. Nicotine can indeed offer a brief sensation of relaxation triggered by the release of the hormone dopamine, but this is short-lived and leaves us wanting more, which is what ultimately leads to addiction and cravings. People with depression are twice as likely to smoke compared to those without depression – which may be a bit of a chicken-and-egg scenario; that is, which came first?[95] But actually the research is now strong enough to say that smoking can increase the risk of depression.[96] On top of that, female smokers carry their own sex-specific risks including increased risk of postpartum depression, earlier menopausal transition and more severe menopausal symptoms.[97]

Alcohol

Many people believe that having an alcoholic drink will help them feel more relaxed. However, leaning on alcohol to take the edge off or unwind after work could actually be doing the opposite. Here's the thing: women who engage in binge drinking are more likely to experience depression and, similarly, women with depression are more likely to engage in binge drinking.[98] I say this without judgement as someone who has regularly done the same in the past – reaching for a glass of wine to relax after work or having a shot of 'Dutch courage' prior to a big social event or a date. However, this can become such a vicious circle and can exacerbate feelings of anxiety and low mood. Alcohol can do this directly, through altering the neurochemicals in your brain and reducing brain-essential B-vitamin levels, but also indirectly through next-day hangxiety (that intense anxiety many experience during a hangover) and by interfering with work, life and relationships. Regardless of what your relationship is with alcohol, it might be sensible to cut down on it (or cut it out) if you're experiencing anxiety or depression.

Movement

While exercise equally benefits men and women when it comes to depression and anxiety, women are typically less active than men and therefore are more likely to be missing out on the brain-protecting effects of exercise. Regular physical activity has not only been associated with a reduced risk of depression and anxiety, but it also improves sleep, quality of life and self-esteem.[99] Regular physical activity during pregnancy can reduce the risk of depression during pregnancy and also in the postpartum period, and help with reducing postpartum depressive symptoms.[100] Even low-intensity activities, such as walking and yoga, have been shown to reduce the symptoms of depression in pregnant women.[101] This holds true during other periods of life including the transition through the menopause. Post-menopausal women who are active report better quality of life and lower levels of anxiety, stress and depressive symptoms compared to post-menopausal women who are inactive.[102]

Sleep

Depression can lead to disrupted sleep, including difficulty falling asleep, staying asleep and waking early, but it can also go the other way and lead to not being able to get out of bed. At the same time, lack of sleep can also increase the risk of depression and make symptoms worse.[103] Age and fluctuating sex hormones can also affect sleep, as we have learned, which can make this a particularly tricky area for women to get a handle on. However, understanding that by prioritising your sleep hygiene routine – particularly around periods of major hormonal transition – may help to offset the risk of low mood. See the next chapter for more on the importance of a good night's sleep.

Mindfulness

Mindfulness-based therapies and stress-reduction programmes are used as a treatment for certain mental health problems including anxiety and depression. However, they can be practised by anyone who wishes to simply protect their mental health and well-being. You might think it's a bit too 'woo-woo' for you, but I assure you that there are many ways to practise mindfulness (see the box overleaf for a few methods I like to use). At the very basic level, mindfulness is simply paying attention to the present moment so it can be used in your everyday life and doesn't require much time.

Simple ways to practise mindfulness

- **Breathing:** There are so many different breathing techniques, and more and more research is emerging regarding their role in reducing anxiety and stress. The 4–7–8 breathing technique, also known as 'relaxing breath', involves breathing in for four seconds, holding the breath for seven and exhaling for eight. Yogic breathing has also been shown to improve mood; in particular, a breathing-based meditation practice known as 'Sudarshan Kriya yoga' helped to improve symptoms in people with severe depression. It should be noted that in this study all patients were on medication at the time, but only those who were allocated to the Sudarshan Kriya yoga treatment arm of the study showed improvements.[104]

- **Body scan:** Often when we are feeling stressed or anxious we hold a lot of tension in our body, so this can be particularly useful to check in with your physical health too. I also find this practice incredibly grounding and like doing it in bed before I fall asleep. Start by closing your eyes and gently mentally scan up through your body – starting with your toes and feet. It can be helpful to squeeze and release each muscle as you move up. Notice the sensations and comfort – or discomfort – that you come across. The aim is not to fix anything, but simply to notice.

- **Mindful walking:** This doesn't really require much explanation and can be practised at any time as you go about the day, although it can be far more immersive if you do it in a green space. Spending time in nature has been found to help with mental health problems including anxiety and depression. Try to do this without music, a podcast or your phone. Pay attention to the sounds around you, the sensations of the wind or the heat of the sun, the smells and sights around you. Bring your attention back to the sensations in your own body and how you feel.

- **Meditation:** Meditation is a form or practice of mindfulness. Learning mindfulness meditation is straightforward enough to practise on your own, but a teacher, course or app can also help you get started, particularly if you're practising meditation for specific health reasons. Apps like Calm, Headspace and Just Breathe all offer simple guided meditations to help ease you into this practice.

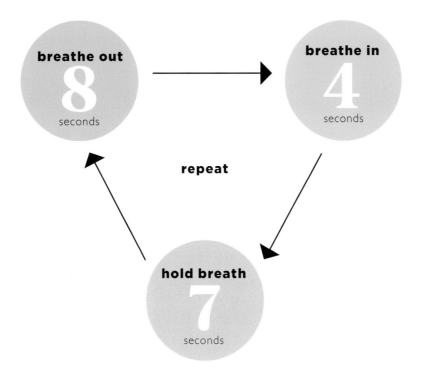

breathe out
8
seconds

breathe in
4
seconds

repeat

hold breath
7
seconds

* * * *

I want to end this chapter by reminding you that it's not all in your head – it's not just that time of the month, part of 'the change' or a normal part of being a woman. Yes, there are certain points across a woman's lifespan where she is more vulnerable to poor mental health, but our biology is not our destiny – and hormones are not the only thing that orchestrate our mood. Our mental health is influenced by multiple factors, and taking the steps outlined in this chapter can absolutely help to protect and improve it. Understanding why these changes to mood may be happening can also be incredibly empowering for women, encouraging them to speak up and ask for help when needed – and ultimately feel less isolated. If you're struggling with your mental health, that should never be dismissed or trivialised simply because of your hormones.

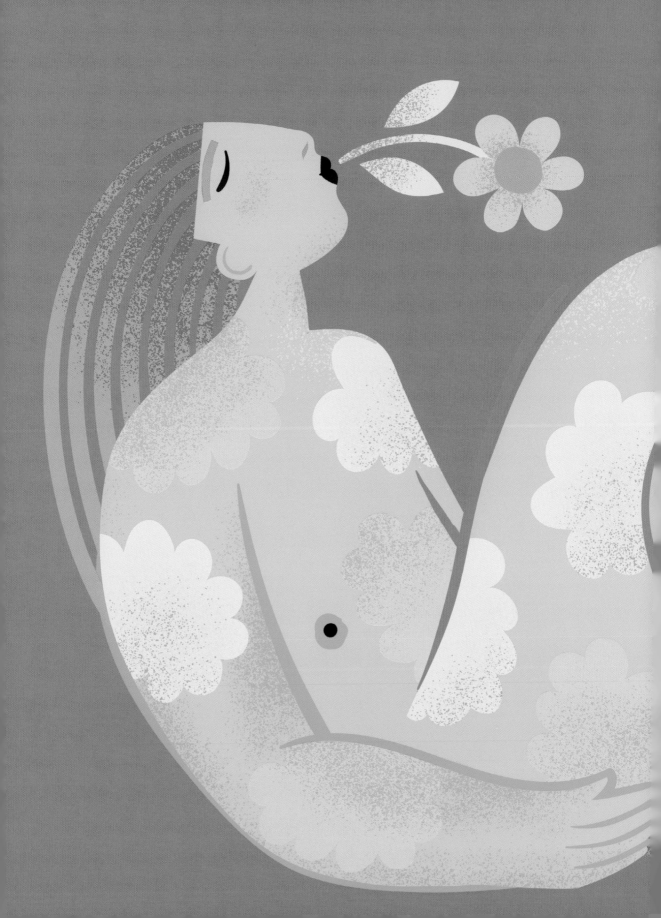

Sleep

Sleep

They say a good night's sleep solves most problems, and I feel that deep in my soul. After years of sleepless nights, I have become a little bit obsessed with sleep – good-quality sleep, that is. In my friendship group, I'm notorious for going to bed early, which is often before 9pm on week nights. I honestly don't get FOMO (fear of missing out) because, in my opinion, sleep is one of the most underrated pillars of health and it affects everything.

However, I wasn't always like this. I averaged a maximum of five to six hours of sleep a night throughout my entire eight years at university – often cutting it to three or four hours during exam season. If only I knew then what I know now: that if I had in fact slept more, I would have consolidated more of what I had learned and possibly performed better. Things didn't improve when I started working as a doctor, because part and parcel of being a junior doctor is doing many night shifts. I recall my first ever night shift, which was on the acute medical unit where we provide rapid assessment and treatment for patients admitted urgently from A&E. I guess you could say I was busy! I was high on adrenaline the whole night and was full of nervous energy right up until handover at 9am the next day. By the time I sat on the Tube to go home, the exhaustion washed over me and I slept the whole journey back – missing my stop and continuing on the line until someone woke me up. I was so frazzled that I ended up leaving my keys on the Tube and not being able to get into the house until my flatmate could meet me on her lunch break. Moral of the story: don't sleep on public transport.

In the last few years, I have really started geeking out on my sleep by tracking it and finding out what little tweaks I can do throughout my day and evening to ensure I make the most of the time I have in bed. For example, by using a WHOOP device, which is designed to track sleep and recovery, I have found that reading before bed, journaling and wearing a sleep mask improve my sleep quality, whereas using my device in bed and drinking alcohol affect the quality of my sleep. What I have also learned, however, is that sleep hygiene practices can be highly individual and what works for one person, may not work for another.

How the Sexes Sleep

It is pretty much undisputed that sleep is essential for health, allowing us to rest and recover – physically, mentally and emotionally – and perform at our best. I am confident that every single person reading this book has experienced at least one bad night of sleep, and that you felt rotten the next day too. One night of poor sleep can impair your concentration and judgement, and make you more prone to mistakes and accidents, but long-term lack of sleep can increase the risk of a wide range of health problems including heart disease and stroke, type 2 diabetes and obesity, depression and risk of death.[1] It also supresses your immune system, making you more susceptible to colds and flu, and lowers your sex drive.[2] Needless to say, this is one aspect of our lifestyle we shouldn't overlook!

While sufficient sleep is vital for everyone, there are important differences between men and women when it comes to catching shut-eye. Surprisingly, women sleep more overall (despite doing more unpaid work and having less leisure time) compared to men.[3] However, women also report poorer sleep quality, including difficulty falling asleep, waking up frequently in the night and having longer wakeful episodes.[4] The latter are often made worse by the fact that many women experience overactive bladder (OAB), which means they typically wake up more times in the night to go for a wee.[5] Women are also more likely to experience heartburn and acid reflux, which can interfere with sleep (and also why I never choose a spicy curry too late in the evening).[6]

We may also be more susceptible to the health effects of sleep loss. A recent study found that older women who experience frequently unconscious wakeful periods, and for longer duration, had nearly double the risk of dying from cardiovascular disease, while the association was less clear in older men.[7]

In addition to sleep disturbances, sex differences also exist in the treatment of sleep disorders. For example, in 2013, the US Food and Drug Administration (FDA) required the manufacturers of Ambien (zolpidem), a popular sleeping pill, to reduce the original dose by half for women. This came about after it was picked up (nearly 20 years after the drug's release) that women were having more adverse effects to the drug than men, including morning sleepiness and impaired driving. As it turns out, women metabolise the drug much more slowly than men, making them more susceptible to the side effects.[8] I should add, however, that other authorities around the world did not change their recommendation and the FDA's was not based on studies showing an actual benefit at this dose – again, we can't just assume women are small (or half-sized) men.[9]

Women are also at higher risk of insomnia, and this sex difference emerges around the time of puberty – oh, hello hormones![10] Similar to mood disorders, sleep issues often coincide with important hormonal and physiological changes throughout a woman's lifespan: puberty, premenstrually, pregnancy and the menopause. Speaking to sleep scientist Dr Sophie Bostock, she has a hunch that women's 'sleep reactivity' – a measure of how easily our sleep becomes disrupted in response to stress – is typically higher, perhaps because of the way our HPA axis is wired and differences in how we respond to stress. For example, while the racing mind is common for men and women, there is evidence that women tend to ruminate and replay things more than men, and that is a characteristic often linked to insomnia.[11]

Of course, biology is not the only driver for this sleep gap between men and women: gender stereotypes are also tied up in this. For example, women disproportionately act as informal caregivers for children, older adults and relatives, which means less time for sleep and more sleep interruptions.[12]

The usual disclaimer applies here: we are speaking in general terms about what happens on average between men and women and this does not apply to every individual. Also, like most other areas of research, studies related to sleep has focused disproportionately on males, which leaves a large, gaping hole in our knowledge.[13]

Getting Back to Basics

Sleep can be broadly divided into rapid-eye movement sleep (REM) and non-rapid-eye movement sleep (non-REM). The latter is broken down into stages 1 to 4, each increasing in depth of sleep. We alternate between the two phases of sleep in 90-minute cycles across the night. Non-REM sleep typically makes up the majority of the total sleep time in adults, but the ratio of REM to non-REM sleep varies throughout the night. For example, we get most of our non-REM deep sleep earlier in the night (stages 3 and 4), whereas REM sleep dominates the final part of the night.[14] Together, non-REM sleep stages 3 and 4 are often known as slow-wave sleep (SWS).[15]

Many people think that the more deep sleep, the better, and that's a sign of a good night's sleep, but actually all phases are important and perform different roles for the brain and body. REM sleep is often called 'dream sleep' as it is the sleep phase where our most vivid dreams occur, but it's also incredibly important for emotional well-being and memory consolidation.[16] Professor Matthew Walker, author of *Why We Sleep*, has referred to REM sleep as 'emotional first aid', which explains why, when we are sleep-deprived, we can be a little more emotional and reactive than usual.[17] Newborns spend more time asleep and, in particular, have a higher proportion of REM sleep, which is believed to play an important role in brain development.[18]

Which hormones affect our sleep?

Sex hormones not only orchestrate reproductive function during the menstrual cycle but have a big influence on sleep and our circadian rhythm – the body's internal 24-hour cycle that regulates bodily functions, from sleeping to waking.

Oestrogen has been shown to decrease the length of time it takes to fall asleep, with fewer awakenings throughout the night, and increase total sleep time (you're thinking, 'what can't this hormone do?' I know!).[19] To add to that, it plays a role in regulating body temperature at night and keeping it low, which is important for a sound sleep, whereas progesterone has anti-anxiety and sedative effects.[20] So it may come as no surprise that sex differences in sleep emerge only after puberty when rates of insomnia in females surpass those in males and persist into adulthood.[21] Women also report more sleep disturbances during periods of major hormonal change such as menstruation, pregnancy and menopause.

Note: If you're waking at night during your period due to leakage/heavy flow, perhaps try absorbent underwear (period pants), cloth pads or a menstrual cup. A good mattress protector is also useful!

Prevalence of insomnia by sex and age[22]

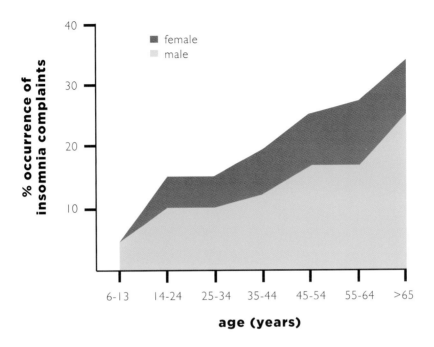

How your sleep changes across your cycle

One of the tell-tale signs for me when I'm due my period is the two to three nights of restless sleep beforehand – and it seems I'm not alone. The most common time for women to report issues sleeping are the days leading up to the period (late luteal phase) and the first few days of the period (early follicular).[23] This is believed to be due to low levels of oestrogen and progesterone during this time, coupled with other premenstrual symptoms such as cramps, headaches and low mood. However, some women also experience sleep disturbance mid-cycle, just after ovulation when body temperature rises about 0.5–1 degree, while others report no difficulty sleeping at any point in their cycle.[24] In addition to the quality of sleep, the type of sleep varies across the menstrual cycle. In the luteal phase, women experience less REM sleep, which is thought to be due to a higher body temperature during this time.[25]

Perhaps start by keeping track of your sleep across your cycle to identify if it's affected at certain points. Then, if you do notice that it is, getting into bed earlier during this part of your cycle will give you a better chance of a good night's sleep. Also focusing on maximising sleep hygiene tips during these points may help offset some of the sleep disturbance and improve sleep quality (more on this later).

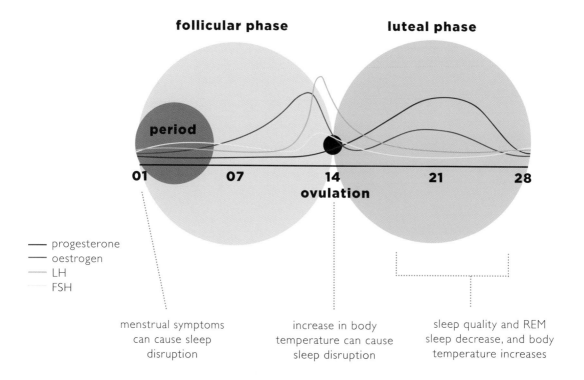

Menstrual cycle + sleep

follicular phase

luteal phase

period

01   07   14   21   28

ovulation

— progesterone
— oestrogen
— LH
— FSH

menstrual symptoms
can cause sleep
disruption

increase in body
temperature can cause
sleep disruption

sleep quality and REM
sleep decrease, and body
temperature increases

Will I sleep better on the pill?

The few studies looking at sleep and oral contraceptives have found no proof of poorer quality sleep or increased sleep disturbance, but the phases of sleep do appear to be altered. Women taking combined oral contraceptives (a combo of oestrogen and progesterone) have more light and less deep, slow-wave sleep, compared to non-pill taking women.[84] However, it's not known how or if these changes affect a woman day to day. Some women may actually find they sleep better on the pill because they aren't experiencing the same fluctuations in hormones as non-pill women, and their body temperature, while slightly higher overall, remains relatively consistent.[85] The impact the pill has on sleep appears to be pretty small, but we need far more evidence to draw hard-and-fast-conclusions.

Restless Nights from Bump to Birth

Pregnancy brings about significant fluctuations in hormones that interfere with sleep, not to mention the small matter of an expanding bump, a tiny kicking human, tender breasts, the constant urge to wee, heartburn, leg cramps, backache – and everything else that comes with pregnancy! About half of pregnant women report poor sleep, and this unfortunately becomes worse by the third trimester.[26] This includes difficulty falling and staying asleep, increased awakenings in the night, restless sleep, daytime sleepiness and also more nightmares compared to non-pregnant women.[27] The amount of REM sleep also decreases in pregnancy, while stage 1 (light sleep) increases.[28] To add to that, about one in five pregnant women will also experience restless legs syndrome (RLS), a very uncomfortable sensation causing an uncontrollable urge to move your legs, in the third trimester, which also makes it difficult to fall asleep. Fortunately, it usually disappears within four weeks of delivery.

Poor sleep during pregnancy is not only frustrating but may influence the type and length of delivery. One study found that pregnant women who slept fewer than six hours at night in their final month of pregnancy experienced longer labours and were four-and-a-half times more likely to have Caesarean deliveries.[29] The authors concluded that, given the results, pregnant women should be prescribed eight hours of sleep per night and that sleep quantity and quality should be assessed throughout the pregnancy. The thing is, as much as we all want a golden eight hours of sleep, it's easier said than done, but practising good sleep hygiene (more on this later) during pregnancy has been shown to improve sleep quality.[30]

Is it looking better for postpartum mums? Unfortunately, these sleep disturbances often continue for the first few weeks after giving birth (and some women sleep even less than they did during pregnancy). However, sleep quality typically recovers after three to five months.[31] I know from my friends and sisters, who have children, that even when the baby is sleeping there seems to be an endless list of jobs to do – from tidying up and putting on the washing to planning the next feeds – so it's not always easy to 'sleep when baby sleeps', but if you can, you should. Remember you do not need to be superwoman; you don't need to do it all – the most important thing is that you and baby are healthy. Ask friends and family to help out and, if you have a partner, share the nights if you can. If you can't switch off or nap, try practising a ten-minute Yoga Nidra session, which is basically a guided meditation practice that puts you into a state of deep relaxation. There appears to be an increasing amount of research validating its effects, and I've found it helps me to recover after a poor night of sleep when I do it around midday the next day.[32] There are lots of free resources and videos online to guide you through the practice.

Is Menopause Disrupting Your Rhythm?

Just as we have seen at other periods of hormonal flux, sleep issues become more common, and worsen, during the menopausal transition. In particular, post-menopausal women often experience difficulty falling asleep, frequent awakening and/or early-morning awakening.[34] That said, objective measures of sleep quality (measured in a sleep lab) have not shown a decrease during the menopause, and some parameters have been found to increase, including more slow-wave, deep sleep, longer sleep duration and better sleep efficiency (the percentage of total time in bed actually spent in sleep).[35] However, this increase in deep sleep may not necessarily be an indicator of better-quality sleep as it may well be a reflection of making up for sleep loss.[36]

The reason why sleep becomes an issue after the menopause seems to be due to a few things: the presence of uncomfortable hot flushes and sweats (vasomotor symptoms), ageing itself, lifestyle factors, coexisting medical conditions and, of course, hormones. After the menopause, we naturally lose the sleep-promoting benefits of oestrogen. However, this can be somewhat replaced with HRT, which has been shown to improve sleep quality and can be used to treat menopausal insomnia (see page 42 to read more about HRT).[37]

Quality versus Quantity

In general, women and men need the same amount of sleep per night – seven to nine hours. Babies, children and teenagers need more to enable growth and development, and people above the age of 65 need a little less, between seven and eight hours per night. Of course, this is based on averages and people fall on either side of the 'recommended' range. It's important to have averages so that we can spot sleep disturbances when they occur, but counting the number of hours spent in bed doesn't necessarily mean you're actually asleep for that length of time – so not only do we need the right quantity of sleep, but we also want good-quality sleep.

There are a number of sleep quality scales and surveys used in research and clinical practice, and sometimes it is measured in a lab using special sleep tests such as polysomnography. Although, these are not easily accessible ways to quickly check how you're sleeping. There are apps and wearable devices that can measure sleep, but they vary in terms of accuracy and, while useful for some people (personally I geek out on this kinda thing), for others they can cause sleep anxiety – leading to worse sleep.[38] The most simple – and perhaps best – metric for measuring how good your sleep was is to see how you feel each day.

Good sleep quality might be described as falling asleep within 10–30 minutes, not waking or waking up one time in the night – and for fewer than 20 minutes – and spending most of your time in bed asleep rather than awake. If your answers aren't really matching up to this, or perhaps they do but you're not waking up feeling well-rested and are falling asleep in the day, you might want to try implementing some of the following sleep hygiene tips into your life. If you have already tried these steps, or you have had trouble sleeping for months and it affects your daily life in a way that makes it hard to cope, you should speak to your GP for further support.

Clean Up Your Sleep Routine

In the same way that you practise personal or oral hygiene, it's good to get into the habit of practising sleep hygiene. Essentially, this is creating a routine of things that support you in meeting your sleep needs and avoiding habits that disrupt your rhythm. These routines add structure to your day, which in itself is helpful to your sleep, but also create boundaries around behaviours that may not be the most helpful anyway, such as checking your smartphone every five minutes of the day (and night). Sleep hygiene advice applies to both sexes, really, as we don't have unique guidance for women (yet). In many ways, the causal drivers behind poor sleep are not that important, because the intervention with the best evidence for improving sleep is the same, whether you're a 15-year-old boy or a 70-year-old woman. I've listed some tips below on what can help and what can hinder your sleep routine:

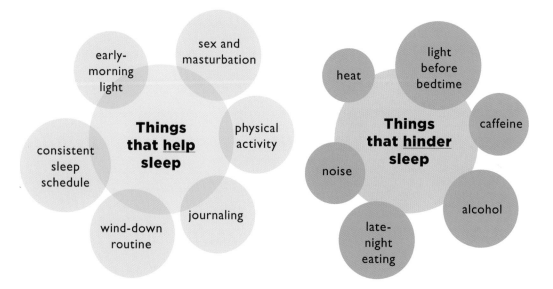

early-morning light

sex and masturbation

Things that help sleep

consistent sleep schedule

physical activity

wind-down routine

journaling

heat

light before bedtime

caffeine

Things that hinder sleep

noise

alcohol

late-night eating

Light exposure

Light is possibly the most influential external factor in our lives that drives our sleep–wake cycle.[39] When we view light, the retina in our eye carries that information to a tiny region of the brain called the suprachiasmatic nucleus (SCN) – also known as the central master clock. This master clock sends signals to other parts of the body to coordinate and regulate the many different body functions that occur in a 24-hour cycle. During the day, when we view light, it sends signals to keep us alert and, in the evening (if levels of light are low), it initiates the production of melatonin, preparing us for sleep. The effects of light on our circadian rhythm depend on the timing. So, if we view light in the morning, this advances the clock, while evening light delays the clock – leading to later sleep and wake times.[40]

To 'hack' this system, aim to get around 30 minutes of light in the morning, even on cloudy or overcast days. You can habit stack (the process of adding a new behaviour to your daily routine by 'stacking' it on top of an existing habit) this with something that you do already – perhaps walking or cycling to work instead of driving or getting the bus, or exercising outside instead of inside a gym (two birds, one stone). It might be tricky to achieve this in the colder and wetter months, and in such scenarios, light boxes or a SAD lamp can be used for 30 minutes a day to replicate this.[41] The intensity of the light emitted from these lamps is measured in lux – the higher the lux, the brighter the light, but in general ~10,000 lux is recommended. Light therapy is generally safe; however, it may not be suitable for people who have an eye condition or are particularly sensitive to light, or those taking medications that increase sensitivity to light, such as certain antibiotics, antipsychotics and the supplement St John's Wort.[42]

In the evening, you want to reverse this process, so dim overhead lights, using low-light lamps instead, and put away all blue-light-emitting devices – that includes most phones, laptops, TVs, tablets and e-readers. The blue light that's emitted from these screens can delay the release of melatonin, increasing alertness and making it harder to fall asleep. If you have no choice, you can use 'night mode' on most devices now, which adjusts the colour balance of the screen, and some people may wish to try blue-light-blocking glasses, although evidence is lacking as to whether they improve sleep quality in the general population.[43] Even if your device is not blue-light-emitting, technology in the bedroom can affect your sleep by making sounds, lighting up, buzzing and blinking, and also the act of using tech before bed can stimulate your mind and make it harder to unwind (especially if you're checking emails or watching TikTok). You want to start the day bright and light, and end the day dark and dim.

Melatonin

Melatonin is a hormone involved in the circadian rhythm, including sleep promotion. It is made naturally in the body, but also can be taken as a supplement purchased over the counter in certain countries (it is a prescription-only medicine in the UK).

Melatonin is produced naturally by a pea-sized gland deep in the centre of the brain known as the pineal gland. One thing I remember about this gland from med school is that it was historically referred to by some cultures as the 'third eye'. Some believe it helped people become enlightened or to spiritually awaken.[44] Melatonin has its own nickname as the 'hormone of darkness' due to its release in response to darkness. As the sun begins to set, melatonin starts to rise, peaking early in the night and then gradually falling in the second half of the night. As we age, the amount of melatonin we produce decreases, and this decline is particularly apparent during the menopause.[45] Melatonin levels also fluctuate across the menstrual cycle, rising in the late luteal phase following the mid-luteal surge in progesterone.[46]

Melatonin supplementation has been shown to be helpful for preventing and reducing symptoms of jetlag and improving sleep in certain sleep disorders such as insomnia.[47] In post-menopausal women with sleep issues, melatonin has been found to be helpful compared to a dummy pill.[48] When it comes to shift workers, studies haven't found conclusive results and, as for healthy adults, melatonin supplementation may marginally improve sleep outcomes, but it does not seem to be especially helpful.[49] As it stands, supplementation for the treatment of insomnia is not currently recommended by the American Academy of Sleep Medicine and the American College of Physicians and, in the UK, it is typically only prescribed for adults over 55 with insomnia for short-term use only – with some other exceptions.

Although considered relatively safe, there are some side effects, including daytime sleepiness, irritability, anxiety, nausea and diarrhoea. It should also be avoided if pregnant or breastfeeding, in certain medical conditions (autoimmune diseases, for example) and with certain medications. If you do wish to try it, experts recommend low doses (as low as 0.3mg up to 2mg) given 1 hour before bedtime.[50] However, buyer beware: supplements are not regulated in the same way as medicines and recent research has found that the actual melatonin content often varies from what is on the label, with some products having as much as 83 per cent less and others containing as much as 478 per cent more than they claim.[51]

The effect of light on melatonin production[52]

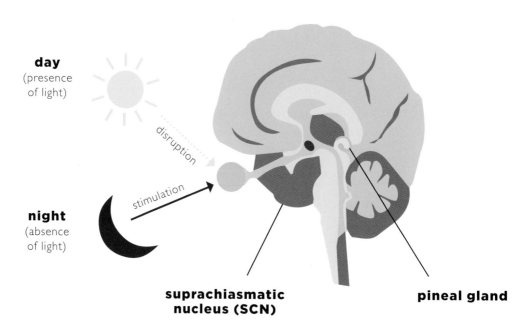

day
(presence
of light)

night
(absence
of light)

disruption

stimulation

suprachiasmatic
nucleus (SCN)

pineal gland

Exercise

Regular exercise has long been associated with better sleep, and it seems that many forms of activity – from yoga and tai chi, to aerobic exercise and resistance training – all have the potential to improve sleep.[53]

One question I'm often asked is: does the time of day matter? It's a commonly held belief that exercising too close to bedtime will keep you awake by increasing adrenaline and raising your core body temperature. However, the research shows that evening exercise does not impair sleep and can actually help people to fall asleep faster and spend more time in deep sleep.[54] There is one important exception: the opposite is true if it is vigorous activity and an hour before heading to bed.[55] The other thing to avoid, for evening gym-goers, is pre-workout drinks with caffeine (or other stimulants), large meals prior to bed and too much screen time.

Basically, once you're not doing HIIT or CrossFit too close to bedtime, when you exercise – in terms of your sleep quantity and quality – it really doesn't matter and, actually, exercising at any time is better than not exercising at all.

Why am I waking to wee?

If you're waking many times in the night to wee, you may have overactive bladder syndrome (OAB) which affects 20 per cent of women and is more common as we get older, especially after the menopause.[56] This is where you have a sudden urge to go to the toilet (you cannot wait), you need to pass urine more often than normal (called frequency) and this occurs several times during the night as well as many times during the day. There is sometimes leakage (urge incontinence), but not always. Practical advice is often to reduce fluid intake, but this can actually make symptoms worse as urine becomes more concentrated which can irritate the bladder. So, the best advice is to drink normal quantities of fluid per day (about two litres). However, cutting down on alcohol and caffeine can help as they can worsen symptoms. The mainstay of treatment is bladder training, which can help you regain control of your overactive bladder so you can hold more urine and don't need to go as often. Some women develop urge incontinence after the menopause, and this is thought to be due to the lining of the vagina shrinking (vaginal atrophy) due to a drop in the level of the female hormone oestrogen. In this case, intravaginal oestrogen can be helpful. There are lots of other medications and treatment options available, so please don't suffer in silence.

Meal timing

Many foods are touted to improve sleep quality but when you eat seems to have more of an impact than what you eat. Just as light and other cues from our environment influence our circadian rhythm, so do our mealtimes. Like the clock in the brain, our gut, liver, pancreas and muscle all have their own 'clocks', known as 'peripheral clocks', and can be influenced by when we eat. So when meal timing is aligned to the daytime, the clocks in these peripheral organs and tissues can run in synchrony with the light-driven timing of the master clock in the brain. We call this 'circadian alignment'. However, when these clocks are operating on a different schedule to the master clock, we call this 'circadian misalignment', which is like jetlag.

Alan Flanagan, a friend of mine and PhD researcher in this field, explains it using the useful analogy of an orchestra and conductor. The conductor is the master clock; it sets the overall timing and rhythm for the symphony to be played. The pieces of the orchestra are the peripheral clocks. The violins and the clarinets could go off playing on their own, but this would sound awful (misalignment). However, if they read their sheet music correctly (get the right signals), then the orchestra comes together and the conductor can ensure it all plays to a well-synchronised symphony (alignment). Think of meal timing as the sheet music for the orchestra.

Importantly, eating at unusual times (say, during shift work and travelling through different time zones) is a major cause of body-clock disruption.[57] Lack of sleep can also disrupt hunger and fullness hormones, ghrelin and leptin, which can cause us to feel hungrier the next day and less satiated, which may lead to consuming more calorie-dense foods.[58] Of course, this is not an issue as a once-off, but over time this could lead to poor health.

Does a warm glass of milk help you to fall asleep?

There is some evidence to say that consuming milk may help with sleep.[59] This is thought to be due to the fact that milk and dairy products contain an amino acid called tryptophan, which melatonin is made from. However, for tryptophan to work its magic it has to cross the blood–brain barrier (the brain's security system), which isn't easy, but research suggests that eating carbohydrates along with foods high in tryptophan may help it to pass through.[60] This is why malted milk or milk sweetened with honey are often recommended as sleep aids. However, there's currently no evidence to suggest that a single glass of milk contains enough tryptophan or melatonin to significantly influence your sleep or treat insomnia. But, if drinking milk before bed is part of your bedtime routine and you feel that it helps your ZZZs, then go for it.

Caffeine

Caffeine gets a bad rap, but it's not all bad and actually has some pretty powerful effects when it comes to mental and physical performance. However, the timing and the dose do matter. Caffeine is a psychoactive stimulant and works through a variety of mechanisms, but mainly through its effects on adenosine. Adenosine accumulates across the day as we are awake; the more we have, the sleepier we feel. Caffeine acts by preventing adenosine binding to its receptor – essentially elbowing it out of the way – and blocking it from doing its job. This increases alertness which, of course, can be a positive thing (depending on the time of day), but it can have knock-on effects on our sleep later on. Here's the thing: caffeine acts fast, reaching peak levels in the blood in about 30 minutes, but can take hours to get rid of. The half-life (time taken to eliminate half of the caffeine in your system) varies from person to person, but on average it is about five hours – although it can be anywhere between two and ten hours – which means that your post-lunch coffee could very well be keeping you up at night.[61] Ideally, you want to have a caffeine cut-off around midday, or around eight hours before going to bed. In terms of how much caffeine you can consume a day, 400mg is considered safe for adults (200mg/day for pregnant women) which is about four to five cups of coffee (depending on who makes it). The other important thing to note is that caffeine is in many other foods and drinks (see table below):

Caffeine levels in food and drink[62]

Drinks/Foods	Volume	Caffeine [mg] Mean [range]
Filtered coffee	125ml	85 [60–135]
Espresso	30ml	60 [35–100]
Soluble instant coffee	125ml	65 [35–105]
Decaffeinated coffee	125ml	3 [1–5]
Tea (leaves or bag)	150ml	32 [20–45]
Iced tea	330ml	20 [10–50]
Hot chocolate	150ml	4 [2–7]
Caffeinated soft drinks	330ml	39 [30–48]
Sugar-free caffeinated soft drinks	330ml	41 [26–57]
Energy drinks	330ml	80 [70–120]
Chocolate bar	30g	20 [5–36]
Milk chocolate	30g	6 [1–15]
Dark chocolate	30g	60 [20–120]

Alcohol

Alcohol is a sedative and can induce feelings of sleepiness and relaxation. For this reason, it's often used as a sleep aid, even though it's anything but. You might have experienced falling asleep faster after a drink; however, while alcohol can cause you to fall asleep faster, the quality and often net quantity of sleep is worse. This is because alcohol fragments our sleep, meaning we wake up more times in the night (which you may or may not be consciously aware of) and reduces the amount of restorative REM sleep we have.[63] Low levels of alcohol will have less of an effect but, unfortunately, even as little as one drink has been shown to impact sleep and recovery.[64] I hate to be the fun police, but it's something to keep in mind if you're depending on alcohol for a restful slumber.

Sleep consistency

Sleep consistency is one of the most important factors for better sleep – as well as improved cognitive performance and health overall.[65]

Ideally, we want to have a relatively consistent sleep schedule: going to bed at roughly the same time most nights and waking up at a fixed time. This sets the body's internal clock to expect sleep at a certain time, night after night. Count back roughly eight hours from the time you need to wake up in the morning and this is ideally when you should be in bed (if not a little before). On the weekends or days off work, try not to shift your sleep schedule too much by sleeping in until late or going to bed later – it may feel good at the time, but you will likely be paying for it, with a feeling akin to jetlag, on Monday morning when that 6am alarm goes off. Of course, sometimes life gets in the way and it would be a pretty boring one if our biggest priority was getting into bed at 10pm every night. So, as with anything we do in life, it's what you do the majority of the time that makes the biggest difference.

Wind-down routine

Having a bedtime routine signals to your brain that you are winding down to go to sleep. Studies of new mothers have also found that a consistent bedtime routine is a helpful tool for improving sleep of the infant or toddler, as well as the mood of the mother.[66]

My friend Michael James Wong, founder of Just Breathe, describes it this way: 'The sun doesn't just switch on and off, and neither should we – so give time, and space, to fully wind down.' Even if you are the type of person who falls asleep once your head hits the pillow, I would still give yourself a window of 30–60 minutes to wind down prior to bed. For example, for me this looks like: doing my skincare routine, brushing my teeth, changing into pyjamas, journaling and reading ten pages of my book. It sounds extensive, but it takes about 20–25 minutes. If reading is not for you, listening to some relaxing music, meditating or Yoga Nidra (see page 120), or having a warm bath may be more up your street.

Journaling

There are many things that keep us up at night, but perhaps one of the most common factors is stress, worry and rumination, which women, on average, do more of than men.[67] For many, this might be overthinking past events or perhaps worrying about all the work you need to get through. One practice that I personally find helpful (and is backed by science) is journaling before bed. I call it my 'brain dump' and this typically involves reflections from the day, things I am grateful for or simply my to-do list. In fact, a recent study in the *Journal of Experimental Psychology* found that writing a to-do list before bedtime helped people to fall asleep nine minutes faster than those who wrote about completed tasks.[68] And it makes sense, right? When we have a task that's unfinished, it plays on our mind more than any task we have completed. Similarly, people who practise gratitude exercises also report better sleep.[69] Night-time journaling doesn't have to be long-winded or airy-fairy – perhaps start by writing your to-do list and ending your practice with something (or someone) you are grateful for.

Environment

The optimal sleep environment should be cool, quiet and dark:

- **Keep it cool:** Ensure the room is cool (around 18˚C). In cold climates, this may involve turning radiators off or down in the bedroom and using a fan in the warmer months. In warmer climates, where there is often air conditioning, this is a bit easier to calibrate. If you experience hot flushes or struggle with your sleep during the luteal phase, perhaps invest in some light, breathable pyjamas and choose sheets made from materials like bamboo or cotton.

- **Keep it quiet:** Unless you live somewhere pretty secluded, it's almost impossible to control all external sounds. Earplugs are the cheapest, simplest solution to drown out noise. Some people enjoy falling asleep to the hum of white noise, which can help to block out variable noises by providing constant, soothing sounds. To be honest, a fan or air purifier can produce a similar effect.

- **Keep it dark:** Block out as much light as possible with heavy curtains or blackout blinds. After night shifts, I often use those portable blackout blinds, meant for babies, or I will tape my curtains to the windowpanes with reusable masking tape to avoid any light leaks. If all else fails, a good, comfortable eye mask is a great investment.

Sex and masturbation

Yep, let's talk about sex, baby. Surprisingly (or unsurprisingly) few studies have actually looked at the relationship between sex and sleep. Although, of those that have, there seems to be a positive relationship between the two – especially between orgasm and subjective sleep quality.[70] This is thought to be due to the release of oxytocin and prolactin, and the suppression of cortisol (a stress hormone), which follows orgasm. This combination promotes feelings of connection and closeness, relaxation and sleepiness. And while orgasm with a partner seems to offer the most benefit. around 50 per cent of both men and women say that an orgasm from masturbation helps them fall asleep and improves their sleep quality.[71]

But what if you don't orgasm? Interestingly, it seems that men find sex – in general – improves sleep and speed of falling asleep, whereas women typically only report sex with orgasm helps.[72] This may be down to the 'orgasm gap' (see below). If orgasm is the pièce de résistance when it comes to boosting sleep through sex, then, in my humble opinion, it's a public health issue that women are missing out here.

Finally, lack of sleep can also totally crush libido in women and make them less likely to have sex.[73] Sleep deprivation over a longer period can also impair ovulation, mess with the menstrual cycle and, ultimately, affect fertility.[74] Men are not free from the effects of sleep deprivation, however, as even one week of restless sleep can reduce testosterone by 10–15 per cent compared to levels found after a normal night's sleep.[75]

The orgasm gap

The orgasm gap describes how, in heterosexual relationships, women on average have fewer orgasms than men. The gap doesn't just exist between heterosexual men and women – one study, inclusive of over 50,000 adults (including those who are lesbian, gay and bisexual) found that 95 per cent of heterosexual men reported they usually or always orgasmed during sex. Gay and bisexual men also fared pretty well, with orgasm success rates of 89 and 88 per cent respectively, with women trailing behind – especially heterosexual women reporting only 65 per cent of the time.[76]

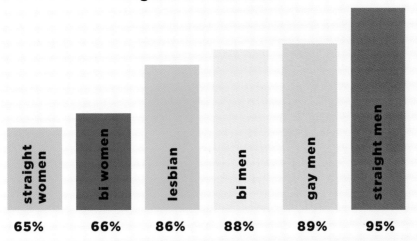

Orgasm success rates[77]

straight women	bi women	lesbian	bi men	gay men	straight men
65%	66%	86%	88%	89%	95%

Rates vary based on sexual orientation, partner gender and whether it's relationship or causal sex – the latter increasing the orgasm gap. For example, lesbian women are more likely than either heterosexual or bisexual women to orgasm during sex, and bisexual women are more likely to orgasm if the partner is a woman.[78] Unfortunately, the research has not been inclusive of non-binary or transgender individuals.

There are so many reasons why this orgasm gap exists, but one of the most important things to acknowledge is that most women need clitoral stimulation, using hands, toys or oral sex, to achieve orgasm. This is rarely – if ever – emphasised in the media, movies or porn, where orgasm seems to be achieved through a few heavy hip thrusts alone. Unfortunately, this can mean women feel like there is something wrong with them when really, as little as 4 per cent of women report penetrative sex alone is enough to achieve orgasm.[79] This insecurity often means that women will fake orgasm to feel normal while also saving their male partner's ego.[80] Women are also less likely to receive oral sex or clitoral stimulation (and therefore reach orgasm) during a casual hook-up than they would in a relationship – essentially due to the fact that women don't feel as entitled to ask and men are less motivated to provide.[81]

This is not to say that all men don't care about female pleasure, but women shouldn't feel like they can't communicate their needs or that their pleasure or orgasm is worth any less than their partner's. As it stands, however, sex education still does not cover sexual pleasure, and female pleasure remains quite a taboo. However, there is some evidence that empowering women and men with clitoral knowledge and evidence-based methods to enhance women's orgasm (see *Becoming Cliterate* by Dr Laurie Mintz for more) can improve sexual pleasure for women.[82] Perhaps reading this might help some more women understand the female anatomy a little more – and what they need in order to achieve orgasm – or perhaps it's something you want to share with your partner? After all, if it's a factor which can improve sleep quality, then I argue this is a public health issue.

Shift Work

As someone who has worked a fair amount of night shifts, I know how difficult it can be to get enough (good-quality) sleep during the day and feel alert during the night. In addition to problems with sleep (and staying awake!), it is now well established that night-shift workers have an increased risk of poor health including cardiovascular disease, depression and even breast cancer, compared to those who don't work nights.[83] Additionally, sleep deprivation can also reduce our alertness and impair performance and concentration – making mistakes more likely to happen.

Shift work is necessary, and our shift workers are key workers doing incredible work, so it's important that we do what we can to support their health inside and outside of work.

My top tips for night-shift workers include:

- For people rotating from day to night shifts, start adjusting your sleep schedule several days before commencing the new shift schedule. If you are on permanent nights, try to keep regularity in your sleep patterns, even on days off.

- Plan for sleep. It seems like a no-brainer, but planning ahead and building sleep into your daily schedule will mean you're more likely to get the sleep you need. Some people like to sleep straight after a night shift and wake up a few hours before their next one (my personal routine), while others like to stay awake a little longer and then wake up closer to their shift start time.

- Usual sleep hygiene tips apply. Keep your bedroom cool, dark and quiet. Use an eye mask or blackout blind, and wear earplugs or try a white noise machine or app. If you live with other people, let them know when your sleep times are, so they can try not to disturb you (I also put a note on my door to warn the postman!).

- Expose yourself to bright light before work and wear sunglasses on the way home after a night shift.

- Exercise can help improve sleep quality and also make you more alert before your shift. Some people like to exercise straight after a night shift (major kudos to you), but I've always been far too tired and prefer doing it after my daytime sleep before my next shift.

- Use caffeine wisely. Having caffeine before work or at the start of your shift will help you feel alert, but try to avoid it for the second half of your shift so that it doesn't impact your sleep when you get home.

- If you do get a chance to nap on your break, try not to sleep for longer than 20–25 minutes to avoid deeper stages of sleep or it may leave you feeling groggier.

- During the biological night, our body digests and metabolises food much less efficiently than during the day, pushing up blood glucose, insulin and cholesterol levels, which can lead to poor health down the line. Practically speaking though, we also need the right fuel to keep us alert and perform at our best. Typically what I advise is:

- Have your main meals before and after your shifts (for example, lunch/dinner before your shift or early in the night and a breakfast when you get home). Ideally you want these meals to be as nutrient-dense as possible with lots of colourful fruit and vegetables, slow-releasing carbohydrates, lean protein and healthy fats – like my Harissa Salmon + Chunky Veg Couscous (see page 191) or DIY Protein Poke Bowl (page 210).

- Either avoid eating between midnight and 6am or, if you feel hungry, opt for low-fat, high-protein snacks such as Greek yogurt and berries, a protein shake or smoothie, or hummus or peanut butter on rye crackers.

- Keep hydrated with water throughout the night or drink decaf hot drinks – dehydration can lead to fatigue and reduce mental alertness.

- Plan ahead and pack your own snacks and drinks – try my Chocolate + Chia Nut Balls (page 220) or Spiced Nuts + Chickpeas (page 223). In my experience, the best treats can be found at the nurses' station on a night shift and they're always super generous with them, but try not to depend on jelly babies and cake to see you through the night – this energy is unlikely to sustain you.

- Finally, on your way home be safe! When you're sleep-deprived it's easy to make mistakes. Avoid driving if you can but, if public transport or walking is not an option, keep the windows open and turn up the radio. If you do feel drowsy when driving, pull over into a rest area or car park and take a nap before continuing.

* * * *

Sleep is not a passive activity, and I would go as far as saying it's the most important thing for our health and well-being. I don't believe we place enough emphasis on it – and the fact that women have poorer sleep quality is, in my eyes, a public health problem. Writing this chapter reinforced that for me, along with how little information is out there to support women during those pivotal stages in their lives where sleep disruption is most common.

I don't want you to finish this chapter feeling deflated though, because understanding when we may be more vulnerable to sleep disturbances allows us to be better prepared. I want you to take the advice in this chapter and start implementing it so that you can get the best-possible-quality sleep – despite the odds.

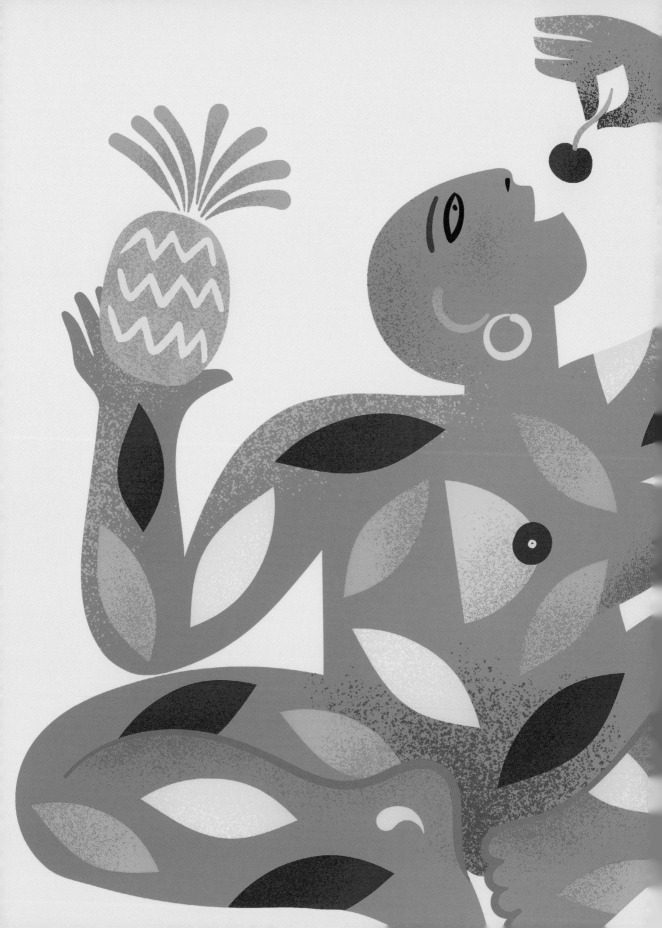

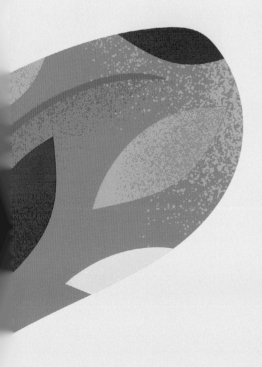

Recipes

A guide to the recipes

The Food Medic blog and books have always focused on delicious food that nourishes you, so it was important to include some everyday dishes in this book. In the following pages there are 50 recipes for breakfast, lunch, dinner, snacks and baking + desserts. You'll spot icons for vegetarian recipes, vegan recipes and also which recipes are a source of protein, fibre, iron and Omega 3, so you can easily find dishes to boost your intake of these nutrients.

Key to icons:

(V) Vegetarian

(Ve) Vegan

(P) Source of Protein: at least 12% of the calories come from protein

(F) Source of Fibre: recipe provides at least 3g of fibre per 100g or at least 1.5g per 100kcal

(I) Source of Iron: recipe provides 15% of the daily Reference intake (RI) per serving

(O) Source of Omega 3: recipe provides at least 0.4g of omega-3 fatty acids per serving

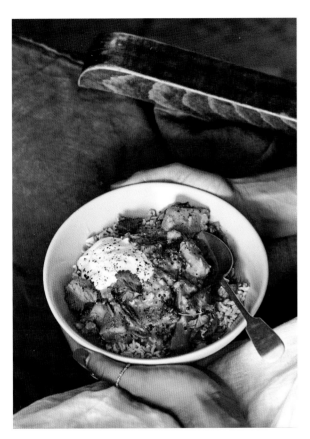
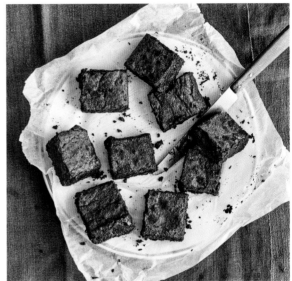
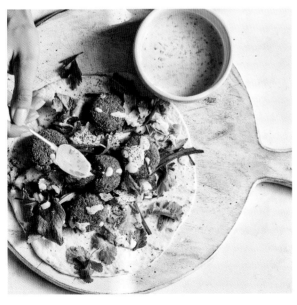
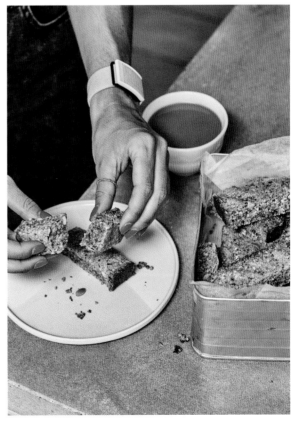

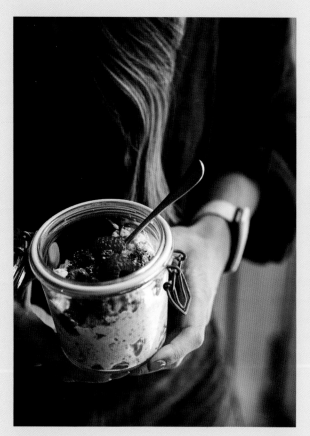

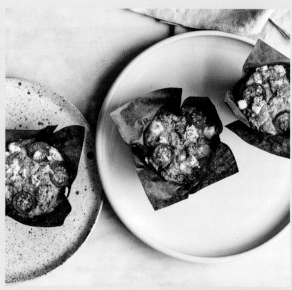

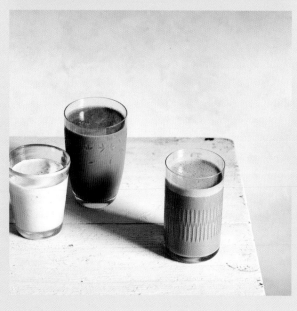

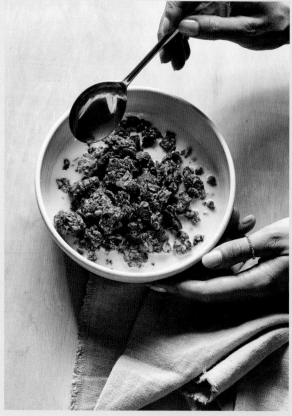

Breakfast

Three smoothies

Breakfast on-the-run

Serves 1

- 1 banana, peeled and chopped, frozen for extra creaminess
- 1 tbsp almond butter (substitute peanut butter)
- 200ml milk (any kind)
- 1 shot (50ml) of strong coffee, cooled
- 1–2 tsp cacao or cocoa powder
- 2 tbsp oats (approx. 20g)
- Ice cubes

This is the ultimate I-don't-have-time-to-make-breakfast meal. It's filling and fuelled with carbohydrates, healthy fats and caffeine to wake you up on your morning commute. It's also a good source of protein, with 16g per serving when using dairy milk or 14g when using soya or pea milk.

Combine the ingredients in a blender and blend until smooth. Pour into a glass to serve.

Tip: For a thicker smoothie, use frozen banana!

Hidden greens green smoothie

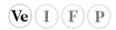

Serves 1

- 2 big handfuls of kale
- ½ avocado
- 1 frozen banana
- 2 tsp flaxseed
- 1 tbsp chocolate protein powder (substitute cacao/cocoa powder)
- 1 tbsp maple syrup

Suggested topping
Chunky granola

I'll let you in on a secret, I'm not a fan of green smoothies or juices – they generally taste like grass (I said grass!) but this smoothie is different. It's still got the greens in there but it's creamy and chocolatey and tastes delicious. Feel free to whizz in whatever greens you've got hanging around your fridge.

Combine the ingredients in a blender and blend until smooth. Pour into a glass to serve.

Ve **P**

PB + jelly smoothie

Serves 1

1 tbsp peanut butter

2 tbsp oats

2 tbsp Greek or soya yogurt

Handful of frozen strawberries (or raspberries)

1 tbsp maple syrup/honey

100ml milk (any kind)

Ice cubes

To top

1 tbsp crushed peanuts

Peanut butter and jelly (or jam, as we call it this side of the pond) is a classic combo. This smoothie packs a punch of protein (20g of protein per serving) with all the flavour of a PB and jelly sandwich.

Combine the ingredients in a blender and blend until smooth. Pour into a glass to serve.

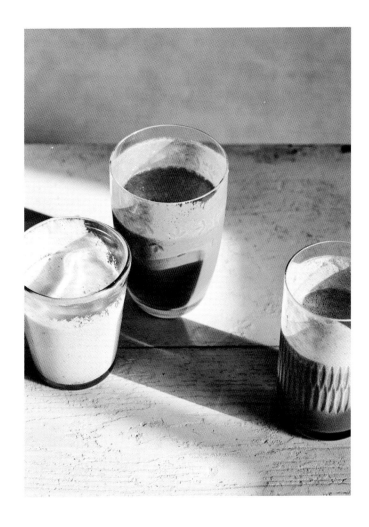

**Makes 4–5
servings**

Chunky granola clusters

The chunkier the granola clusters the better in my book – but feel free to adapt to your liking. Serve with milk, yogurt, or on top of a smoothie bowl. Warning: incredibly moreish – not many people can stop at one serving.

175g rolled
porridge oats

50g wholemeal flour

20g ground/milled
flaxseed

30g almonds, with
skins, roughly
chopped

60g soft brown sugar

1 tsp ground
cinnamon

1 banana, peeled
and mashed

3 tbsp maple syrup

3 tbsp coconut
oil, melted (or
melted butter)

Preheat the oven to 150°C fan/325°F/gas mark 3. Line a baking tray with baking parchment.

Combine all the ingredients in a bowl and mix well.

Spread the mixture in little clusters on the baking tray. Bake for 35–40 minutes (it may need a little longer, based on the size of the clusters and how crunchy you like your granola), stirring halfway, until golden.

After cooling, store in an airtight container.

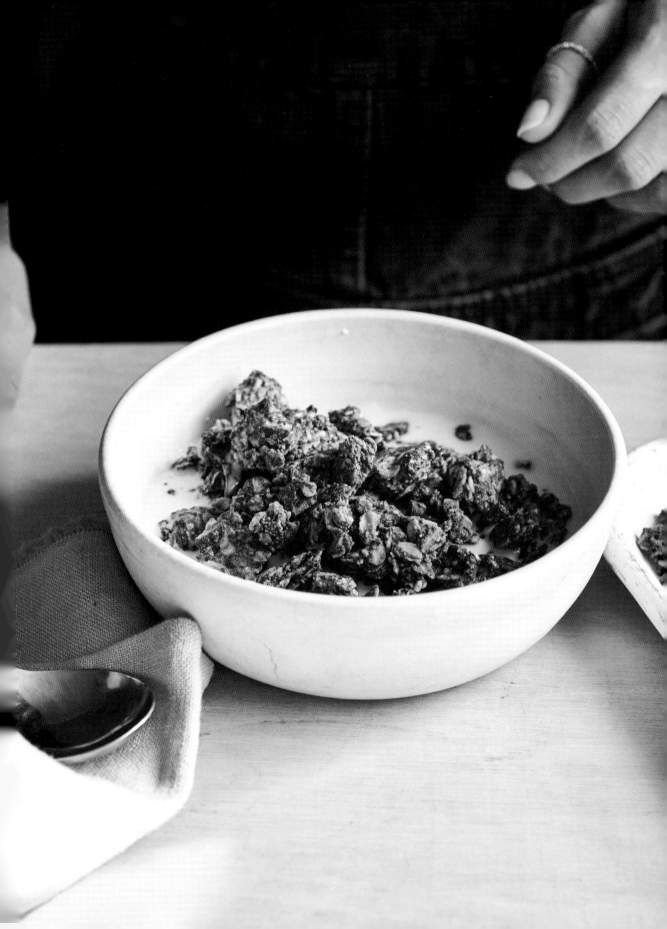

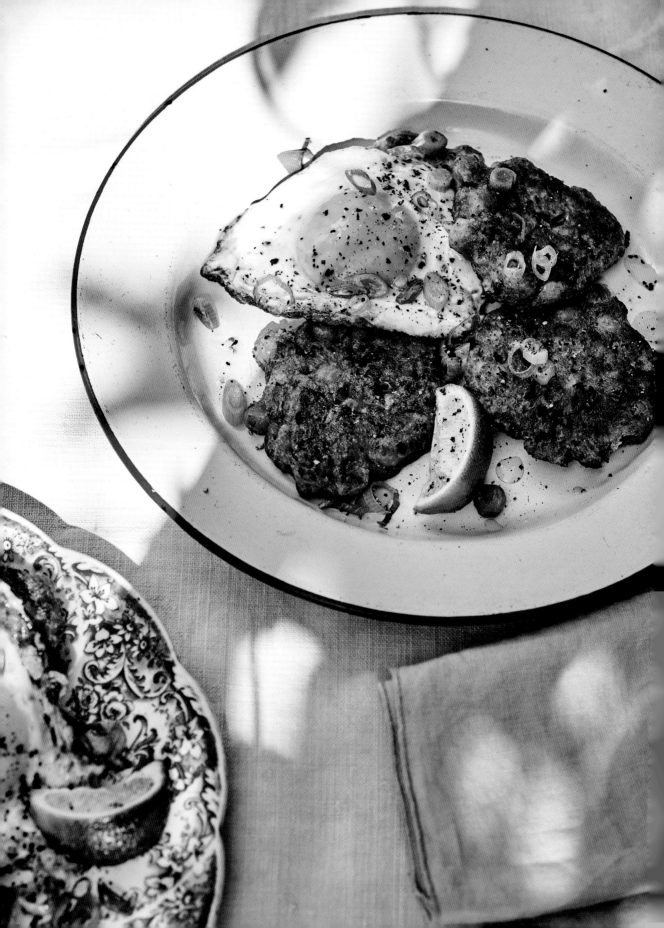

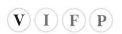

Chickpea fritters with eggs

Serves 4

A classic Saturday-morning brunch recipe. I like mine served with a soft poached egg on top, but for a vegan alternative you could add some smashed avocado and salsa – yum. Leftover fritters (a rare occurrence) also make an awesome lunch the next day.

1 x 400g tin of chickpeas, drained

130g wholemeal flour

1½ tsp cumin seeds

4 spring onions, very finely chopped, plus a few extra to serve

2 garlic cloves, crushed

1cm piece of fresh root ginger, peeled and finely grated

15g fresh coriander or parsley, finely chopped

200ml milk

1 tsp fine sea salt

Olive oil, for frying

4 eggs

1 lime, cut into wedges

Put all the ingredients, apart from the oil, eggs and lime, into a large bowl and mix together.

Cover the base of a large non-stick frying pan with a thin layer of olive oil and set over a medium–high heat. In batches, place heaped tablespoons of the batter into the pan and gently flatten into small rounds, taking care not to overcrowd the pan. Fry for 3–5 minutes on each side, until crisp and deeply golden brown. Remove to a plate lined with kitchen paper.

Poach or fry the eggs to your liking. Serve on top of the chickpea fritters, with a little more sliced spring onion scattered on top and the lime wedges to squeeze over the fritters.

Serves 2

Good-for-your-gut overnight oats

I call this good-for-your-guts oats because of the unique gut-health-promoting ingredients. You may not have heard of, or used, dairy kefir before – it's a fermented milk drink which is like yogurt but thinner in consistency, a little more tart in flavour and has a slight 'fizz' to it. It's quite easy to make at home using kefir grains but it's also easy to find in the yogurt section of most supermarkets. If you can't find it, you can sub with milk. While the research on fermented foods and human health is limited at the moment, kefir contains live microbes which can support gut health and appears to be better tolerated by those who suffer from lactose intolerance. Porridge oats, flaxseed/chia seeds and apple are also sources of fibre which help to feed and fertilise the microbes in our gut. In fact, one portion provides 13g of fibre, which is almost halfway to our 30g/day recommended target.

40g oats

150ml kefir*

2 tbsp natural live yogurt

1 tsp flaxseed or chia seed

1 apple, grated

½ tsp ground cinnamon

Handful of blueberries or raspberries

You can substitute milk, but you may need to reduce the fluid to 100–120ml.

Combine all the ingredients in a bowl and leave overnight (or for at least 4 hours in the fridge). Top with extra berries in the morning if you wish.

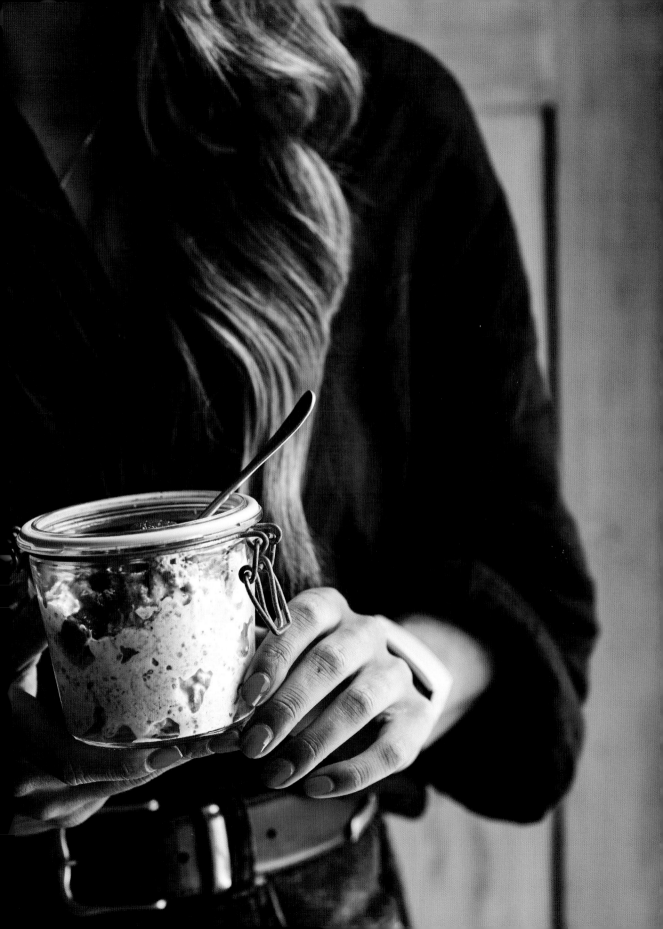

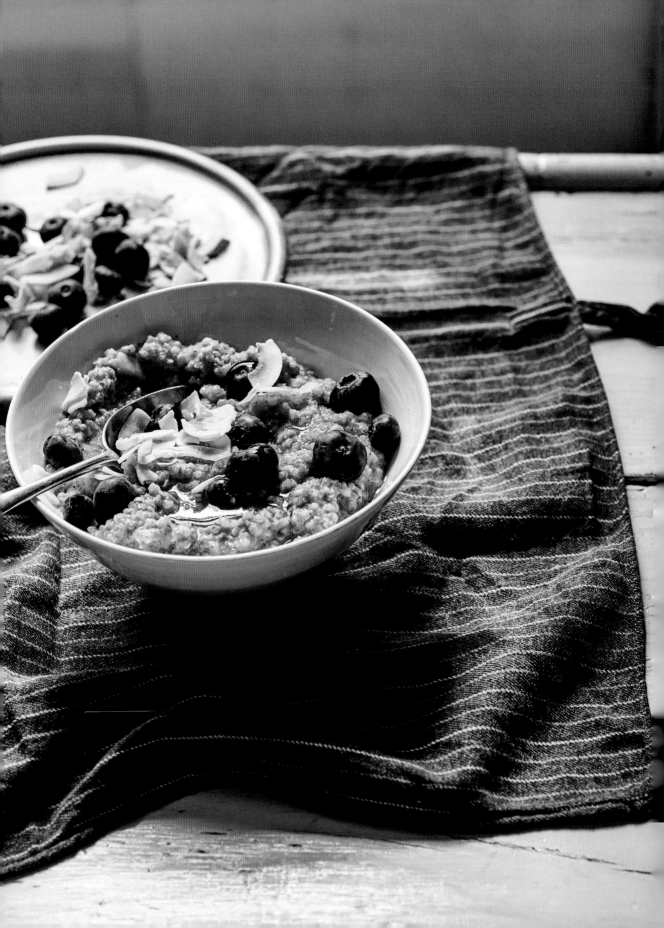

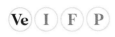

Serves 2-3

Coconut, quinoa + oat porridge

Quinoa, pronounced 'keen-wa', is a pseudo-grain with an impressive nutritional profile as a complete plant protein (meaning it contains all nine essential amino acids) and a good source of fibre. In addition to the protein boost, it adds a nutty taste and texture to this dish, which makes a nice change from a classic bowl of porridge.

185g quinoa (any colour)

40g jumbo oats

1 x 400ml tin of coconut milk (light)

1 tsp ground cinnamon

½ tsp vanilla extract

1 tbsp maple syrup (optional)

Pinch of salt

To top

Toasted coconut flakes, blueberries and flaked almonds

Rinse and drain the quinoa.

Put the quinoa, oats, coconut milk, cinnamon, vanilla extract and maple syrup into a saucepan. Bring to the boil over a medium heat, then cover, reduce the heat and simmer for 15 minutes, until all the liquid has been absorbed and the quinoa is light and fluffy. Season with a pinch of salt.

Fluff with a fork and serve with toasted coconut flakes, blueberries (or whatever fruit you have) and flaked almonds.

Store leftovers in the fridge for 3–4 days.

Sheet pancakes

Makes 1 large pancake, to serve 6

These are pancakes – but not as you've known them before. They're perfect when cooking for a crowd or for mornings when you need a pancake fix but don't necessarily want (or have) all the hands-on time. Divide them up and serve straight away or pack them into lunchboxes for a special breakfast on-the-go.

500ml plant milk

2 tbsp lemon juice

200g wholemeal flour

80g oats (blended into oat flour)

1½ tbsp baking powder

Pinch of salt

2 tbsp maple syrup

2 tsp vanilla extract

To top

fruit of choice (or chocolate chips)

Preheat the oven to 200°C fan/425°F/gas mark 7 and line a flat 24cm × 18cm baking sheet with baking parchment.

Combine the milk and lemon juice and mix. This will curdle to make a form of buttermilk.

In a large bowl, combine the dry ingredients. Add the 'buttermilk', maple syrup and vanilla extract to the dry ingredients and whisk gently until combined. Set aside for 5–10 minutes.

Pour the mixture on to the baking sheet and top with whatever fruit you're using (or chocolate chips). Bake for 25 minutes, until a skewer comes out clean.

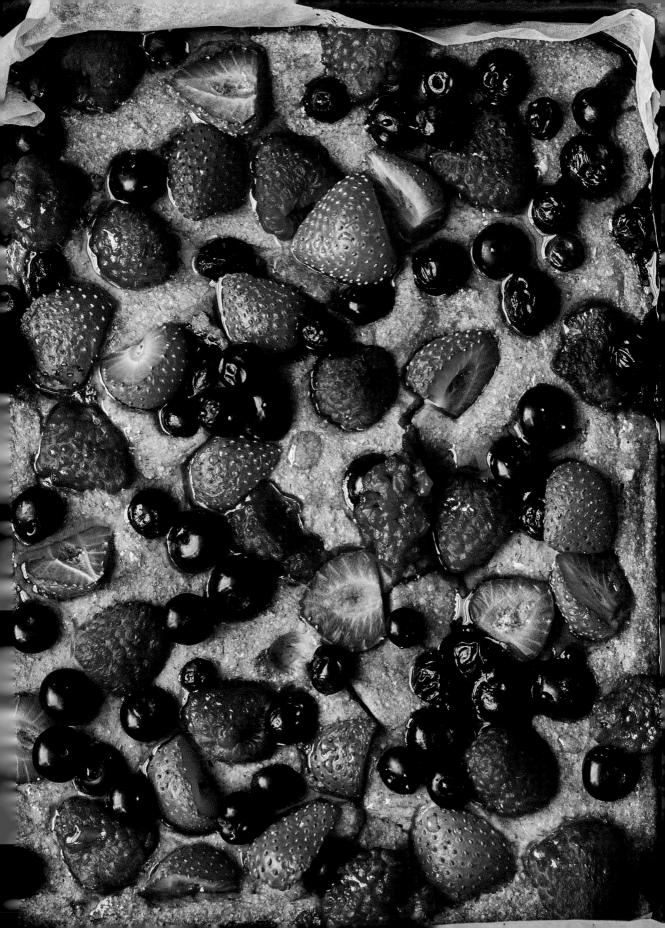

Serves 1

Coffee, chocolate + banana oatmeal

If you're a mocha fan – this one is for you. The deep rich flavour of coffee blended with creamy oats and banana gives you instant fuel and satisfaction until lunchtime. Of course you can skip the coffee or opt for decaf if caffeine is something you're limiting in your diet or if you're cooking for kids.

1 banana, peeled and halved lengthways

40g oats

½ tbsp cacao or cocoa powder

¼ tsp ground cinnamon

40ml strong coffee

150ml milk

1 tsp coconut oil

1 tsp maple syrup

1 square of dark chocolate, chopped or grated

Mash one half of the banana, then chop the other half and set aside.

Put the oats, cacao/cocoa, cinnamon, coffee, mashed banana and milk into a small saucepan and cook for 4–5 minutes, until thick and creamy. Add more milk if needed.

Melt the coconut oil and maple syrup in a frying pan over a medium heat and fry the other half of the banana for 2–3 minutes on either side until golden.

Transfer the porridge to a bowl and top with the caramelised banana and dark chocolate.

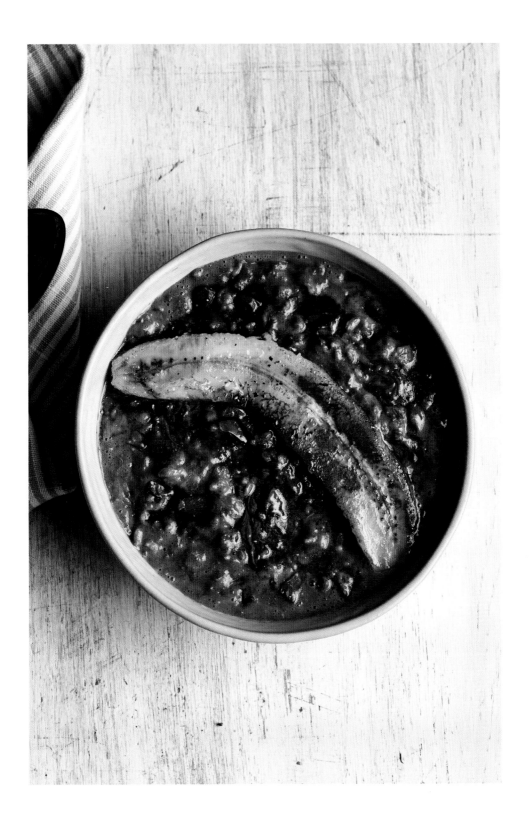

Breakfast quesadilla 3 ways

Quesadillas are really having a moment thanks to TikTok, and I am here for it. With the right filling, they can be a quick, balanced meal at any time of the day. They're super versatile too, so they can be sweet or savoury, and are suitable for most dietary types and preferences.

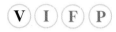

Scrambled egg, avo + rocket quesadilla

Serves 1

2 eggs
I tbsp chopped fresh chives
Salt and black pepper
Olive oil
½ avocado, sliced
Handful of rocket
I large wholewheat tortilla wrap
sriracha sauce (optional)

Beat the eggs in a bowl with a fork. Add the chives and a pinch of salt and pepper. Heat a splash of olive oil in a non-stick pan over a medium heat and pour in the egg mixture. Cook for 2–3 minutes, stirring, until just about set. Remove from the heat.

Place the eggs, sliced avocado and rocket on one half of the wrap (add some sriracha, if you like) and fold over.

Place the folded wrap in a frying pan over a medium heat. Toast for 2–3 minutes, until golden on both sides. Cut in half before serving.

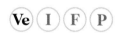

Almond butter, raspberry + granola quesadilla

Serves 1

I large wholewheat tortilla wrap
I tbsp almond butter
Handful of raspberries
Handful of granola

To serve

Greek yogurt or coconut yogurt alternative

On one half of the tortilla spread the almond butter. Top with the raspberries (squashing them down with the back of a fork), and sprinkle the granola on top. Fold over the other half of the tortilla.

Place the folded wrap in a frying pan over a medium heat. Toast for 2–3 minutes, until golden on both sides. Cut in half, and serve with a dollop of Greek yogurt.

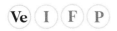

Black bean + corn quesadilla

Serves 1

2 tbsp black beans, drained and rinsed

1 tbsp sweetcorn

1 tomato, diced

¼ avocado, chopped

¼ red onion

Juice of ½ lime

Pinch of chilli flakes

1 tbsp chopped fresh coriander (optional)

Salt and black pepper

Handful of cheese (or vegan alternative)

1 large wholewheat tortilla wrap

Combine all the ingredients in a bowl except for the cheese and the tortilla. Season with salt and pepper.

Place the bean mixture on one half of the wrap. Sprinkle the cheese on top. Fold over the other half of the tortilla.

Place the folded wrap in a frying pan over a medium heat, and toast or 2–3 minutes, until golden on both sides. Cut in half before serving.

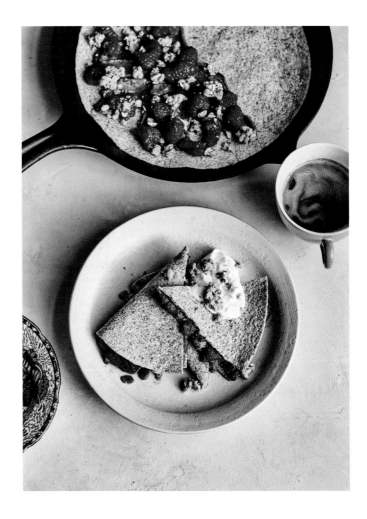

Makes 12

Sweet potato, feta, tomato + spinach breakfast muffins

These muffins can be made in advance, for fuss-free breakfasts for the next few days. The sweet potato keeps them really moist and adds a lovely sweet flavour that works great with the salty feta.

70ml extra virgin olive oil

250ml whole milk

2 tbsp freshly squeezed lemon juice

¾ tsp fine salt

250g wholemeal flour

2½ tsp baking powder

200g feta, crumbled

170g sweet potato, peeled and coarsely grated

Large handful of spinach leaves, roughly chopped

Salt and black pepper

2 eggs, beaten

18 cherry tomatoes, halved

Preheat the oven to 190°C fan/400°F/gas mark 6 and line two 6-hole muffin tins with 12 paper cases.

Put the olive oil, milk and lemon juice into a bowl, whisk to combine and set aside.

Put the salt, flour, baking powder, most of the feta, the grated sweet potato, spinach and a large pinch of black pepper into a mixing bowl and combine.

Pour in the beaten eggs and the milk mixture and quickly fold everything together, taking care not to overbeat. Divide evenly between the 12 muffin cases and top with the remaining feta and the halved cherry tomatoes.

Bake for 24–26 minutes, until golden and a skewer inserted into the centre comes out clean. Remove to a wire rack to cool.

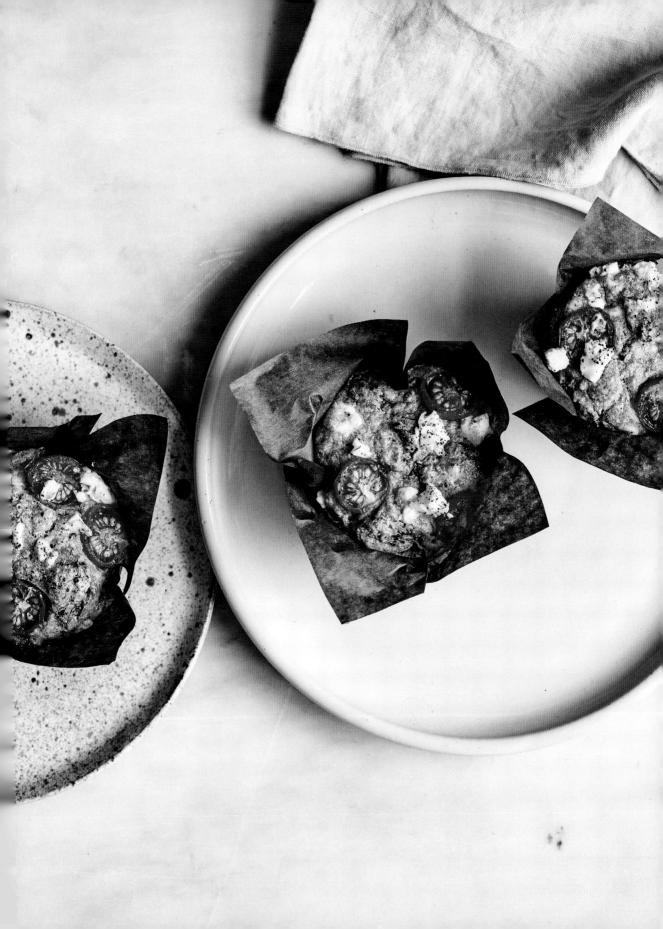

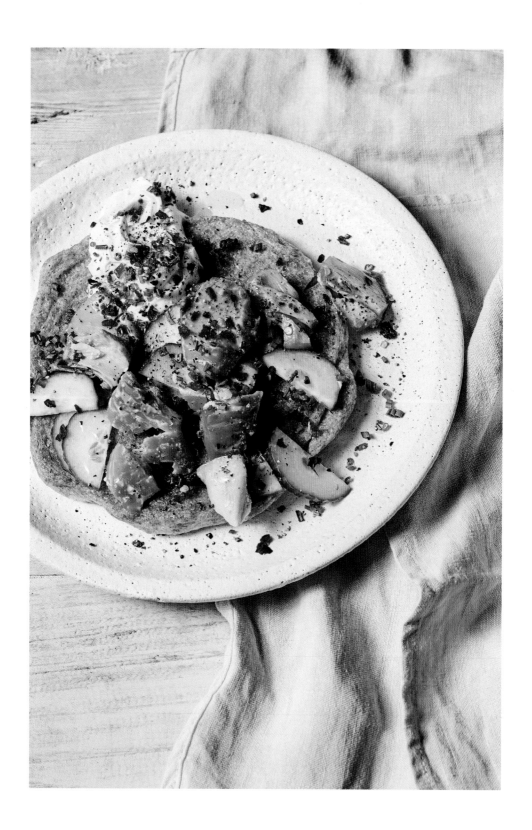

Serves 2

Savoury pancakes with hot smoked salmon, crème fraîche, cucumber + chives

Breaking the pancake rules again, but this time making them savoury, not sweet – trust me on this one. Paired with hot smoked salmon, crème fraîche and cucumber, this is such a delicious breakfast option. However, you can play around with the toppings: poached egg, eggs Benedict, smashed avo, creamy mushrooms – the list is endless.

These pancakes can also be made sweet by adding 1 tablespoon of sugar and 1 teaspoon of vanilla extract to the batter, and serving with maple syrup and fruit or whatever sweet toppings you want.

80g wholemeal flour

2 tsp baking powder

Salt and black pepper

130ml milk

2½ tsp apple cider vinegar or white wine vinegar

¼ cucumber, halved lengthways and sliced thinly into half-moons

¼ tsp dried chilli flakes

Extra virgin olive oil, for frying, plus extra to serve

160g hot-smoked salmon, at room temperature

Crème fraîche, to serve

10g fresh chives, roughly chopped

In a bowl combine the flour, baking powder and a large pinch of salt. Stir in the milk and vinegar until smooth. Set aside.

Put the sliced cucumber into a bowl with the dried chilli flakes and a large pinch of salt. Combine and set aside.

Heat 1 tablespoon of olive oil in a large non-stick frying pan and set over a medium heat. Once hot, pour in half the batter. The pancake should be large, about 14–16cm across. Fry the pancakes one at a time, adding more oil as needed, for 3–4 minutes on one side, until bubbles appear on the surface, then flip over and fry for another 2–3 minutes until both sides are golden.

Remove and keep covered and warm while you fry the remaining pancake. Use a second frying pan if you want them both ready to serve at the same time.

To serve, plate up the pancakes and drizzle generously with extra virgin olive oil. Top with the cucumber, hot-smoked salmon, and a dollop of crème fraîche, and scatter over the chives. Season with a little salt and pepper and serve immediately.

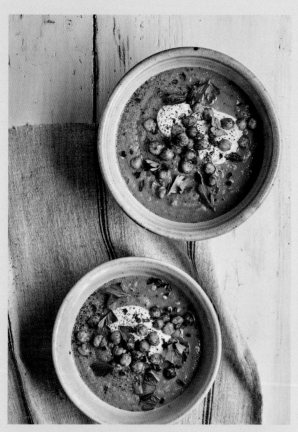

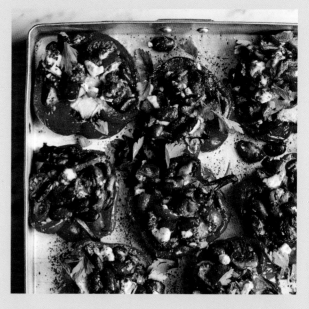

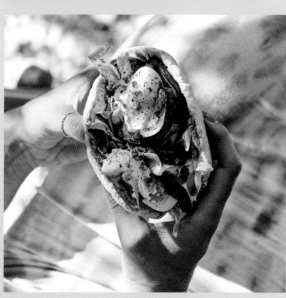

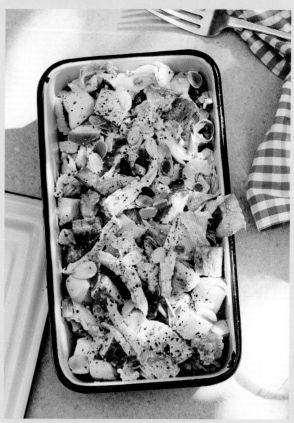

Lunch

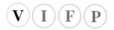

Serves 2

Aubergine, soft-boiled egg + hummus pitta pockets

This recipe is inspired by a brunch spot in London. Honestly, I dream about this meal an unhealthy amount, so it just had to go into the book. I get that aubergine is a bit like Marmite – either you hate it or love it – but when it's cooked well it can be the most delicious thing. Bundle it up into a pitta with creamy hummus and a soft-boiled egg and you have got yourself a nutritious, incredible lunch that will keep you coming back for more.

2 eggs

2 tbsp olive oil

1 large aubergine, cut into 1cm thick discs

Salt and black pepper

2 pitta breads

4 tbsp hummus (see page 219 for my Hummus 5 ways)

Large handful of mixed salad leaves

For the herb oil

25g fresh coriander

15g fresh flat-leaf parsley

1 green chilli, seeds removed

1 garlic clove, peeled

½ tsp ground cumin

¼ tsp ground cardamom (optional)

3 tbsp extra virgin olive oil

For the herb oil, put the coriander, parsley, chilli, garlic, cumin, cardamom (if using) and ¼ teaspoon of salt into a food processor and blitz for a minute or two until everything is very finely chopped, but not quite a paste. Transfer to a bowl and stir in the olive oil. Set aside.

Bring a saucepan of water to a rolling boil. Gently lower in the eggs and cook for 7 minutes. Remove to a bowl of iced water. Once cool, peel the eggs and set aside.

Dip a pastry brush into the olive oil and brush it over both sides of the aubergine slices. Set a large non-stick pan over a medium–high heat. Add the aubergine slices and fry for 3–5 minutes on each side, until golden and softened. Remove to a plate and season with salt and pepper.

To serve, toast the pitta breads, spread the hummus on one side, and fill with the salad leaves and aubergine slices. Cut the boiled eggs into quarters and add to the pitta bread. Drizzle over a teaspoon or two of the herb oil, and serve immediately.

Keep any remaining herb oil in a sealed jar in the fridge, and use within 2 days.

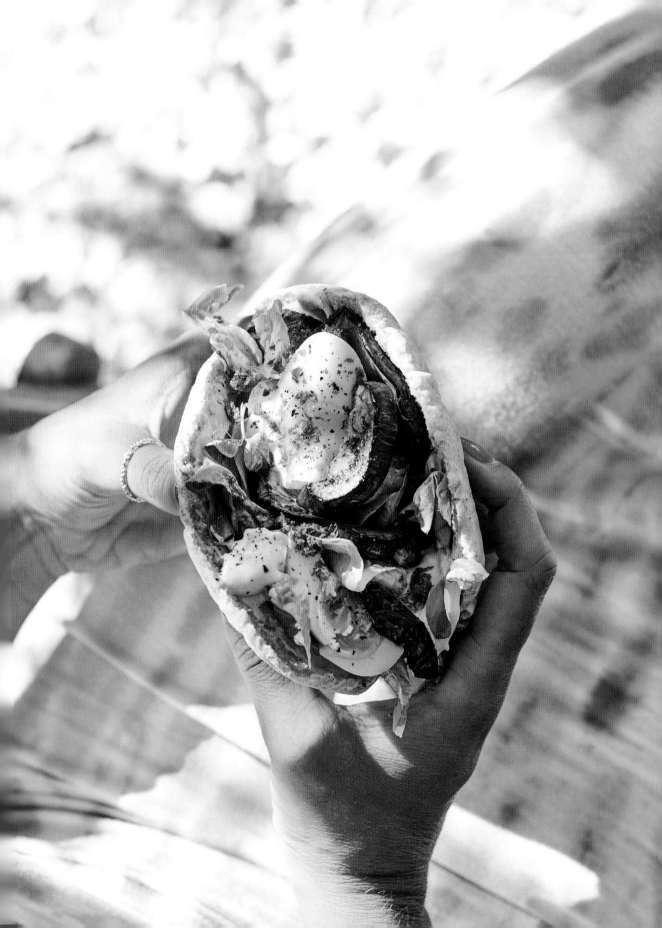

Serves 12

Squash, spinach, pesto + goat's cheese frittata

Perfect at really any time of the year, but this recipe screams autumn to me. I love it as it is, but you could add chorizo if you like for a smoky flavour.

300g butternut
squash, peeled,
deseeded, and cut
into 2cm pieces

2 tbsp extra virgin
olive oil

200g spinach

1 red onion, peeled
and thinly sliced

150g baby plum
tomatoes

Salt and black pepper

12 eggs

80g soft goat's cheese

3 tbsp pesto, bought
or homemade

Preheat the oven to 200°C fan/425°F/gas mark 7.

Put the squash into a large roasting tray, toss with 1½ tablespoons of the olive oil and season well. Roast for 20–25 minutes, until golden and almost tender.

Ten minutes before the squash is ready, stir in the spinach, onion and tomatoes with the remaining ½ tablespoon of olive oil and a pinch of salt and pepper. Roast for another 10 minutes, then remove and set aside.

Meanwhile, crack the eggs into a bowl, whisk and season well. Put about half the spinach, squash, tomatoes and onion into an ovenproof frying pan or a quiche dish measuring about 24–26cm. Pour over the beaten eggs and finish with the remaining half of the vegetables and the goat's cheese scattered on top so you can see their colour.

Cook in the oven for 35–40 minutes, until the frittata has souffléd up and the top is just firm to the touch. If it is still uncooked in the centre, cover with foil to prevent burning and cook until just firm.

Let the frittata cool a little, drizzle over the pesto and serve immediately.

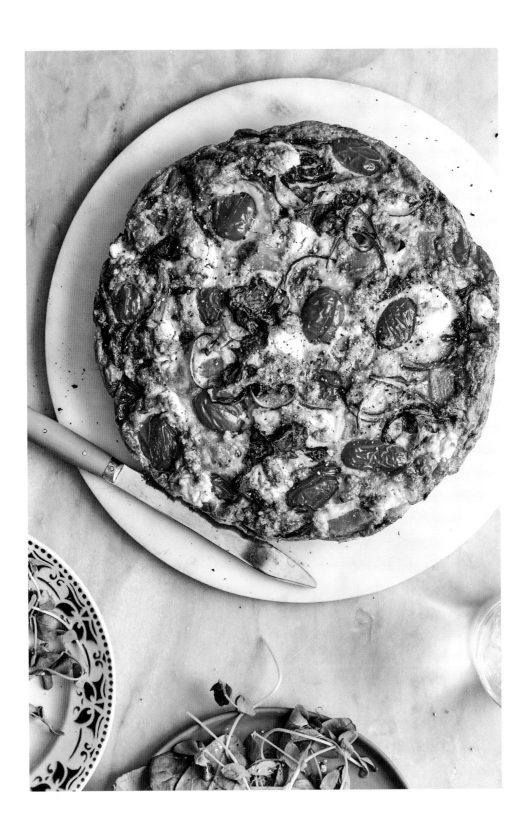

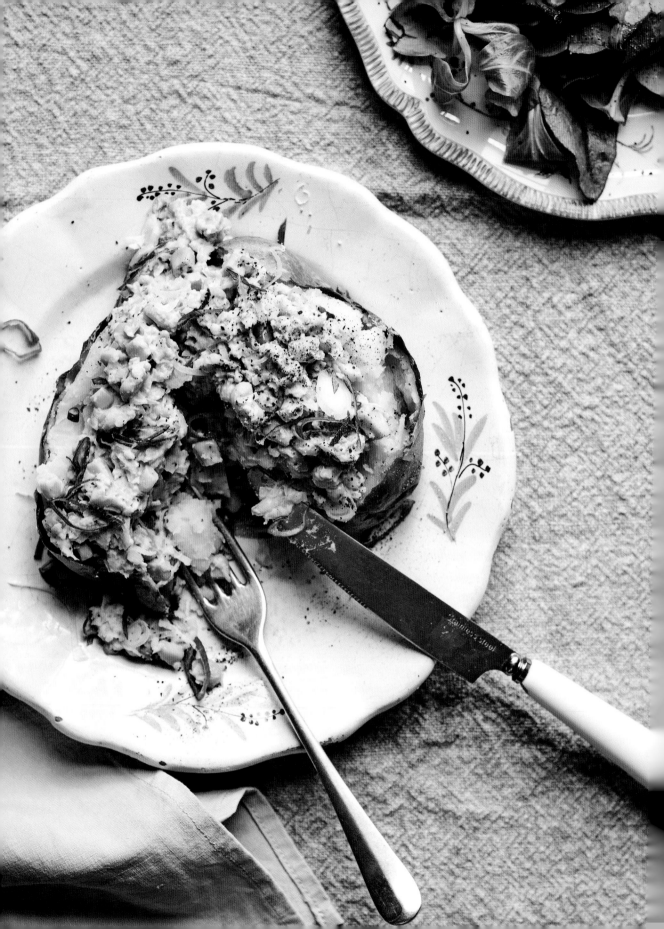

Chickpea 'chuna' baked potatoes

Enough for 3–4 baked potatoes, depending on size

Tuna baked potatoes are a classic lunchtime meal – and I take no issue with it, but I am severely allergic to tuna and so they are off the menu for me. This vegan option is such a good alternative. While shooting this recipe for the book, the team were so confused because the taste and texture are remarkably close to tuna – don't believe me? Well, you'll have to try it. The mixture is also incredible in sandwiches with some salad.

1 x 400g tin of chickpeas, drained and rinsed

2–3 tbsp vegan mayonnaise or hummus

4 spring onions, finely chopped

1 small tin of sweetcorn

Juice of ½ lemon

1 sheet of nori seaweed, crushed (optional)

Salt and black pepper

Put the chickpeas into a mixing bowl and mash them with the back of a fork. Add the rest of the ingredients, and mix to combine. Alternatively, you can use a food processor – starting with the chickpeas, pulse a few times, then add the remaining ingredients, pulsing again a few times until the desired consistency is reached (a little bit of chunk is good).

Serve inside a baked potato with a side salad.

Tip: add 1 tbsp chia seeds for an omega-3 boost.

Serves 6

2 tbsp olive oil

1 onion, finely chopped

2 garlic cloves,
    finely chopped

750g carrots, peeled
    and roughly chopped

1 tsp ground cumin

½ tsp ground coriander

½ tsp ground cinnamon

½ tsp ground ginger

½ tsp salt

1.2 litres vegetable
    stock

1 x 400g tin of
    chickpeas, drained
    and rinsed

To serve

yogurt (optional),
    chopped fresh parsley
    or coriander, chilli
    flakes (optional)

For the spicy
    chickpeas

1 x 400g tin of
    chickpeas, drained,
    rinsed and dried

1 tsp extra virgin
    olive oil

½ tsp ground cumin

½ tsp ground cinnamon

Pinch of salt

Creamy carrot + chickpea soup

This recipe is the definition of comfort in a bowl. The addition of the chickpeas helps to thicken the soup, while also providing a source of protein (which is often missing from veggie soups!), plus the chickpea croutons on top also add a little bit of crunch and texture.

Heat the oil in a large saucepan over a medium heat. Add the onion and cook, stirring occasionally, for 3–4 minutes. Add the garlic, carrots, spices and salt and cook for 5 minutes.

Stir in the stock and the chickpeas. Cover and bring to the boil. Reduce the heat and simmer, stirring occasionally, for 40–50 minutes until the carrots are tender.

Using a hand blender, blend the soup until smooth.

Serve topped with a dollop of yogurt, the herbs and/or chilli flakes (if using), and some spicy chickpeas.

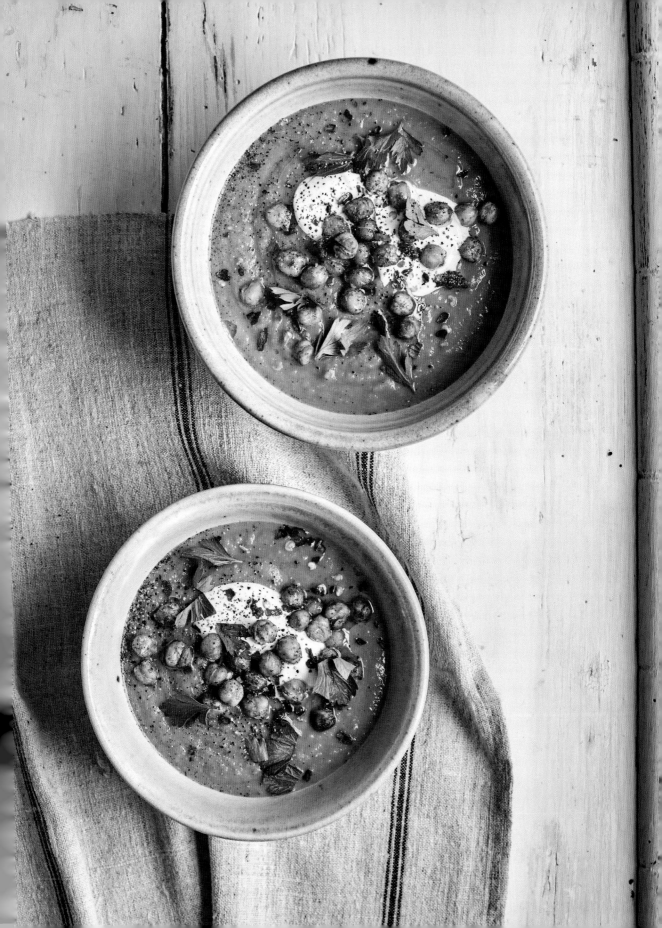

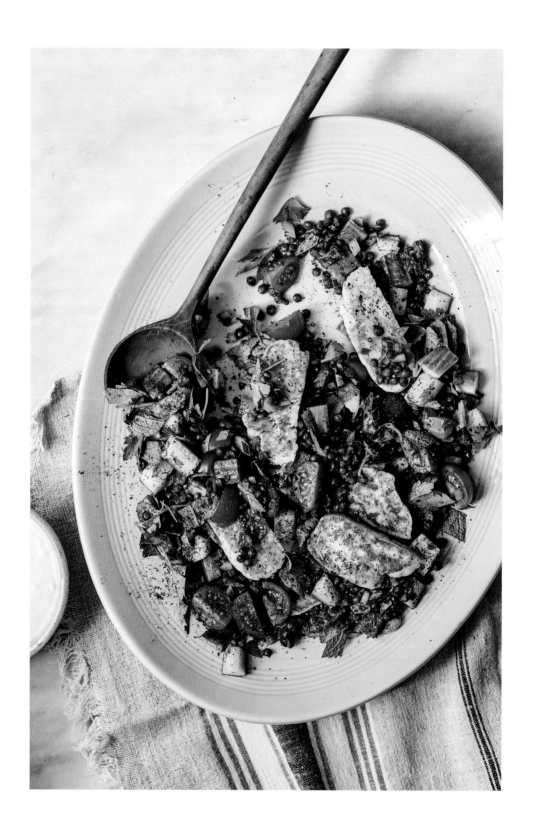

Serves 12

6–8 slices of halloumi

For the tabbouleh

250g tinned or
  packet lentils

Juice of ½ lemon
  (use other half
  for the dressing)

½ cucumber, seeds
  removed and diced

Handful of cherry
  tomatoes,
  quartered

Handful of fresh
  mint, chopped

Handful of fresh
  flat-leaf parsley,
  chopped

½ red onion, finely
  chopped

1 tbsp sumac

For the tahini
  dressing

100g natural yogurt

1 tbsp runny tahini

1 tbsp extra virgin
  olive oil

Juice of ½ lemon

¼ tsp garlic granules

Salt and black pepper

Lentil tabbouleh with grilled halloumi + tahini dressing

This version of a tabbouleh offers a twist, using lentils as the base instead of the traditional bulgur. Lentils are one of my storecupboard must-haves because of their versatility and great nutritional profile, providing protein, fibre and a number of vitamins and minerals including iron and folate. I've paired this salad with halloumi, but it would also work well with feta, roast chicken, or fish.

To make the tabbouleh, combine the ingredients in a bowl. In a separate small bowl, combine the ingredients for the dressing.

Fry the halloumi in a dry non-stick frying pan until golden on both sides.

Toss the tabbouleh with the dressing, add the halloumi then divide between two plates and serve with extra lemon wedges if you like.

Serves 4

2 Romaine lettuce
  hearts, leaves
  washed

2 avocados, diced

2 apples, diced

2 celery stalks,
  trimmed and sliced

4 spring onions,
  finely chopped

2 tbsp flaked almonds
  (or pecans/walnuts)

1 rotisserie
  chicken, or 4
  cooked chicken
  breasts, shredded
  (using a fork)

For the croutons

2 slices of sourdough
  bread, torn

Olive oil

Pinch of salt

For the dressing

120ml kefir (or
  live yogurt)

2 tbsp mayo (or
  vegan alternative)

1 tsp apple cider
  vinegar or
  lemon juice

1 garlic clove,
  crushed or grated

1 tbsp fresh chives,
  chopped

Pinch of salt and
  black pepper

Torn chicken salad with creamy kefir dressing

This recipe was a bit of an accident – or maybe experiment is a better word. After cooking for friends I had some leftover roast chicken and fancied making a Caesar salad of sorts, but I didn't have all the ingredients. So I played around making my own creamy dressing with kefir from the fridge, and it worked an absolute treat. You can make the dressing in a batch and use it for salads across the week or as a dip for crudités. This salad may feel a little experimental for some people, but trust me – your gut will thank you.

Preheat the oven to 200°C fan/425°F/gas mark 7. Put the torn bread on a baking tray, drizzle with olive oil and add the pinch of salt. Cook in the oven for 10 minutes, until lightly browned, then remove and leave to cool.

Meanwhile assemble the salad. Tear or shred the romaine lettuce and put it into a bowl with the avocados, apples, celery, spring onions, almonds, chicken and the croutons.

To make the dressing, combine all the ingredients in a small bowl and whisk until smooth. Drizzle over the salad and mix through.

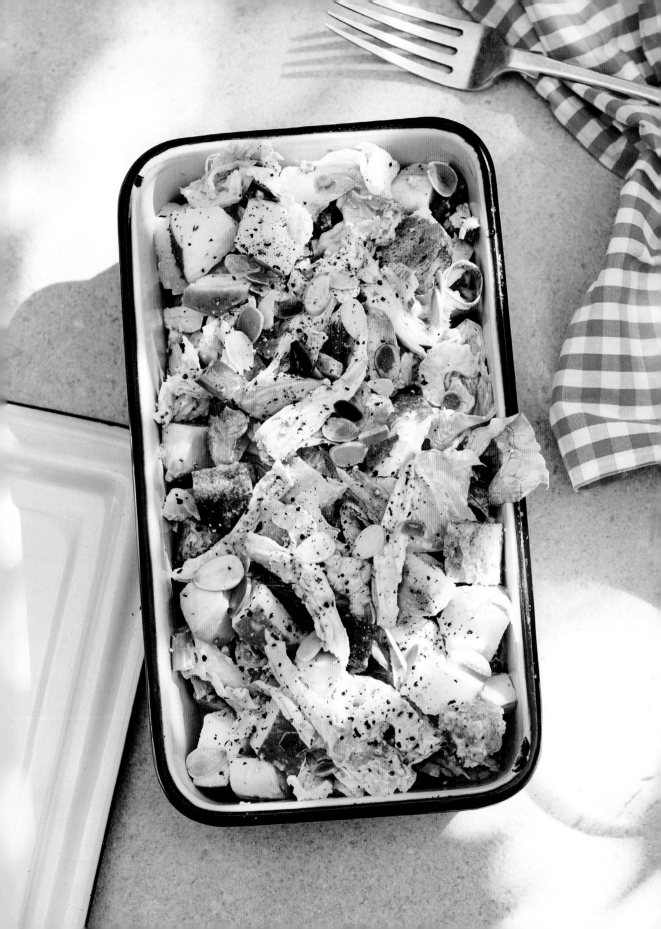

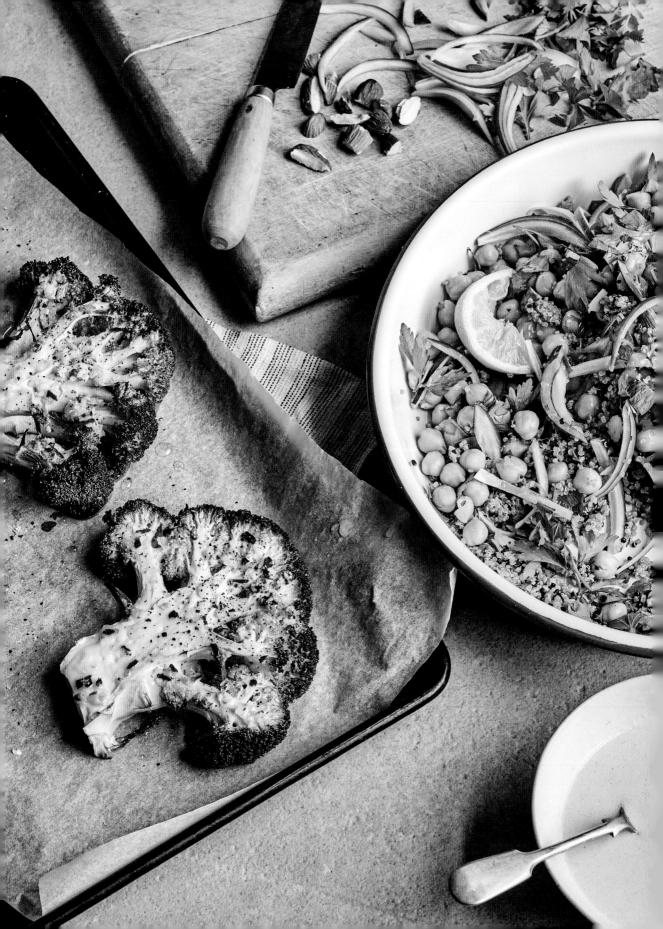

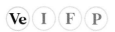

Serves 2

Charred broccoli, chickpea + quinoa salad bowl

One of my favourite ways of cooking broccoli is roasting it – it's seriously good and totally trumps the boiled alternative. This salad is totally plant-based but you won't miss the meat, I promise. For those worried about protein, the chickpeas and quinoa are both great sources.

250g cooked quinoa (or cook from scratch 1 cup quinoa to 2 cups water)

1 x 400g tin of chickpeas, drained and rinsed

40g almonds, roughly chopped

Handful of fresh flat-leaf parsley, chopped

½ red onion, very thinly sliced

For the broccoli steaks

1 large head of broccoli, sliced into thick 'steaks'

1 tbsp olive oil

1 garlic clove, crushed

Pinch of chilli flakes

For the dressing

Juice of 1 lemon

1 garlic clove, crushed or grated

2 tbsp tahini

2 tbsp water

Salt and black pepper

Preheat the oven to 180°C fan/400°F/gas mark 6 and line a baking tray with baking parchment. Place the broccoli on the tray in a single layer. Combine the oil, garlic and chilli flakes in a small bowl, then brush or drizzle over the broccoli. Roast for 25 minutes, until tender and a little charred.

To make the dressing, combine the lemon juice, garlic, tahini and water in a bowl and mix well to form a smooth dressing. Season with salt and pepper.

Combine the quinoa, chickpeas, chopped almonds, parsley and red onion in a bowl. Drizzle the dressing over the salad and toss. Divide between two bowls and serve the broccoli steaks on top.

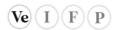

Serves 4

1 tbsp olive oil

1 onion, peeled and diced

2 garlic cloves, crushed or grated

1 tbsp tomato purée

2 tsp cumin

1 tsp smoked paprika

½ tsp cayenne pepper

1 x 400g tin of black beans, drained and rinsed

1 x 400g tin of red kidney beans, drained and rinsed

600ml veg stock

1 x 400g tin of chopped tomatoes

1 bell pepper, chopped

1 small tin of sweetcorn, drained

Salt and black pepper

For the quick guac

1 small avocado

1 lime

Pinch of salt

Pinch of chilli flakes

For the tortilla chips

Large tortilla wraps (approx. 1 per person)

1–2 tbsp olive oil

Salt

Spicy mixed bean soup with quick guacamole + chips

This warming soup is super satisfying and is packed full of good stuff from the mixed beans and colourful veggies. The guac loaded on top makes it a little more special, especially when paired with homemade tortilla chips – such a fun lunch for the whole family.

To make the tortilla chips, preheat the oven to 200°C fan/425°F/gas mark 7. Brush both sides of the tortillas with the oil, then cut into triangles. Arrange in a single layer on a baking tray (or two) and bake for 6–8 minutes (flipping once). Remove, sprinkle with salt and set aside.

Heat the oil in a large pot over a medium–high heat, then add the onion and cook, stirring often, for 3 minutes, or until translucent. Add the garlic and cook for a further 1–2 minutes. Stir in the tomato purée and the spices.

Next, add the black beans, kidney beans, stock, chopped tomatoes, pepper and sweetcorn. Bring to the boil, then reduce the heat and simmer for 15–20 minutes, stirring occasionally. Taste and season with salt and pepper.

Meanwhile make the quick guac by smashing the avocado in a bowl with a fork, together with the lime juice, salt and chilli flakes.

Serve in bowls, topped with the guac, with a handful of tortilla chips on the side.

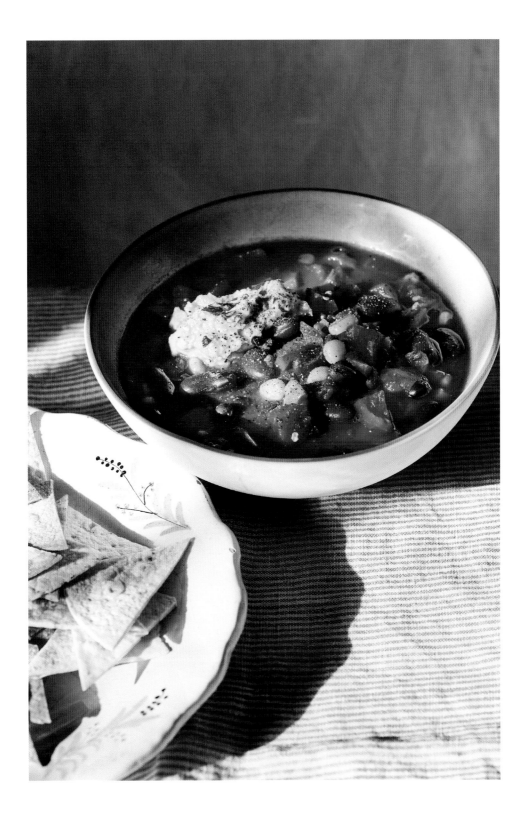

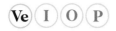

Crispy tofu fried rice

Serves 4

This is a super easy, extremely moreish tofu rice dish. One batch serves 4, so it's great for a family dinner or you can portion it out for the week. If tofu ain't your thing, chicken, salmon or tuna are all great protein swaps for this dish.

3 tbsp vegetable oil

350g firm tofu, drained and cut into 2cm cubes

4 garlic cloves, crushed

Salt and black pepper

2 eggs, beaten (optional)

2 tbsp soy sauce

½ tsp roasted sesame oil

1½ tbsp lime juice

1 red chilli, deseeded and thinly sliced

800g cooked jasmine rice

1 red onion, very thinly sliced

Small handful of fresh Thai or regular basil leaves, to serve

Put 1 tablespoon of the vegetable oil into a large wok or pan and set over a high heat. Once very hot, add the tofu and stir-fry for 4 minutes, then add the garlic and stir-fry for another 30 seconds, taking great care not to burn the garlic. Season with salt and pepper and remove to a bowl.

Add the remaining 2 tablespoons of oil to the pan. Once hot, add the beaten egg (if using) and scramble for 30 seconds until just cooked. Add the soy sauce, sesame oil, lime juice and most of the chilli, and stir-fry for another 30 seconds.

Add the cooked rice and toss together, then spread the rice out over the base of the pan. Fry for 30 seconds then toss together. Repeat this process a few more times, until the rice begins to crisp up. If you are not using eggs, simply fry the rice in the hot oil with all the same seasoning ingredients, as above.

Add most of the red onion slices and toss together. Taste and adjust the seasoning with salt and pepper if necessary. Don't use more soy sauce, as this will make the rice soggy. Stir in the cooked tofu.

Serve with the remaining chilli and red onion scattered over, and finish with the basil leaves.

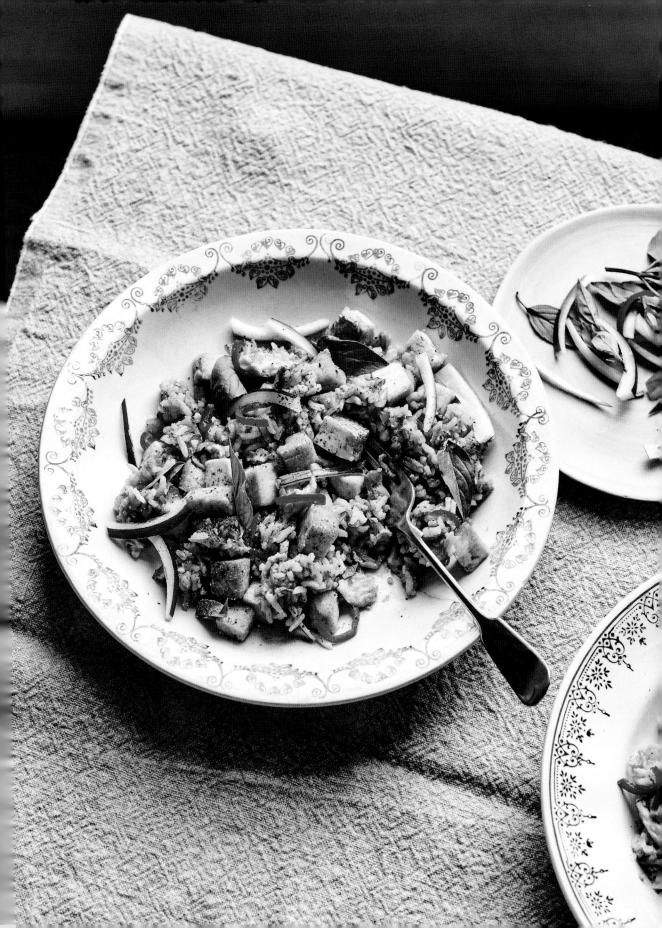

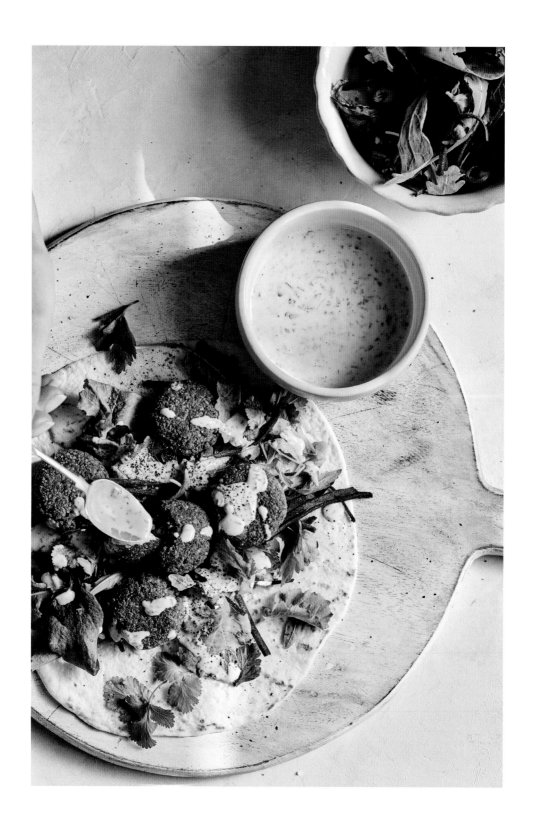

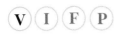

Makes 16–18 falafel, serving 4

225g dried chickpeas, soaked overnight

1 cooked beetroot, drained

2 garlic cloves

½ small red onion, peeled and roughly chopped

15g fresh coriander, leaves only

20g fresh parsley, leaves only

Large pinch of ground cardamom (optional)

½ tsp ground cumin

½ tsp smoked paprika

¼ tsp baking powder

4 tbsp plain white flour

Salt and black pepper

4 tbsp tahini

1 tbsp fresh lemon juice

Sunflower or other vegetable oil, for frying

For the tortilla chips

Wraps or pitta breads,

Rocket or other salad leaves

Beetroot falafel wrap with green tahini dressing

Always in the mood for falafel. I've featured it in all my books. This version has beetroot in there, and when fried they're super crispy on the outside but soft on the inside. You can bake them, however, if you would rather not fry them in oil, and they will still taste great. The green tahini dressing is non-negotiable, though, as it brings the recipe to another level altogether. So I must insist that you don't skip that step.

Drain the chickpeas and put them into a food processor with the beetroot, garlic, onion, coriander, half the parsley, all the spices, the baking powder, flour and half a teaspoon of salt. Blitz until everything is finely ground. Using your hands, firmly press the mixture into slightly flattened small golf-ball shapes, about 1 heaped tablespoon each. Place on a tray, cover and refrigerate.

Finely chop the rest of the parsley and combine with the tahini, lemon juice, 70ml of water and salt and pepper to taste. Add a little more water if it is too thick.

Pour 1cm of vegetable oil into a frying pan and set over a medium–high heat. Once hot, add the falafel in batches. Don't overcrowd the pan, as it will bring the temperature down. Fry for 3–4 minutes on each side, until golden brown, then drain on kitchen paper. Keep warm while you cook the remaining falafel.

Serve the falafel wrapped in wraps or pitta breads, with some salad leaves and the green tahini drizzled over.

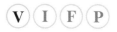

Mushroom, tomato, kidney bean + feta stuffed peppers

This recipe is pretty impressive but it's actually incredibly easy and super versatile. While this combo works a treat, feel free to make this dish your own; the kidney beans can be swapped out for another bean or chickpeas, or perhaps you could swap the feta out for some halloumi cubes or vegan cheese.

4 red peppers, halved and deseeded

3 tbsp extra virgin olive oil

Salt and black pepper

300g mushrooms (e. g. button, shiitake, portobello), thinly sliced

1 onion, finely chopped

3 garlic cloves, crushed

1 x 400g tin of kidney beans, drained and rinsed

150g cherry tomatoes, roughly chopped

100g feta cheese, crumbled

20g fresh flat-leaf parsley, leaves only, finely chopped

Preheat the oven to 200°C fan/425°F/gas mark 7. Line a baking tray with baking parchment.

Put the peppers on the lined baking tray and coat with 1 tablespoon of the olive oil. Season well with salt and pepper and place in the oven for 15–20 minutes, or until beginning to soften, but still holding their shape.

Meanwhile, put the remaining oil into a pan and set over a medium–high heat. Add the mushrooms and onion and fry for 10 minutes, until the onion is translucent and the mushrooms are golden. Add the garlic and fry for another 2 minutes, until aromatic. Add the kidney beans, tomatoes, feta and most of the parsley. Combine and season to taste with salt and pepper.

Remove the peppers from the oven and divide the mixture between them. Return them to the oven for 12–15 minutes, until golden. Scatter over the remaining parsley and serve immediately.

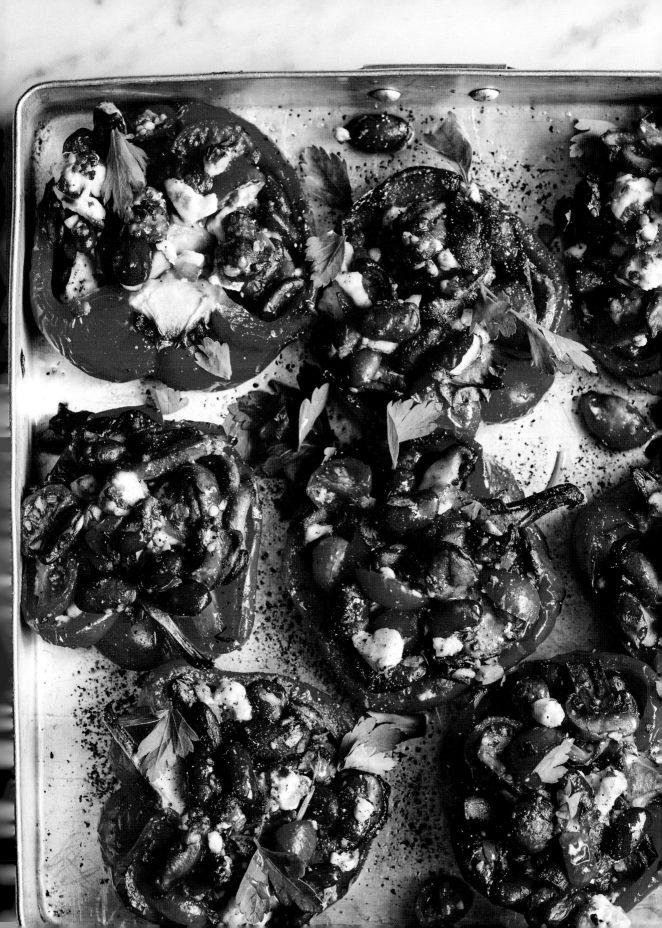

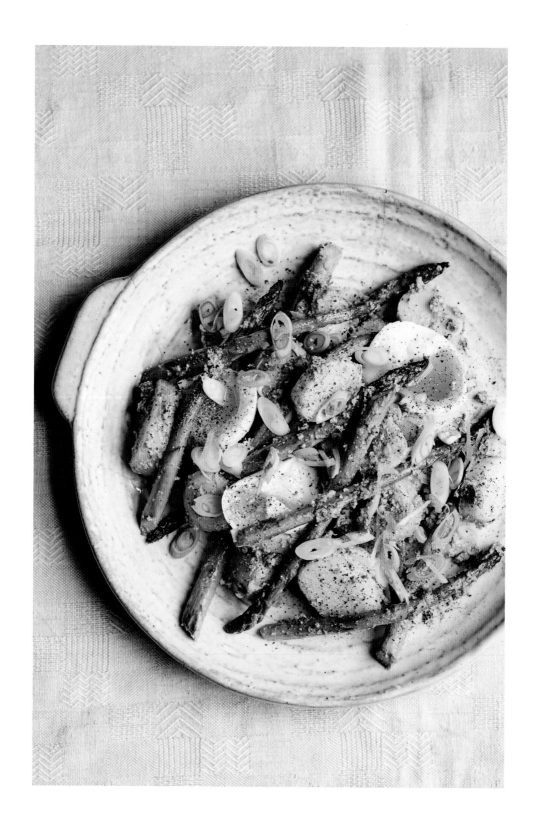

Serves 2

Egg, potato + cashew pesto salad

Potatoes in a salad are totally underrated – maybe because potato salads at salad bars are typically a bit bland and mushy, or because the dish has a reputation for not being healthy. Well, this salad is certainly not bland or mushy, and it's pretty much a balanced meal, with protein from the egg, healthy fats from the pesto dressing and complex carbohydrates from the potatoes. If asparagus is not in season or unavailable when you're making this dish, courgettes, peas or green beans would be fab too.

500g baby potatoes, washed and cut into 1cm slices

Salt and black pepper

2 eggs

250g asparagus, woody ends removed

1 tbsp olive oil

2 spring onions, chopped

For the cashew pesto

80g cashew nuts

4 tbsp olive oil

Handful of fresh basil leaves

1 tbsp Parmesan (or nutritional yeast)

1 garlic clove

Zest and juice of 1 lemon

Put 1 large and 1 smaller pan of water on to boil. Add the potatoes to the larger pan with a pinch of salt and simmer for 10–12 minutes, until tender.

Soft-boil the eggs in the smaller pan for 6–7 minutes (longer for a harder yolk). Lift the eggs out and place in a bowl of cold water. Peel once cooled, then cut into halves.

Toss the asparagus with the oil. Heat a frying pan over a medium heat for 2 minutes. Add the asparagus and cook for 4–5 minutes, until tender.

To make the pesto, simply put all the ingredients into your food processor (except the lemon zest).

Put the potatoes and asparagus into a large serving bowl and stir through the pesto. Add the halved eggs and scatter over the spring onions and lemon zest. Season with salt and pepper.

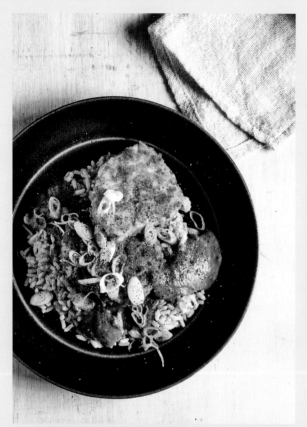

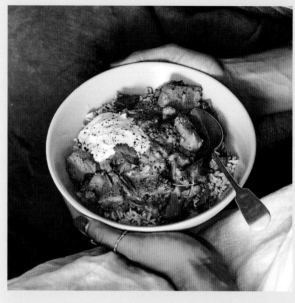

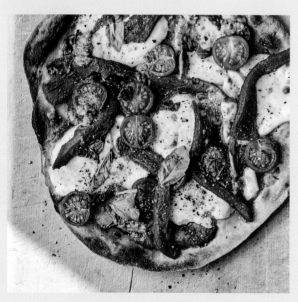

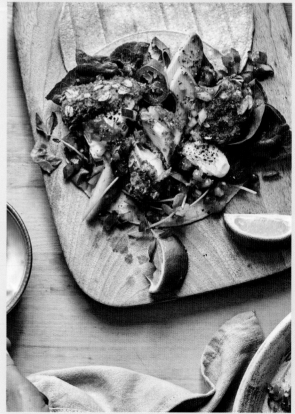

Dinner

Serves 2

1 large sweet
  potato, washed
  and chopped
  into chunks
2 tbsp olive oil
½ tsp paprika
½ tsp ground cumin
½ tsp chilli powder
Pinch of salt
1 bell pepper, sliced
1 x 400g tin of black
  beans, drained
  and rinsed
1 small tin of
  sweetcorn
  (about 160g)
250g cooked
  brown rice
2 good handfuls
  of spinach
Handful of cherry
  tomatoes, halved

For the dressing
Juice of 1 lime
1 tbsp olive oil
1–2 tbsp water
1 avocado, pitted
1 garlic clove
Handful of fresh
  coriander
1 small jalapeño
  pepper, seeded and
  finely chopped
Pinch of sea salt

Sweet potato + black bean burrito bowls with avocado dressing

These throw-together veggie burrito bowls are packed full of nutrients and are perfect for last-minute dinners or meal prep lunches. The pickled red onion is optional, but trust me – it's super simple to make and can be used for other meals across the week.

Preheat the oven to 180°C fan/400°F/gas mark 6. Toss the sweet potato chunks with a tablespoon of olive oil, the paprika, cumin, chilli powder and salt. Place in a large ovenproof dish and cook in the oven for 15 minutes. Remove from the oven and add the sliced pepper and the remaining oil. Toss together, then return the dish to the oven and cook for another 15–20 minutes, or until the pepper slices are crisp and tender and the sweet potato chunks are tender. Remove from the oven and stir through the black beans and sweetcorn.

To make the dressing, combine all the ingredients in a small blender and blend, until smooth. Add more water if necessary for a more pourable dressing.

Divide the brown rice, spinach, tomatoes and the roast sweet potato and black bean mixture between two bowls. Add some pickled red onion, if using, and drizzle the dressing on top.

For the pickled red onion (optional)

250ml white wine vinegar or apple cider vinegar

1 tbsp white sugar

1 garlic clove, peeled

1 tsp salt

1 tsp peppercorns

2–3 small red onions, peeled and very thinly sliced

To make the pickled red onion

Put the vinegar, sugar, garlic, salt and peppercorns into a small saucepan. Place over a medium heat and stir until the sugar has dissolved. Cover and bring to the boil.

Next add the onions and cook for 1–2 minutes to soften. Make sure all the onions are submerged by pressing them down with the back of a spoon.

Take the pan off the heat and set aside to cool at room temperature.

Once cool, transfer the onions and liquid to a glass jar with a lid. Store in the fridge, where the pickle will keep for up to 3 weeks.

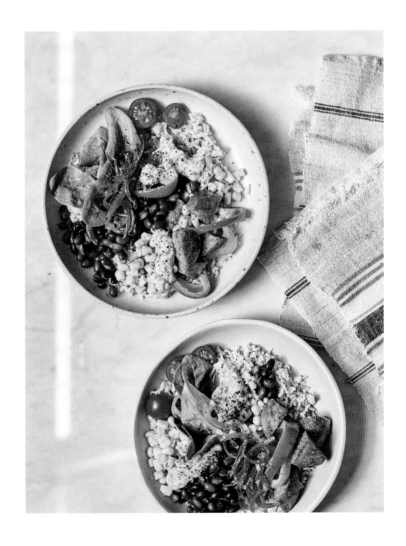

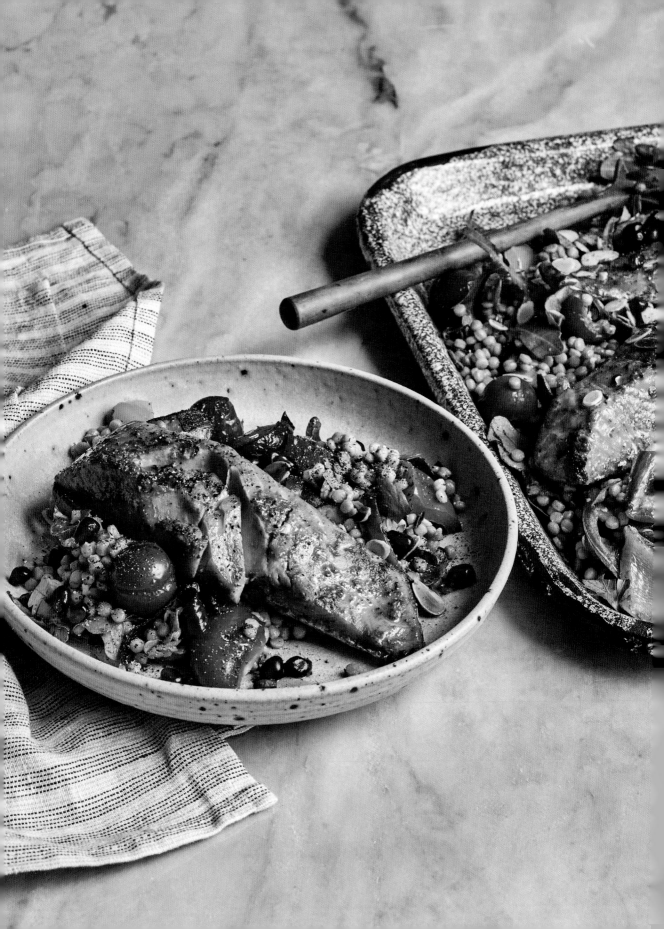

Serves 4

Harissa salmon + chunky veg couscous

This recipe is for people who don't really like to cook – or don't have the time. I usually opt for this when I'm late home from work and want to pop something into the oven which will look after itself while I soak in the bath. It's an incredibly nourishing dish and really brings me back to life after a long day ... PS: Feel free to swap out any of the veg for whatever you have in the fridge – no rules apply here! This is also quite delicious stuffed inside roasted pepper halves.

3 tbsp rose harissa

Zest and juice of 1 lemon

1–2 tbsp olive oil

4 salmon fillets

2 bell peppers (different colours if possible), chopped

2 courgettes, sliced

1 red onion

4 garlic cloves

150g cherry tomatoes

250g giant couscous

300ml vegetable stock

50g flaked almonds

2 good handfuls of rocket

Handful of fresh parsley, roughly chopped

150g pomegranate seeds

Preheat the oven to 180°C fan/400°F/gas mark 6.

Mix 2 tablespoons of harissa with the lemon zest and a tablespoon of olive oil. Rub this mixture all over the salmon fillets and lay them on a baking tray. Allow to marinate for 30 minutes (or overnight).

Put the peppers, courgettes, red onion and garlic on a separate baking tray. Drizzle over the rest of the olive oil and stir in the remaining harissa. Give it all a toss and roast for 30 minutes. Add the cherry tomatoes for the final 10–15 minutes. Place the salmon in the oven at this time too.

Put the couscous into a large bowl, pour over the stock, cover, then set aside for 10–15 minutes. Stir.

Squeeze the garlic pulp from the skins and mash with a fork, then add to the couscous with the almonds, the rocket and the rest of the roasted vegetables. Squeeze the lemon juice on top and stir in the parsley. Sprinkle pomegranate seeds on top before serving with the salmon fillets.

Crispy cod tacos

Serves 4

This is one of my go-to dinner party dishes, because everyone can build their own tacos and add their favourite fillings. Fish is usually a safe option for most people in terms of food preference, but for veggies or vegans you could use tofu or cauliflower, and for a meat option chicken works really well too.

12 corn tacos

1 small head of lettuce, shredded

2 avocados, peeled, pitted and sliced

For the crispy cod

4 skinless cod fillets (approx. 500g)

1 egg

60 ground almonds

40g oats

2 tbsp fajita seasoning

For the salsa

2 large tomatoes, finely chopped

½ red onion, diced

1 garlic clove, grated

1 tbsp extra virgin olive oil

Salt and black pepper

Additional extras

Sour cream, fresh coriander, jalapeños, lime wedges, grated cheese

Preheat the oven to 220°C fan/475°F/gas mark 9 and line a baking tray with baking parchment.

Slice the fish fillets into large chunks.

Whisk the egg in a bowl, then put the ground almonds, oats and fajita seasoning into another bowl. Dip each fish finger into the beaten egg and then into the almond and oat mix so that they are fully coated, and lay them on the baking tray. Bake for 10 minutes. Warm the taco shells in the oven for a few minutes while the oven is still warm.

For the salsa, combine all the ingredients together in a bowl.

Lay out the lettuce, salsa, avocado and additional extras.

Grab a taco shell and load it up with crispy cod and all your favourite toppings

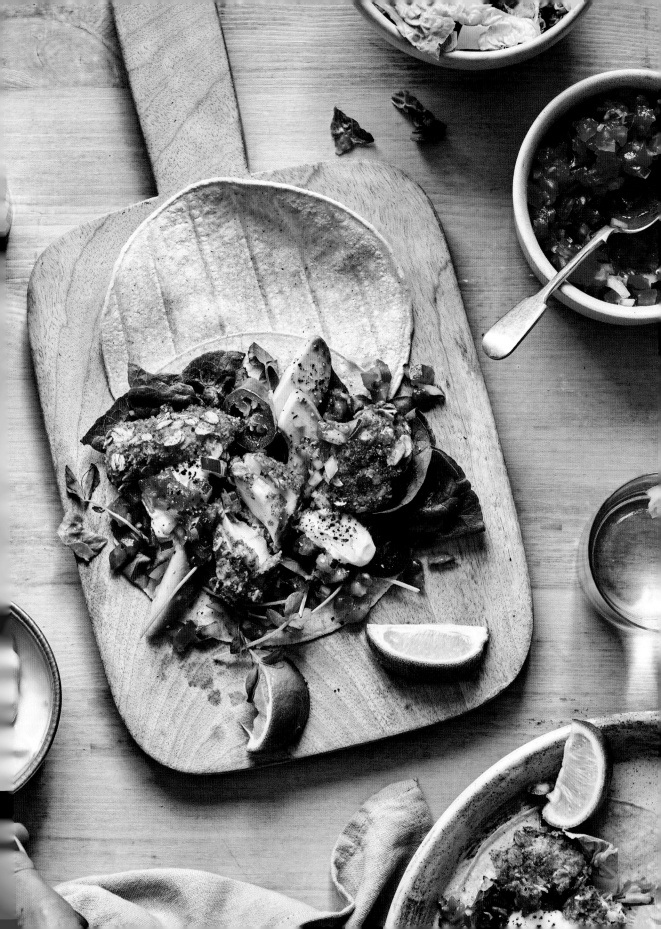

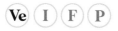

Serves 2

Creamy vegan Alfredo with mushrooms + broccolini

The secret to the creaminess of this sauce is silken tofu. Unlike regular tofu, which most people are familiar with, silken tofu is unpressed and has a softer, jelly-like consistency which works perfectly in sauces and smoothies. In addition to consistency, the tofu also adds protein to this pasta sauce, as well as other important nutrients such as calcium and iron. This gorgeous recipe is also made in under 10 minutes – no fasta pasta.

1 tbsp olive oil

400g mushrooms, sliced (I used chestnut mushrooms)

2 garlic cloves, peeled and crushed

100g broccolini

200g fettuccine

300g pack of silken tofu

Juice of 1 lemon

1 tsp salt

2 tbsp nutritional yeast (optional)

Handful of fresh flat-leaf parsley, leaves only, chopped

Heat the oil in a large, deep frying pan, then add the mushrooms and fry for 5–6 minutes, until softened and golden. Add the garlic and broccolini and gently fry for a further 2 minutes.

Meanwhile, cook the pasta as per the packet instructions. Drain, reserving the pasta water.

Put the tofu, about 100ml of the pasta water, the lemon juice, salt and nutritional yeast into a blender and blend until smooth. Pour into the pan with the mushrooms and broccolini, heat through for 3–4 minutes, then add the pasta and finish by adding the parsley.

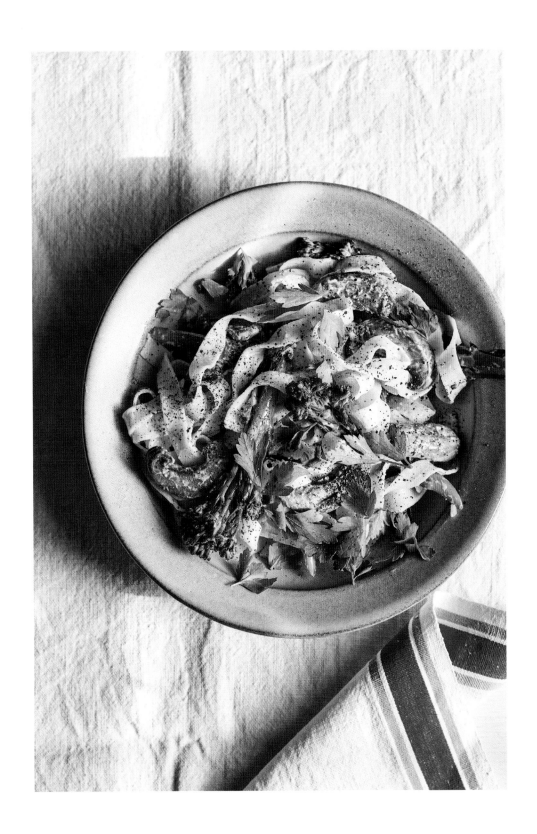

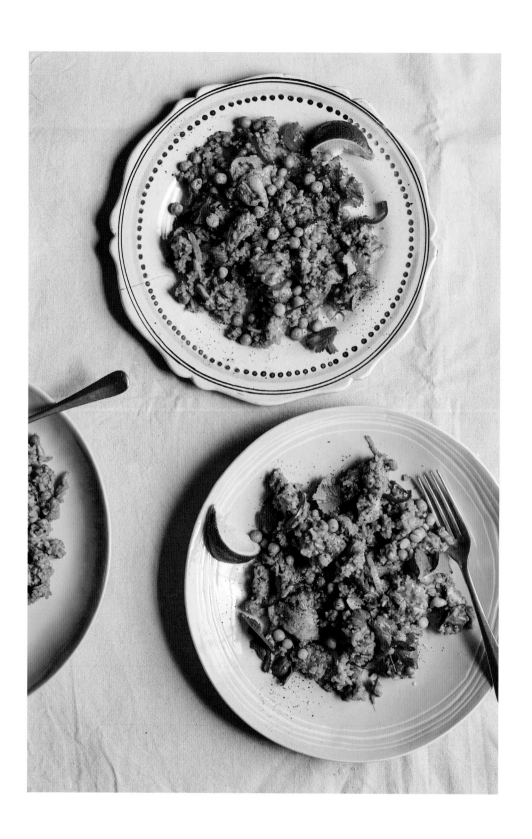

Chicken biryani

Serves 6

Comforting and bursting with aromatic spices, try this easy biryani for a weekday meal that's ready in no time.

3 tbsp olive oil

1 onion, thinly sliced

1 tbsp whole cumin seeds

4 boneless chicken thighs, cut into bite-size pieces

5 tbsp tomato purée

5 tbsp Greek yogurt

100g frozen peas

5 garlic cloves, crushed

2 red chillies, deseeded and finely sliced

1 tbsp garam masala

1½ tsp ground turmeric

350g basmati rice, rinsed until water runs clear

1 litre chicken stock

1 tsp fine sea salt

2 tbsp unsalted butter

Large handful of fresh coriander leaves, finely chopped, plus more to garnish

1 lime, cut into wedges

Put the oil into a large pan with a tightly fitting lid and set over a medium heat. Add the onion and cumin seeds and sauté for 10 minutes, stirring frequently, until translucent.

Add the chicken, tomato purée, yogurt, peas, garlic, most of the chillies, the garam masala and turmeric and cook for another 5 minutes, until sizzling and aromatic.

Stir in the rice, stock and salt (omit the salt if your stock is already salted), bring to the boil, then reduce the heat a little and simmer for 10–15 minutes, until most of the stock has been absorbed. Stir frequently to prevent the rice sticking and burning. Turn off the heat, place the lid on top and leave to steam for 10 minutes.

Stir the butter and most of the coriander through the mixture. Serve with the remaining coriander and sliced chillies scattered over and lime wedges on the side.

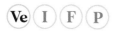

Tofu katsu with rice

Serves 4

This katsu with its creamy, golden sauce and crunchy tofu gives Waga's a run for its money. I've used cornflakes in the coating for added crunch but also because they are fortified with iron – a nutrient which can often be tricky to obtain from plant-only diets.

400g firm smoked tofu, drained

4 tbsp olive oil, plus more for frying

1 onion, finely chopped

2 carrots, peeled and cut into 1cm pieces

3 garlic cloves, crushed

3cm piece of fresh root ginger, peeled and finely grated

1 tbsp mild curry powder

1 tsp garam masala

¾ tsp ground turmeric

1 tbsp plain white flour, plus 50g for coating

400ml vegetable stock

2 tbsp soy sauce

Salt and black pepper

100ml milk of your choice

50g fresh breadcrumbs

50g cornflakes, crushed

Cooked rice, to serve

3 spring onions, finely chopped

Wrap the drained tofu in a clean tea towel and place a heavy book or chopping board on top. Set aside to drain further while you make the curry sauce.

Put 2 tablespoons of the oil into a pan and place over a medium heat. Add the onion, carrots, garlic and ginger and cook gently for 8 minutes, stirring frequently, until the onion is translucent, taking care not to let anything burn. Add the curry powder, garam masala, turmeric and flour and stir-fry for 2 minutes. Gradually stir in the stock and soy sauce and bring to the boil. Reduce the heat and simmer for 10 minutes, stirring frequently, until thickened and the carrots are cooked through.

Using a handheld or upright blender, blitz the sauce until completely smooth, adding a little water if it is too thick. Season well with salt and pepper.

Slice the block of tofu into 4 steaks of even thickness. Put the 50g of flour for coating into one bowl, the milk into a second bowl and the breadcrumbs and cornflakes combined into a third bowl. Coat each tofu steak with flour, then dip into the milk. Finally coat with the breadcrumb mixture on all sides. Put the remaining 2 tablespoons of oil into a large non-stick pan and set over a medium–high heat. Fry the tofu steaks for 2–4 minutes on each side, until golden and crispy.

Serve the sauce over the rice, with the tofu katsu on top and the spring onions scattered over.

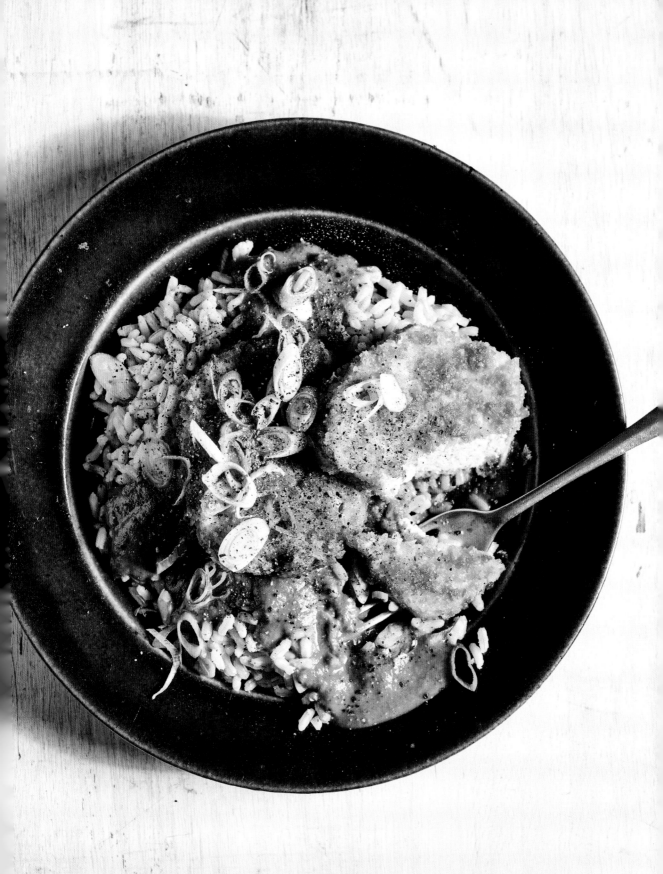

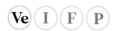

Makes 4 large burgers

Carrot + black bean veggie burgers with harissa mayo

I've had many veggie burgers that have been totally underwhelming and extremely dry, BUT these burgers will not let you down. They are thick, flavoursome and moist (I hate that word too) and when loaded up with harissa mayo they just go that extra mile *chef's kiss*. They also provide 16–17g of plant-based protein per serving, depending on whether you use quinoa, rice or both.

100g grated carrot

1 x 400g tin of black beans, drained

2 garlic cloves, crushed

4 tbsp harissa paste

1½ tsp ground cumin

1¼ tsp sweet smoked paprika

150g cooked quinoa or brown rice (or a combination of both), cooled

30g Parmesan, finely grated, or nutritional yeast, if vegan

2 tsp maple syrup

Salt and black pepper

1 tbsp olive oil

To serve

6 tbsp mayonnaise, or vegan mayo if you prefer

Wholemeal burger buns

Lettuce leaves,

1 beef tomato, sliced

Spread the grated carrot on a few sheets of kitchen paper, then roll it up and press firmly to extract as much moisture as possible. Transfer to a large mixing bowl.

Put three-quarters of the black beans and the garlic into a food processor and blitz, until almost smooth. Transfer to the bowl of carrot. Add the remaining whole black beans, half the harissa, the cumin, paprika, cooled quinoa or rice, Parmesan or nutritional yeast, maple syrup and 1 teaspoon of salt. Thoroughly combine. Taste for seasoning and adjust if necessary.

Preheat the oven to 200°C fan/425°F/gas mark 7.

Divide the mixture into 4 portions of equal size (about 140g per burger) and shape into burger patties. Put the oil into a large non-stick pan and set over a medium–high heat. Fry the burgers for 3–4 minutes on each side, until golden. Turn them very gently, as they are quite fragile at this stage. Transfer to a baking tray and bake in the oven for 15 minutes.

Combine the remaining harissa with the mayonnaise. To serve, divide the harissa mayo between the halved burger buns. Layer on the lettuce and tomato, then add the burger patties (handling them carefully) and place the remaining burger bun halves on top.

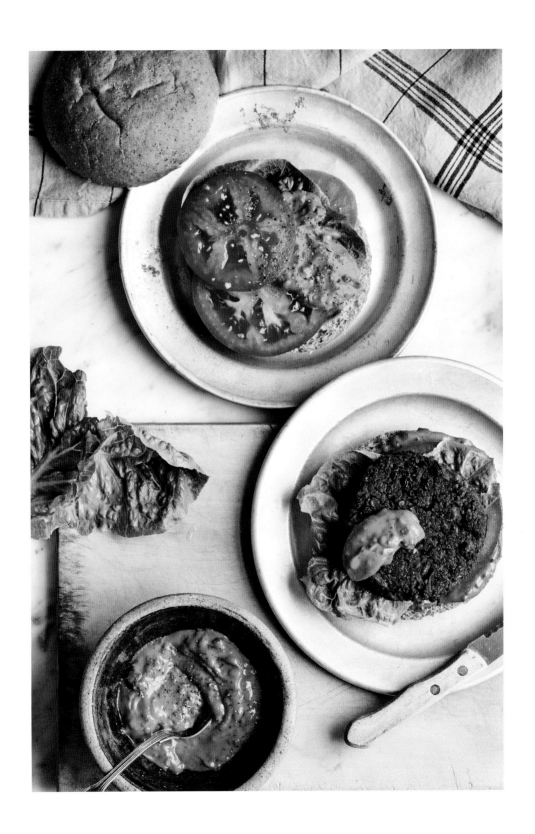

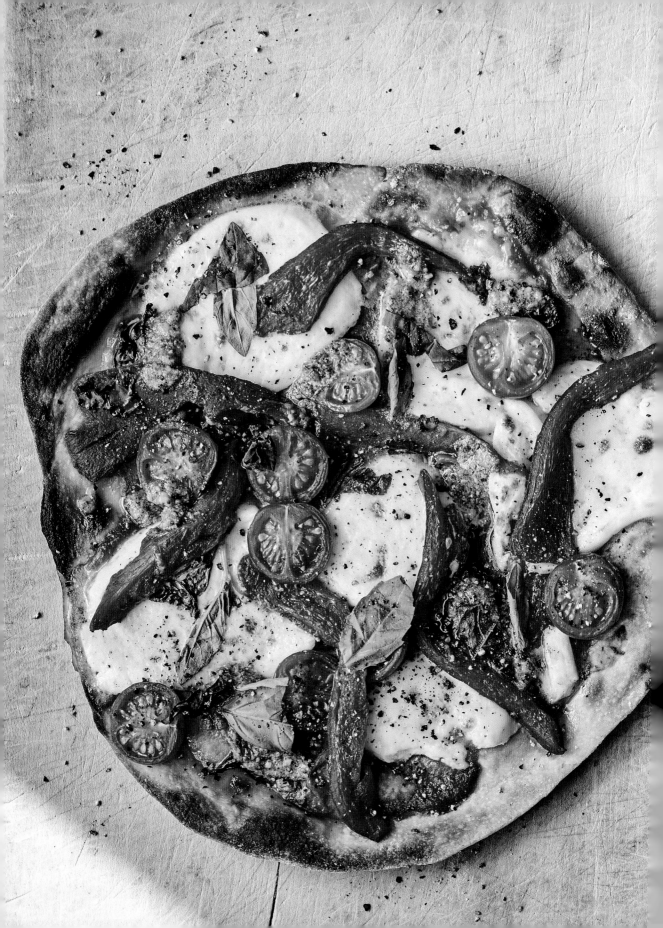

Quick flatbread pizzas

Serves 3

I rarely have the patience to make pizza from scratch but this easier flatbread version is the perfect trick for beginners (or people who want to skip to the good bit). Below are topping ideas, but use whatever your favourite combinations are.

100g plain white or white spelt flour, plus more for dusting

¼ tsp fine sea salt

1 tbsp extra virgin olive oil

50ml water

Toppings suggestions

- Sauces:
  tomato sauce, truffle oil, pesto
- Cheese:
  mozzarella, Parmesan, ricotta, Taleggio, Gorgonzola, feta
- Vegetables:
  onions, cherry tomatoes, any blanched green vegetables, spinach, dried or fresh chillies, any fresh herbs, olives, sun-dried tomatoes, rocket, radicchio, fried mushrooms, grilled veg such as peppers, aubergines, courgettes
- Meat and fish:
  anchovies, tuna, prawns, cured meats

In a large bowl combine the flour and salt. Add the oil and all but 2 tablespoons of the water and bring together into a dough. Add the remaining water a bit at a time, bearing in mind you may not need all of it, to form a smooth and soft dough. It should not be sticky. Knead for 2 minutes. Cover and set aside for 15 minutes to rest.

Divide the dough into 3 pieces of equal size. Dust your work surface with flour, then one by one roll out each ball of dough into a thin round measuring about 22cm. Dust with flour as you go to ensure the dough does not stick.

Place a non-stick frying pan over a medium heat. Place a flatbread on the dry pan and cook for about 1 minute on each side, until just cooked through for a softer flatbread pizza, or if you prefer your flatbread a little more crispy, cook for a further 30 seconds on each side, until slightly blistered, taking care not to let it burn. Remove to a plate and cover with a clean tea towel while you make the rest.

To make the pizzas, top the warm flatbreads with your favourite toppings and cook under a hot grill for 3–5 minutes, until slightly blistered. Serve immediately.

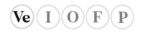

Ve I O F P

Makes 16 balls, serving 4

Walnut, chia + kidney bean meatballs

Walnut, chia + kidney bean meatballs

These (no)meatballs are not only an incredibly tasty alternative to the OG meat versions but they are little nutrition powerhouses packed with protein, fibre and omega-3 fatty acids. Dog-ear this page for meat-free Monday.

2 tbsp olive oil, plus more for greasing

1 onion, peeled and very finely chopped

3 garlic cloves, crushed

½ tsp ground cumin

½ tsp sweet smoked paprika

1 x 400g tin of kidney beans, drained

1 tbsp ground chia seeds

80g walnuts

2 tsp fresh thyme leaves

50g Parmesan, grated, plus more to serve

Salt and black pepper

320g spaghetti

200g tomato sauce, homemade or shop-bought

Small handful of fresh basil leaves, to serve

Put the oil into a pan and set over a medium–high heat. Add the onion and sauté for 8–10 minutes, until soft and translucent. Add the garlic, cumin and paprika and fry for another minute, until aromatic. Set aside.

Preheat the oven to 210°C fan/450°F/gas mark 8. Line a baking sheet with baking parchment and drizzle over a little oil.

Put the kidney beans, ground chia seeds, walnuts, thyme and Parmesan into a food processor. Pulse on and off until coarsely ground. Season to taste with salt and pepper and pulse once more to combine. Stir through the onion mixture.

Using damp hands, shape the mixture into 16 balls of equal size, approximately 28g per ball. Place the balls on the baking tray and drizzle over a little more olive oil. Bake in the oven for 20 minutes, until golden.

Meanwhile, cook the spaghetti in boiling salted water according to the packet instructions, until al dente. Drain, then return it to the pan with the tomato sauce to heat through. Serve the spaghetti with the meatballs on top and the basil and a little more Parmesan scattered on top.

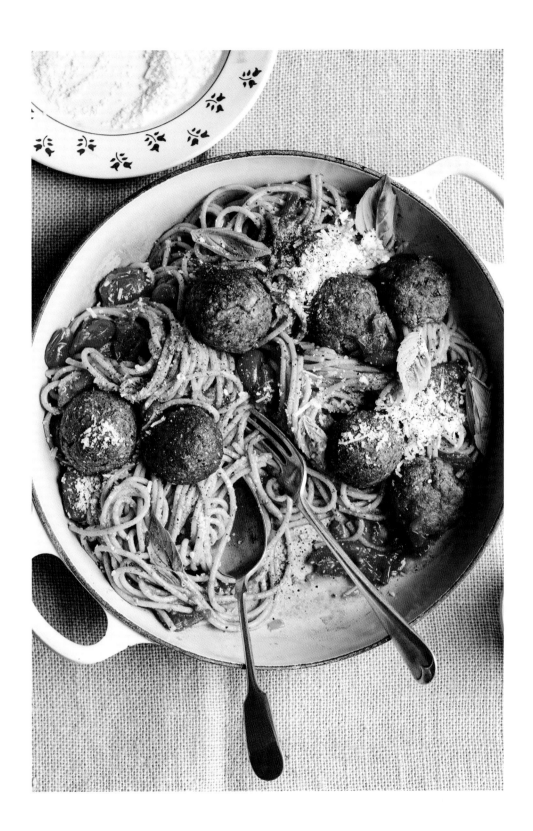

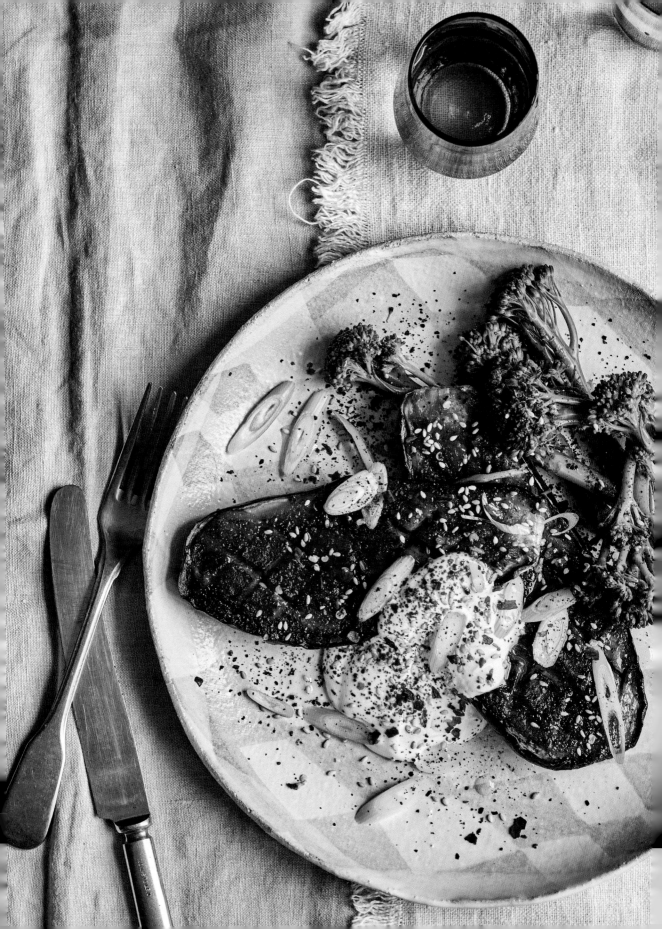

Serves 4

Miso-glazed aubergine with broccoli + yogurt

Long-term Food Medic followers will recall the viral sticky soy-roasted aubergine from my first book. So I simply had to bring back another version. This recipe will convert people who have yet to find a love of aubergine (or eggplant) – trust me. The sticky and sweet miso topping and the yogurt combo is like dinner and dessert wrapped up in one.

2 large aubergines, halved lengthways

Olive oil, to coat

200g tenderstem broccoli

3 tbsp white miso

3 tbsp mirin

100g natural or Greek yogurt, or plant-based alternative

2 spring onions, thinly sliced on the diagonal

2 tsp sesame seeds

Dried chilli flakes, to serve

Preheat the oven to 200°C fan/425°F/gas mark 7. Score the flesh side of the aubergines, taking care not to cut through the skin. Drizzle over a little olive oil and rub into the flesh. Place on a baking tray in the oven for 15–20 minutes, until the flesh is tender.

Meanwhile, blanch the broccoli in boiling salted water for 3 minutes, until just tender. Drain and set aside.

Combine the miso and mirin together and spread evenly over the flesh of the aubergines. Return the aubergines to the oven and cook for a further 8–15 minutes, until the miso is bubbling and beginning to colour and the aubergine flesh is soft. Watch carefully, as it can burn quickly.

Serve the aubergines with the broccoli on the side, a dollop of yogurt and the spring onions, sesame seeds and a pinch of dried chilli flakes scattered on top.

Serves 4

Sweet potato lentil coconut curry

Fuss-free, warming and full of flavour – comfort food at its best.

2 tbsp olive oil

1 red onion, peeled and roughly chopped

1 tbsp mustard seeds

Handful of fresh curry leaves

5 garlic cloves, crushed

½ tsp dried chilli flakes

1 tsp ground cumin

2 sweet potatoes, chopped into bite-size pieces (no need to peel)

150g red lentils

400ml coconut milk

500ml vegetable stock

150g spinach, washed

2 tbsp lemon juice

Salt and black pepper

To serve

Cooked rice

Yogurt

Large handful of fresh coriander leaves, to serve

Put the oil into a large high-sided pot and set over a medium heat. Add the onion and sauté for 5 minutes, until beginning to soften. Add the mustard seeds, curry leaves, garlic, chilli flakes and ground cumin. Fry for 3–4 minutes, stirring now and again, until aromatic.

Add the sweet potatoes, lentils, coconut milk and stock and bring to the boil. Simmer for 30–35 minutes, stirring frequently to prevent the lentils from sticking to the bottom, until the sweet potatoes and lentils are cooked through. Add the spinach and cook for another 5 minutes, until wilted down.

Stir in the lemon juice and season to taste with up to a teaspoon of salt and a grinding of black pepper, bearing in mind that your stock may already have been salted.

Serve with rice on the side, a dollop of yogurt and the coriander leaves scattered over.

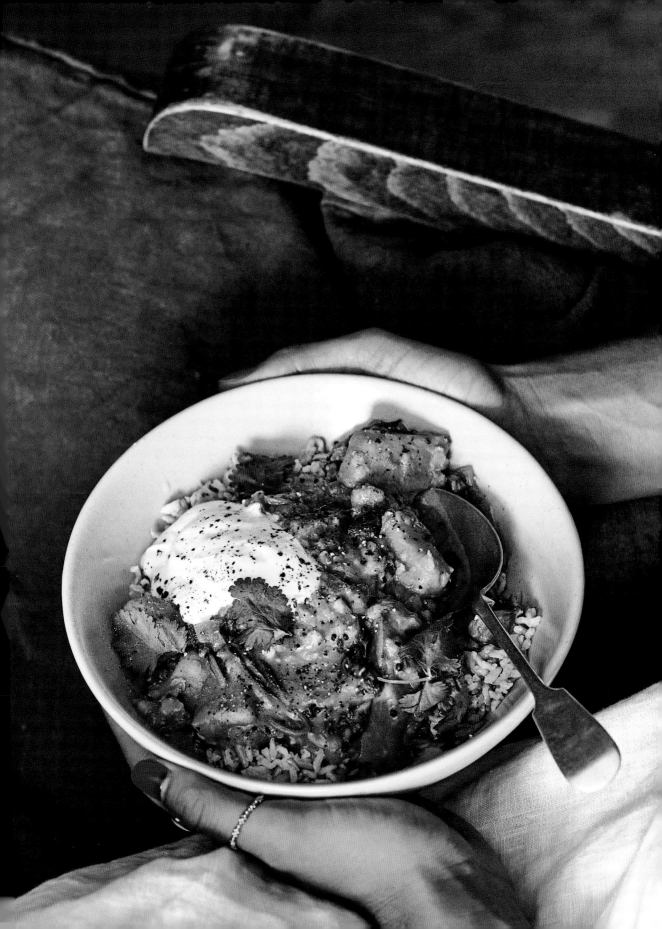

DIY protein poke bowl

Serves 2

My best mate and I love a poke bowl on a Friday night when we catch up. Poke is a Hawaiian dish which traditionally uses diced raw fish with a sticky rice base. The beauty of a poke bowl is that they're super customisable, convenient, nutritious and filling. So how this works is basically like a pick 'n' mix poke bowl. Choose your protein, grains, greens and toppings and drizzle the dressing over each.

For the dressing

2 tbsp soy sauce

1 tbsp sesame oil

½ tbsp rice wine vinegar

Juice of ½ lime

To garnish

1 sheet of nori seaweed, chopped

1 tbsp sesame seeds

Lime wedges

Make the dressing by whisking the ingredients together in a bowl.

Choose your protein, grains, greens and toppings from the suggestions below, and divide between bowls.

Drizzle dressing over each bowl and finish with your choice of garnish.

Protein (1 palm-sized portion each)	Grains (250g)	Toppings
tuna	wholegrain rice	1 avocado, stone removed, peeled and chopped
salmon fillet	sushi rice	1 mango, stone removed, peeled and chopped
chicken	quinoa	¼ cucumber, thinly sliced
tofu	**Greens (1 large handful)**	6 radishes, trimmed and sliced
prawns	Spinach	1 carrot, shredded
falafel	kale	100g edamame, shelled, cooked according to packet instructions
2 soft-boiled eggs	mixed leaves	

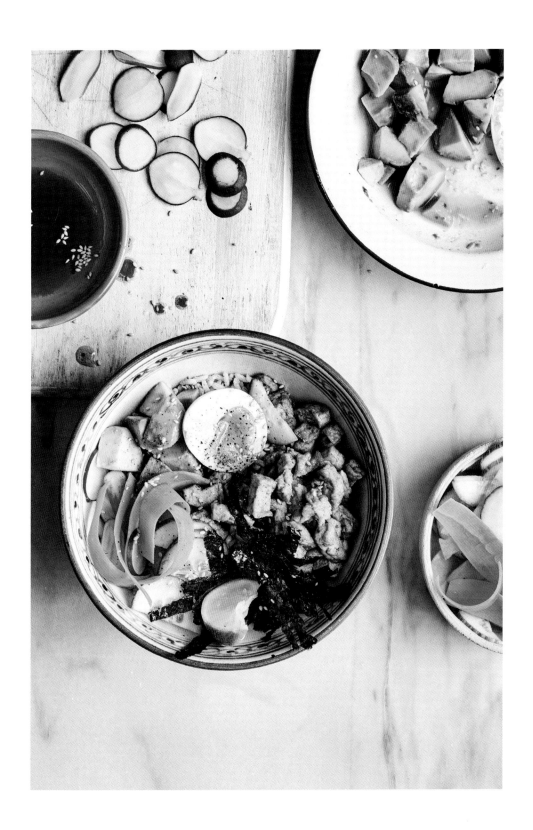

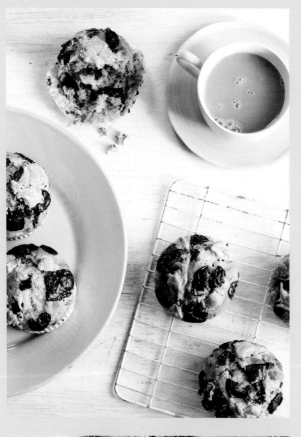

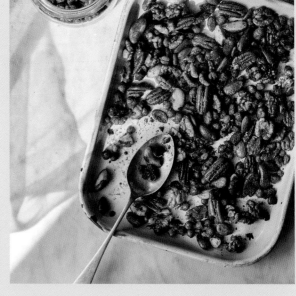

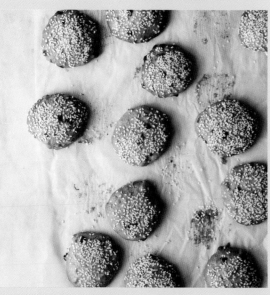

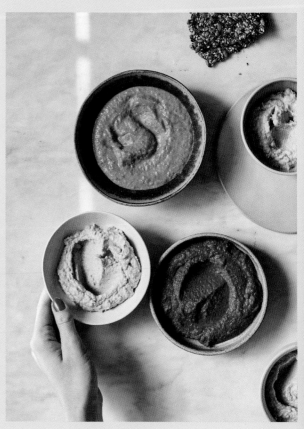

Snacks

Tahini + chocolate cookies

Makes 12

Tahini is traditionally used in savoury meals and snacks, but it works as a great alternative to peanut butter and actually I almost prefer the saltiness it provides to the cookies. These can also be made vegan using chia eggs.

50g oats

90g plain flour

Pinch of salt

1 tsp baking powder

150g brown sugar

125g tahini

1 tsp vanilla extract

1 egg, whisked*

60g apple sauce (smooth recommended)

80g dark chocolate chips

40g sesame seeds, to top

* To make vegan, swap for 2 chia eggs (2 tablespoons of chia seeds mixed with 4 tablespoons of water and left to sit for 5 minutes)

Preheat the oven to 180°C fan/400°F/gas mark 6 and line a baking tray with parchment paper.

Combine the dry ingredients in a bowl.

Add the tahini, vanilla, egg and apple sauce to the dry ingredients and stir to combine. A cookie dough should form – if it's too dry, add a splash of water or milk, or if not dry enough, add a little more flour. Fold in the chocolate chips.

Scoop out heaped tablespoons of the mixture. Roll each one into a ball and dip into the sesame seeds. Place on the baking tray and press down slightly.

Bake for 15–18 minutes, until golden but not brown. Allow to cool on a wire rack for 10–15 minutes.

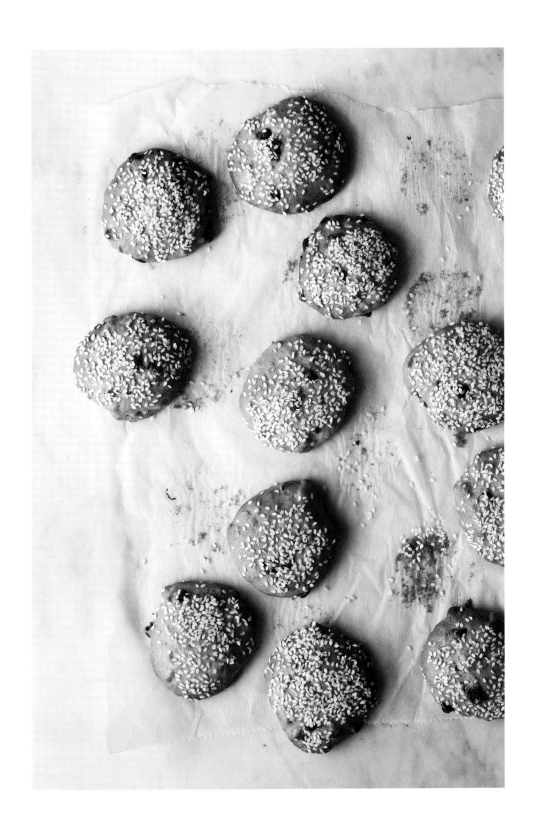

(Ve) (I) (O) (F) (P) # Omega-3 crackers

Serves 12

Omega-3 fatty acids play an important role in many bodily processes, including inflammation, heart health and brain function. Walnuts, chia seeds and flaxseeds are some of the best sources of the omega-3 fatty acid alpha-linolenic acid (ALA).

100g walnuts
80g chia or flaxseeds
75g sunflower seeds
75g pumpkin seeds
50g sesame seeds
240ml water
¼ tsp salt

Preheat the oven to 170°C fan/375°F/gas mark 5. Line a baking tray with baking parchment.

Blitz the walnuts in a food processor to form a crumb.

Transfer the walnuts to a bowl with the rest of the ingredients and leave for 15 minutes, until the water has been absorbed.

Spoon the mixture on to the baking tray and spread out to about ½cm thick. Use the tip of a knife to score the shape of the crackers.

Bake for 25 minutes. Remove and gently turn over the crackers so you can cook the other side. Carefully peel off the paper, then put the crackers back on the baking tray and return them to the oven. Bake for a further 20 minutes, or until golden brown and firm.

Break up the squares – it's OK if they're a little oddly shaped or odd sizes! Leave to cool, then store in an airtight container for 7–10 days.

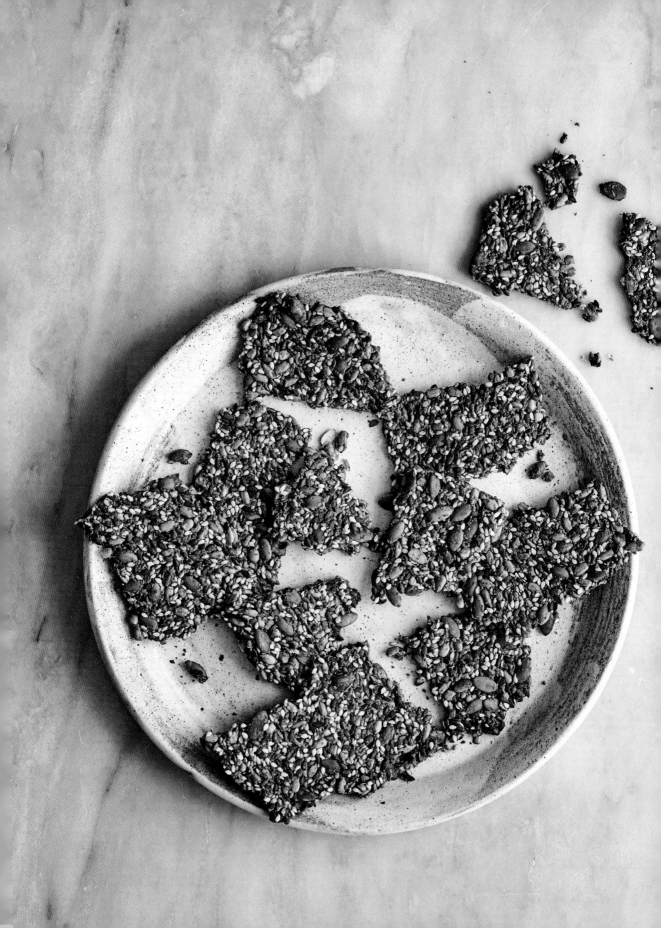

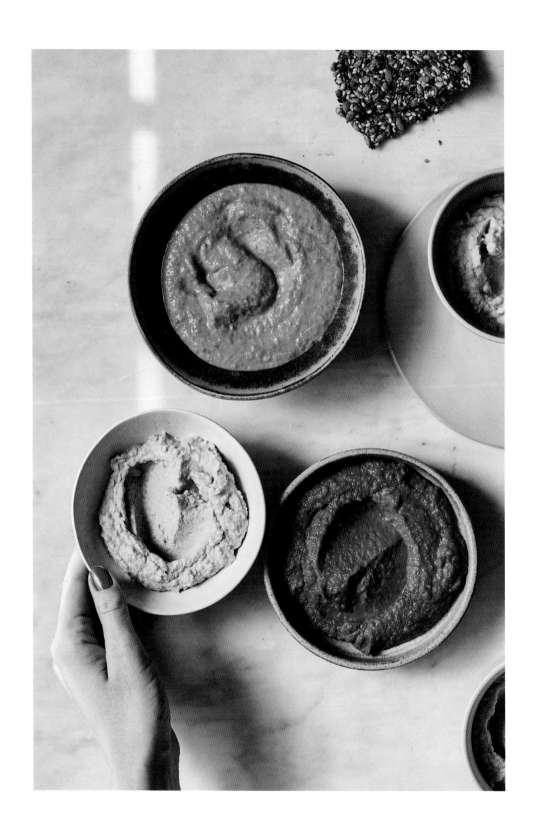

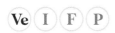

Hummus 5 ways

Serves 4

Classic hummus

- 1 x 400g tin of chickpeas, drained and rinsed
- 2 garlic cloves, peeled
- Juice of 1 lemon
- 2 tbsp tahini
- 2 tbsp olive oil
- 3–4 tbsp water (you can also use the liquid from the chickpeas)
- 1 tsp ground cumin
- Good pinch of salt

Additional extras

Avo-hummus: add an avocado*

Beetroot hummus: add 1 cooked beetroot*

Roast pepper: add 2 roast peppers from a jar*

Golden turmeric + ginger: add 1 tsp turmeric powder and 1 tsp fresh grated ginger

I always have hummus in my fridge – it's so great as a quick snack with some rye crackers or carrots, or inside a pitta with some roasted veg or dolloped on top of a salad for a bit of oomph. I've given you 5 different flavour suggestions to take your hummus game up a level. Some tips for super creamy hummus that I learned from my friend and cookbook writer Jordan Bourke:

1. Chickpea skins are edible, but if you want creamy hummus, peel the chickpeas and discard the skins. It helps to soak the chickpeas in a bit of hot water with some baking soda, which takes the chickpea skins right off. It does require a little bit of work, so feel free to skip this step.

2. Add an ice cube while blending – ICE? The ice cubes almost whip the hummus into a creamier texture. Try it!

Put all the ingredients into a food processor and blitz until smooth. Add more water, a little at a time, if it looks too thick.

Season, and transfer to a bowl.

Note: when adding extras to your base hummus, you may need to add an extra tablespoon of water or olive oil to achieve the right consistency.

Makes 16–18 balls

Chocolate + chia nut balls

No-bake with a few ingredients. My kinda recipe! Feel free to swap the cacao powder for chocolate protein powder to increase the protein content of this snack. They also carry really well if you're out and about, at work or out on a hike.

50g raw cashew nuts

50g raw hazelnuts or pecan nuts

1 tbsp almond butter

1 tbsp chia seeds

7 Medjool dates, pitted

2 tbsp raw cacao or cocoa powder

Pinch of sea salt

Put all the ingredients into a food processor and blitz until the mixture comes together when pressed between your fingers.

Shape into little balls, roughly 1 heaped teaspoon per ball. Keep refrigerated in an airtight container. They will keep for 1 week.

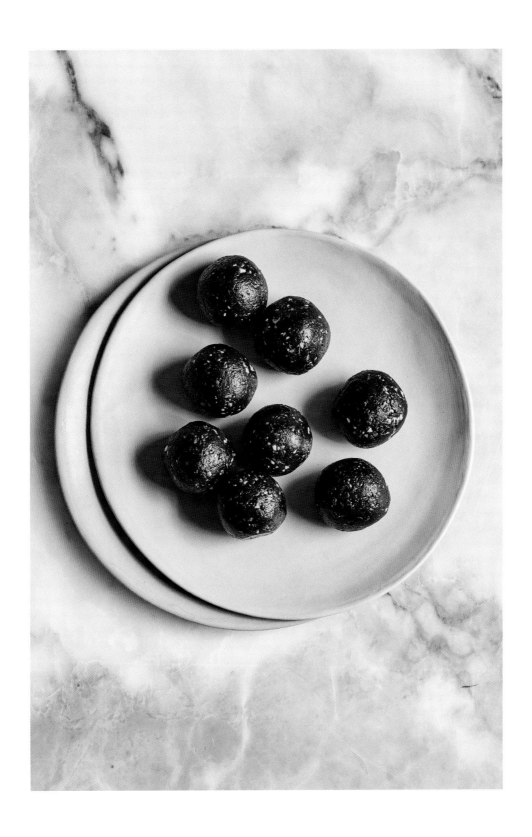

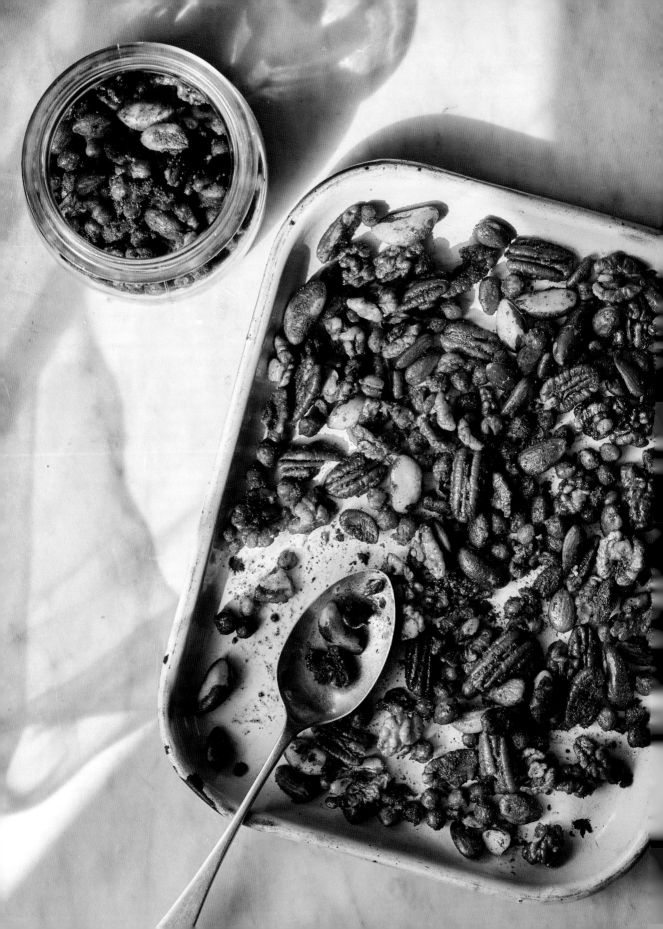

Serves 8

Spiced nuts + chickpeas

This sweet and salty nut and chickpea mix is full of protein, fibre and healthy fats. It's the perfect snack on the go, or served with pre-dinner drinks when entertaining.

1 x 400g tin of chickpeas, drained

1½ tsp sweet smoked paprika

1 tsp ground cinnamon

2 tsp ground cumin

3 tbsp olive oil

2 tbsp brown sugar

1½ tsp sea salt

300g mixed nuts

Preheat the oven to 200°C fan/425°F/gas mark 7. Line a baking tray with baking parchment.

Place the drained chickpeas on a clean tea towel, then fold over and gently pat dry. The drier the chickpeas, the crispier they will become when roasted.

Put the chickpeas into a bowl with half the spices, half the oil, half the sugar and the salt. Combine, then transfer to the baking tray and roast for 25 minutes. Meanwhile, put the nuts into the same bowl and combine with the remaining spices, oil and sugar.

After 25 minutes, add the nuts to the baking tray, mix in and bake for a further 6–8 minutes, until the nuts are a shade darker. Take care not to let them burn.

Remove and leave to cool a little before serving. Store in an airtight container at room temperature.

Ve

Makes 12–14

On-the-run
fruit + nut bar

I've called this on-the-run fruit and nut bar because I'm forever looking for easy-to-carry (and eat) snacks when I'm out on a longer run. One bar offers 25g of carbohydrates, which is great pre-workout or intra-workout fuel for those workouts/runs lasting >1 hour. PS: Don't worry if you've not worked out, as these energy bars are great at any time of the day.

200g rolled oats

100g roasted
   hazelnuts, finely
   chopped

50g pumpkin seeds

Pinch of sea salt

150g Medjool
   dates, pitted

1 ripe banana, peeled

60g unsalted butter
   or coconut
   oil, melted

80g cashew nut
   butter

50ml brown
   rice syrup

Zest of ½ lemon

Preheat the oven to 200°C fan/425°F/gas mark 7. Line a 24cm x 16cm tin with baking parchment.

Put the oats and hazelnuts into a food processor and pulse on and off, until they resemble breadcrumbs. Transfer to a bowl with the pumpkin seeds and salt, and mix together.

Put the dates and banana into the food processor (no need to clean it) and blitz, until smooth. Transfer to a bowl, then add the melted butter together with the cashew nut butter, brown rice syrup and lemon zest, and mix together until smooth.

Add the date mixture to the oats and thoroughly combine, ensuring all the oats are coated. Spread the mixture out in the lined tin and firmly compact into place with the back of a wet spoon (wetting the spoon prevents the mixture sticking). Bake for 15–18 minutes, until golden. Remove and leave to cool for 10 minutes, then slice into bars and leave to cool completely. Once cool, carefully transfer the bars to an airtight container. They will keep for a week in the fridge.

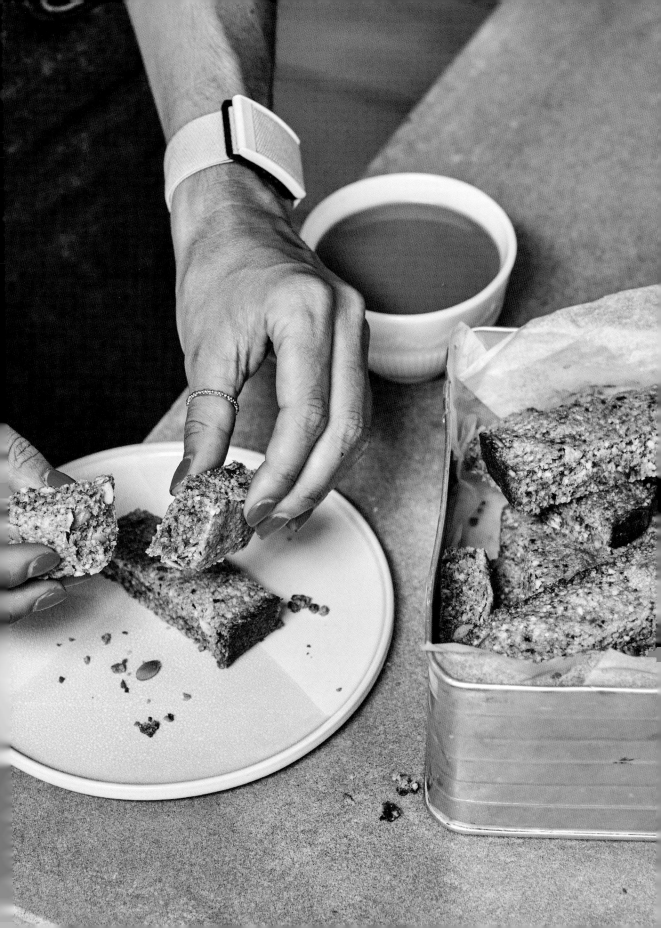

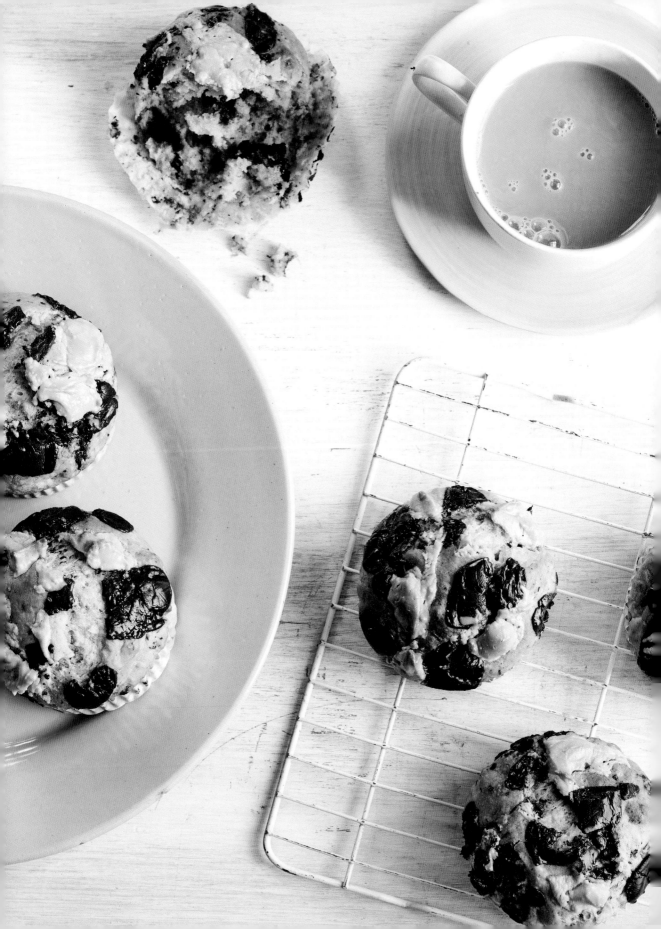

Ve

Makes 6

Chocolate, banana, peanut butter muffins

I love how simple these muffins are to make because they taste so damn good, with three of my favourite flavours in one recipe – banana, peanut butter and chocolate. One batch makes 6 muffins, enough to see you through the week, or you can freeze some for another day.

180g plain white or white spelt flour

1½ tsp baking powder

Pinch of sea salt

1 large banana, peeled and mashed

1 tsp vanilla extract

150ml milk

100ml maple syrup

1 tsp apple cider vinegar or white wine vinegar

100g dark chocolate, 70%, roughly chopped

4 tbsp peanut butter

Preheat the oven to 200°C fan/425°F/gas mark 7 and line a muffin tray with 6 paper cases.

In a large bowl, combine the flour, baking powder and salt. In a separate bowl, mix together the mashed banana, vanilla, milk, maple syrup, vinegar, three quarters of the chocolate and half the peanut butter. Add this to the flour mixture and stir to combine.

Divide the mixture evenly between the 6 muffin cases. Scatter over the remaining chocolate and drizzle over the rest of the peanut butter. Bake for 18–20 minutes, until golden and a skewer comes out mostly clean. Remove and leave to cool on a wire rack.

The muffins will keep in an airtight container in the fridge for up to 2 days.

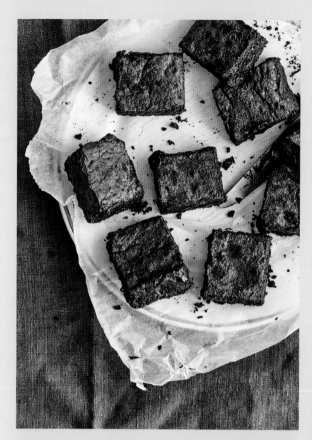

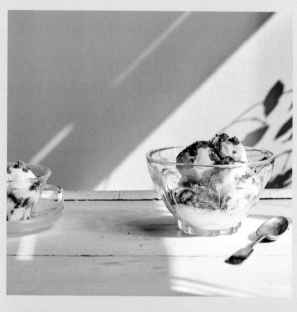

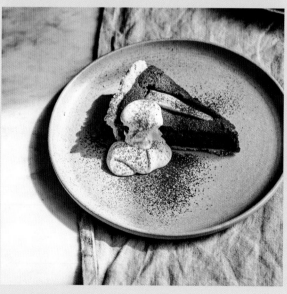

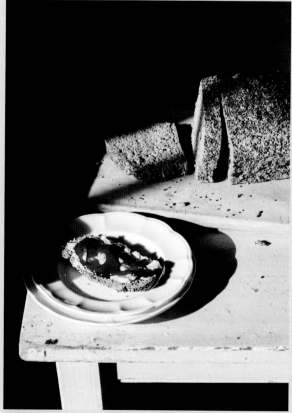

Baking
+ Desserts

Serves 6

Frozen yogurt with granola + mixed berries

Froyo is one of my favourite summer desserts. It can be made with or without an ice-cream maker and with only a handful of ingredients. I like mine served with granola and mixed berries, but chopped nuts, sliced banana, chocolate chips and peanut butter are also delicious toppings.

Zest of ½ lemon,
  plus 2 tbsp juice
1 litre Greek yogurt,
  or dairy-free
  alternative
130g caster sugar
Large pinch of
  fine sea salt

To serve
Granola
Mixed berries

Put the lemon zest, juice, yogurt, sugar and salt into a large bowl and whisk until the sugar has completely dissolved. It should not feel grainy to the touch.

Churn in an ice-cream maker, until frozen. If you do not have an ice-cream maker, pour the mixture into a wide, flat dish and place in the freezer. After 40–60 minutes, when the edges begin to freeze, mash them up with a fork and stir them into the mixture. Return to the freezer and repeat this process three or four more times, until almost completely frozen, then transfer the frozen yogurt into a food processor and blitz, until completely smooth, to remove any ice crystals.

Return the mixture to the tray and store in the freezer, until ready to serve. It will freeze completely solid after a few hours, so you will need to remove it from the freezer at least 30 minutes prior to serving to achieve the desired consistency.

To serve, scoop into glasses or bowls and top with granola and mixed berries.

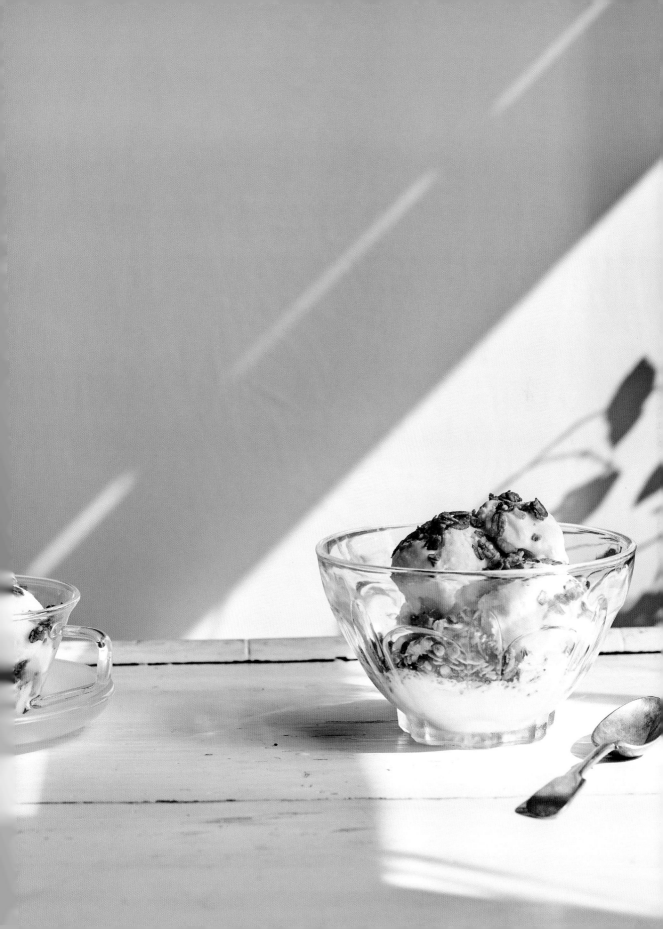

Serves 10-12

Blueberry, almond + cinnamon cake

This is basically a giant blueberry muffin. Lots of people ask why I use sugar in my recipes and not an unrefined alternative. Here's the thing: 'unrefined sugar' is a term used in the wellness world to describe sugar that is naturally present in food, rather than being refined or added, such as honey, maple syrup and coconut sugar. Although it may seem like a healthier than table sugar, it's not necessarily... to the body sugar is sugar, and these foods contain simple sugars which the body breaks down and absorbs in the form of glucose, fructose or galactose – just as it does with refined sugar. While unrefined sugars can contain more micronutrients, the amount is pretty insignificant when we take into account portion sizes – you would need to eat A LOT to get any measurable benefit. So really, we should treat them in the same way. I would rather you make and eat a cake with a sugar that you like best, rather than one you feel you need to use because it's 'healthier'.

225g unsalted
  butter, softened

225g caster sugar

225g plain white or
  white spelt flour

100g ground almonds

2 tsp baking powder

Large pinch of
  sea salt

1 ½ tsp ground
  cinnamon

3 eggs, beaten

125ml milk

200g blueberries

Yogurt, to serve

Preheat the oven to 180°C fan/400°F/gas mark 6 and line a 23cm round springform tin with baking parchment.

Cream together the butter and sugar for 5 minutes with an electric whisk or in a food mixer, until pale, light and fluffy. In another bowl, combine the flour, ground almonds, baking powder, salt and cinnamon. Fold a third of this dry mixture into the butter and sugar, followed by a third of the beaten egg and a third of the milk. Repeat with the remaining flour mixture, egg and milk, until evenly combined.

Scrape the batter into the lined cake tin and dot a third of the blueberries over the top. Bake for 30 minutes, then gently remove the cake from the oven and dot the remaining blueberries over the top. Return the cake to the oven and bake for a further 25–30 minutes, until just firm and a skewer inserted into the centre comes out mostly clean. If the cake is browning too quickly, cover it with foil.

Remove from the oven and leave to cool for 10 minutes, then turn out on to a wire rack and leave to cool completely. Don't worry if the cake sinks a little in the middle, this is exactly as it is meant to be – a moist, dense, rustic cake, laden with berries.

Serve in thick slices, with yogurt on the side.

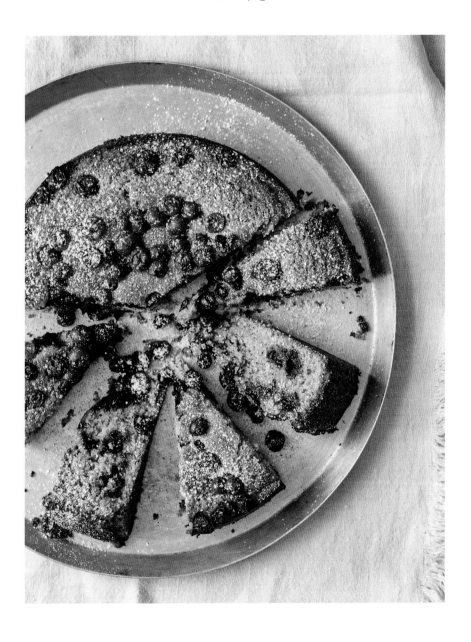

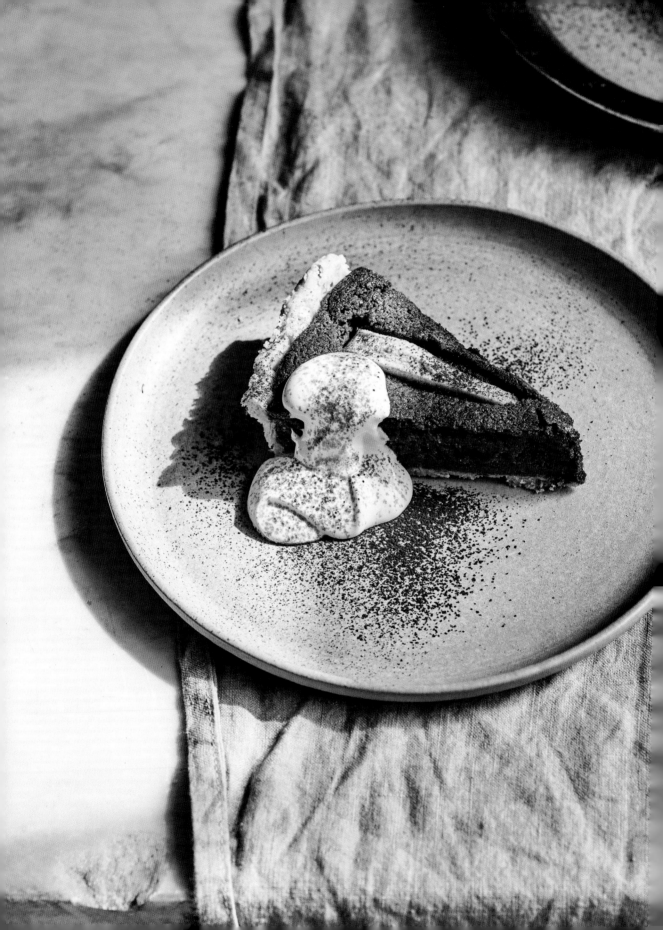

Chocolate + pear tart

Serves 10–12

Save this one for date night or your next dinner party. It looks so impressive and slices like a dream! This recipe also goes a long way too.

320g ready-rolled shortcrust pastry

200g unsalted butter

175g light muscovado sugar

2 tsp vanilla bean paste or extract

Zest of ½ lemon

Pinch of salt

275g ground almonds

3 eggs, beaten

3 tbsp plain white or white spelt flour

100g dark chocolate, minimum 70%

1 pear, peeled, halved lengthways and cored

Cocoa powder, to dust

Yogurt, to serve

Preheat the oven to 180°C fan/400°F/gas mark 6.

Line a 24cm fluted tart tin with the pastry and prick the base with a fork. Line with baking parchment, fill with baking beans, and bake blind for 20 minutes. Remove the paper and beans and bake for a further 5 minutes, until the tart shell is cooked through and biscuity.

Meanwhile, put the butter, sugar, vanilla, lemon zest and a good pinch of salt into a food processor and blitz, until light and fluffy. Add the ground almonds, together with the eggs and flour, and beat together, until thoroughly combined. Melt the chocolate in a heatproof bowl set over a pan of simmering water and fold into the mixture.

Transfer the mixture to the baked tart shell and smooth out. Slice the pear halves lengthways into thin slivers and position in a circle around the top of the tart filling. Bake for about 35 minutes, until the tart has firmed up around the edges, but retains just a little wobble towards the centre.

Leave to cool completely, then turn out of the tin on to a platter. Sift over a little cocoa powder. Serve in slices, with yogurt on the side.

Banana, flax + walnut bread

Serves 8-10

One can never have too many banana bread recipes, right? I've loaded this one up with walnuts and flaxseeds, which adds a boost of essential omega-3 fatty acids.

220g unsalted
butter, at room
temperature

150g light
brown sugar

4 ripe bananas;
peeled, 3 mashed
and 1 left whole

1 tsp vanilla extract

3 eggs, beaten

100g walnuts

2 tbsp flaxseeds,
plus an extra
2 tsp for the top

150g wholemeal flour

2 tsp baking powder

Preheat the oven to 180°C fan/400°F/gas mark 6. Grease a 20cm x 10cm loaf tin and line with baking parchment.

Beat together the butter and sugar, until light and fluffy, at least 5 minutes. Fold in the mashed bananas, vanilla, eggs, walnuts, flaxseeds, flour and baking powder, until thoroughly combined.

Transfer the mixture to the loaf tin and level the top. Scatter over the remaining 2 teaspoons of flaxseeds and gently pat down so they stick to the surface. Cut the remaining banana in half lengthways, and lay on the surface of the loaf. Bake for 50–60 minutes, until golden and firm and a skewer comes out clean. Cover with foil if the loaf browns too quickly.

Remove and leave to cool for 10 minutes, then turn out on to a wire rack.

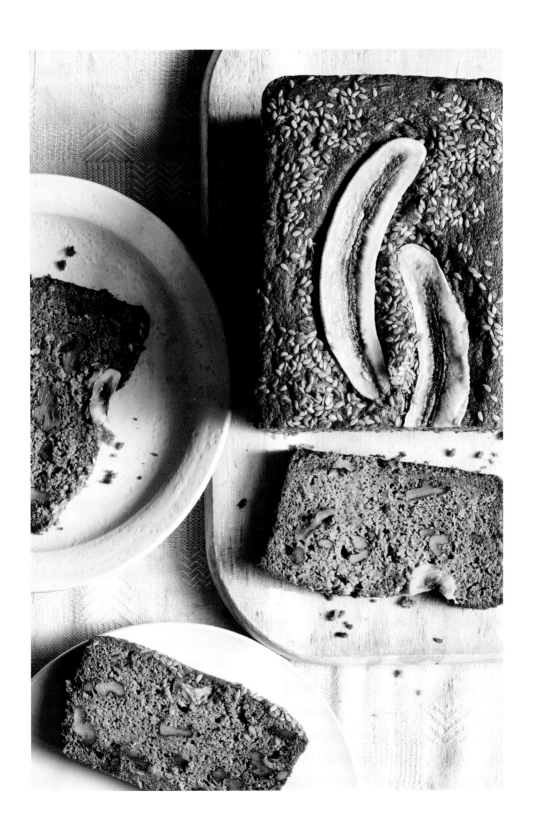

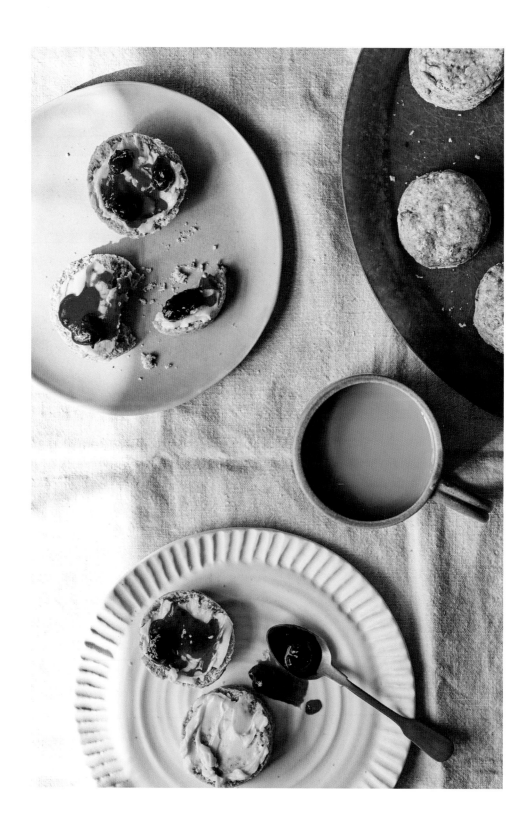

Wholemeal scones

Makes approx. 12

This recipe is a nod to the Irish soda bread my mother and grandmother used to make. Soda bread is one of those utterly simple recipes that requires no yeast or rising time. You can make this as a loaf, but I quite like mine as scones, so that they are easily freezable when making a big batch. Best served with Irish butter and jam, or savoury with cheese and homemade soup.

175g wholemeal flour, plus extra for dusting

1 tbsp caster sugar (optional)

Pinch of salt

175g plain flour

1 tsp baking powder

50g butter (or vegan alternative)

200ml buttermilk (or vegan alternative*)

A little milk or egg, to glaze (optional)

Preheat the oven to 200°C fan/425°F/gas mark 7. Lightly dust a flat baking sheet with flour (any kind).

Put the wholemeal flour, sugar and salt into a large mixing bowl. Sift the plain flour and baking powder into the bowl. Mix together.

Now rub in the butter, using your fingertips. Finally, stir in the buttermilk, to make a soft dough. Turn out on to a lightly floured surface and gently knead for a few seconds. Flatten the dough out and cut out scones (approximately 10) using a scone cutter or an upside-down glass. Place on the baking tray. Brush with a little milk or egg to glaze, if you like.

Bake for 15–20 minutes, until golden (it may need longer if the scones are larger). Remove and leave to cool on a wire tray.

To make vegan buttermilk, add 1 tbsp apple cider vinegar or lemon juice to a plant milk.

Quinoa + chia loaf

Makes 1 loaf

Your gut bugs (and taste buds) will thank you for this bread. Homemade bread can be laborious to make, but that's not the case with this speedy loaf. It's gorgeous with a sweet or savoury topping, dipped in soup or with butter or peanut butter.

200g wholegrain flour

300g plain white or white spelt flour

1 tsp baking powder

1 tsp bicarbonate of soda

1 tsp sea salt

2 tbsp chia seeds, plus more to scatter over

100g cooked quinoa, cooled

1 tbsp maple syrup

520ml water

Preheat the oven to 200°C fan/425°F/gas mark 7. Lightly grease a 23cm x 13cm loaf tin and line with baking parchment.

In a bowl, thoroughly mix together the flours, baking powder, bicarbonate of soda, salt, chia seeds and most of the quinoa. Add the maple syrup and water and mix to combine.

Pour the mixture into the lined loaf tin and scatter over the remaining quinoa and chia seeds. Bake for 50 minutes, then carefully remove the loaf from its tin and continue to bake on its side for a further 10 minutes until it sounds hollow when tapped.

Remove the loaf from the oven and leave to cool completely before slicing.

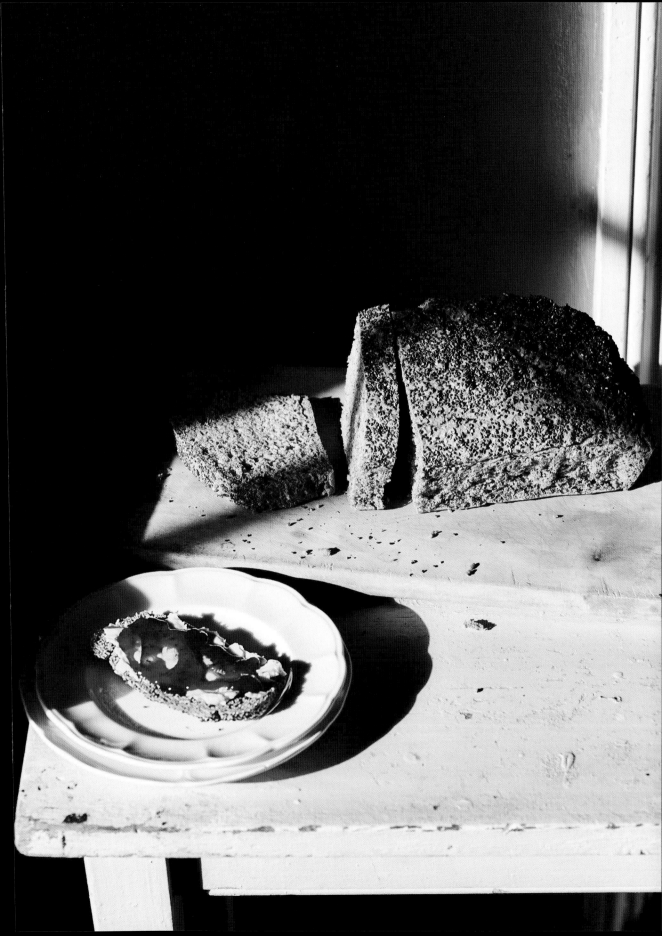

Espresso brownies

If you haven't gathered already, I love my coffee! This recipe calls for only a small amount, so don't fret if you're not a fan, and of course it can be subbed with decaf.

Makes 12–16 brownies, depending on size

200g dark chocolate, 70%, roughly chopped

200g unsalted butter, cubed, plus extra to grease

3 eggs

120g caster sugar

90g light muscovado sugar

3 tbsp espresso or very strong coffee

120g plain white or white spelt flour, sifted

20g cocoa powder, sifted

¼ tsp fine sea salt

Preheat the oven to 170°C fan/375°F/gas mark 5. Grease a 24cm × 16cm baking tray and line with baking parchment.

Put the chocolate and butter into a heatproof bowl over a pan of barely simmering water, ensuring the base of the bowl does not touch the water. Heat gently, stirring occasionally, until the butter and chocolate have melted. Remove and leave to cool.

Meanwhile, use an electric whisk or stand mixer to whisk the eggs and both sugars, until pale and creamy, for at least 5 minutes. Once the melted chocolate and butter has cooled to room temperature, pour it into the egg and sugar mixture with the espresso and whisk on high for another 2 minutes, until glossy.

Fold in the flour, cocoa powder and salt, until thoroughly combined. Transfer to the lined tin and bake for 25–30 minutes, until set and slightly crusty on top and a little gooey in the centre. Remove and leave to cool completely in the tin.

Once cool, transfer to a board and cut into squares. Store in an airtight container for up to 3 days.

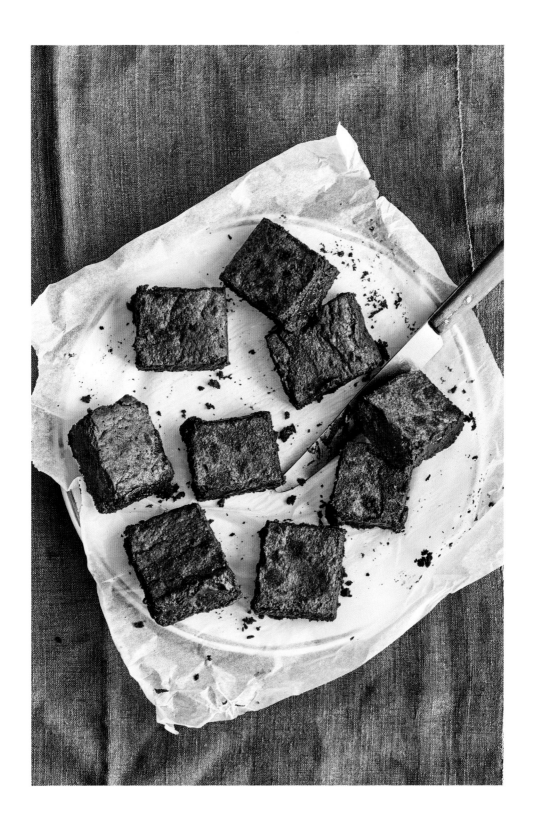

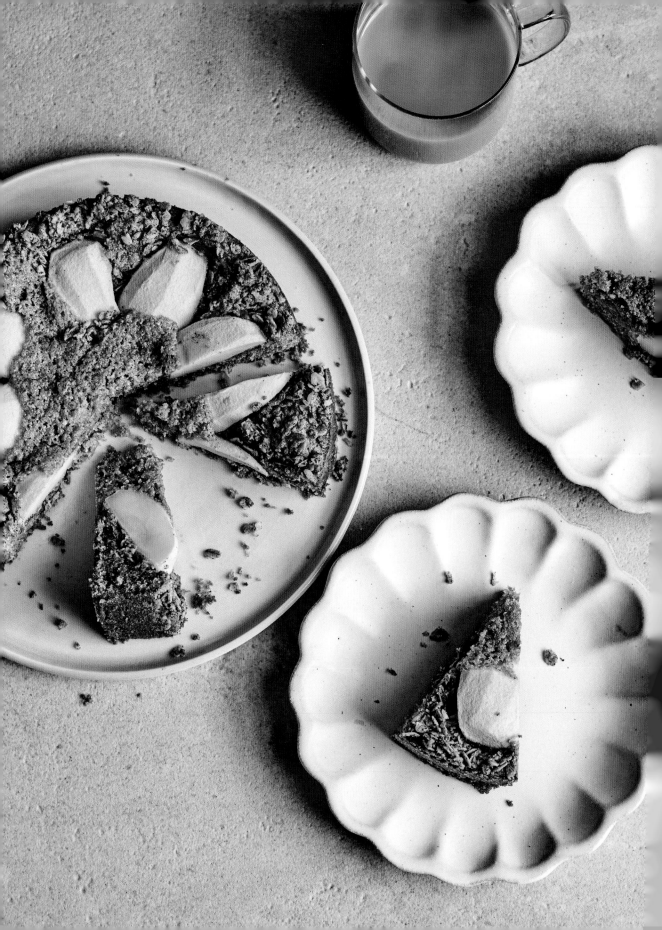

Apple crumble cake

Serves 10–12

Apple crumble was the first recipe I ever learned to make – honest! My mother would make it every Sunday, and so by the time we were school age we all knew how to make the perfect crumb topping. This is not a crumble recipe, however, and is a little more sophisticated, yet still reminiscent of my childhood – Mum, I hope you approve!

180g unsalted butter, at room temperature

150g caster sugar

2 eggs

150g wholemeal flour

2 tsp baking powder

½ tsp fine sea salt

Zest of 1 lemon, plus 1 tbsp juice

1½ tsp ground cinnamon

60g rolled oats

30g brown sugar

2 eating apples

Yogurt, to serve

Preheat the oven to 180°C fan/400°F/gas mark 6. Grease a 20cm round springform tin and line it with baking parchment.

Using an electric mixer, beat 150g of the butter and the sugar together, until light and fluffy. Beat in the eggs, until fully incorporated, then fold in the flour, baking powder, salt, lemon zest and juice and half the ground cinnamon, until fully combined. The mixture will be quite stiff. Transfer to the lined tin and flatten out. Bake for 10 minutes.

Meanwhile, put the oats, brown sugar and the rest of the cinnamon into a bowl and rub in the remaining 30g of butter until you have a crumb consistency. Peel and quarter the apples, then cut away the cores.

Remove the cake from the oven and scatter the crumble over the top, then gently position the apple quarters on top of the cake, curved side facing up, taking care not to press down too firmly.

Bake for a further 30–35 minutes, until golden and a skewer inserted into the centre comes out clean. If the cake is browning too quickly, cover it with foil.

Remove and leave to cool for 10 minutes, then turn out on to a wire rack. Serve while still a little warm, with yogurt dolloped on top.

Appendix 1:
Polycystic Ovary
Syndrome and Endometriosis

Polycystic Ovary Syndrome (PCOS)

PCOS is *the* most common reproductive hormone disorder, affecting 5–10 per cent of women of childbearing age.[1]

Symptoms include	Criteria for diagnosis
• irregular or absent periods • difficulty becoming pregnant (reduced fertility) • dark or thick facial and/or body hair (hirsutism) • acne or oily skin • hair loss from the scalp (alopecia) • having a higher body weight* or difficulty losing weight • depression and anxiety *Though some people with PCOS have a 'normal' BMI (18.5–24.9kg/m2).*	At least two of the following three (Rotterdam) criteria must be met:[2] • Irregular or absent periods. • Evidence of excess androgens (or 'male hormones'), either on a blood test or clinical signs such as excess body/facial hair and/or acne. • Presence of multiple follicles or cysts on the ovaries. (Note: You may have multiple cysts on your ovaries and not necessarily have PCOS, unless symptomatic.)

What causes PCOS?

Multiple factors seem to play a role, including hormones, genetics, environment and lifestyle, as well as how these factors interact with one another. Insulin resistance – where cells are less responsive to insulin – is a common feature in many women with PCOS (the risk is greater if their BMI is greater than 30). Higher levels of insulin in PCOS can interfere with sex hormones, leading to excess testosterone production, which, in turn, causes anovulation (failure of the ovaries to produce eggs) and irregular periods.

How is it treated?

- **Lifestyle:** Weight management, nutrition (see below), regular physical activity (including resistance training), stress management and sleep optimisation.

- **Medication:** A number of medicines are available to manage different symptoms associated with PCOS, such as insulin resistance, irregular/absent periods and ovulation.

Nutrition

- **Carbohydrates:** A low-glycaemic index (GI) diet, which provides a slower release of energy, has been shown to reduce insulin resistance, improving hormone levels and regulating periods in those with PCOS.[3]

- **Omega-3 fatty acids:** This type of fat appears to play a role in reducing inflammation and improving insulin resistance; the opposite is true of diets high in saturated fats and trans fatty acids.[4] Flaxseed (30g/day), which is rich in omega-3, has been shown to improve hormone levels in women with PCOS.[5]

- **Protein:** Research related to protein consumption for women with PCOS is limited, but this may also help with hormone and blood glucose regulation.[6] As this is a filling and satisfying nutrient, eating enough protein is seen to be beneficial for those trying to lose weight.[7]

A note on glycaemic index and glycaemic load

The glycaemic index (or GI) ranks carbohydrates on a scale from 0 to 100, according to the extent to which they raise blood sugar (glucose) levels after eating. Glycaemic load (GL) is a measure that takes into account the amount of carbohydrate in a portion of food, together with how quickly it raises blood glucose levels. In general, high-GI foods are simple and refined carbohydrates, such as white bread, sweets and dried fruit, and low-GI foods are usually complex carbohydrates, like oats, brown rice and rye bread. The GI of a food also depends on the type of food, ripeness, processing, storage, cooking method and other foods that it is eaten with.

Supplements

- **Inositol:** Myo-inositol, either used alone or with D-chiro-inositol (in a ratio of 40:1), may help with improving insulin sensitivity, decreasing testosterone, supporting ovulation and regulating menstrual cycles.

- **Vitamin D** deficiency has been associated with insulin resistance in women with PCOS, and women with PCOS are more likely to be deficient in this vitamin.[8] Combined treatment with vitamin D and calcium has also been shown to be effective in women with PCOS.[9]

Other supplements that have less evidence to back them up include:

- **Chromium picolinate:** May help with insulin sensitivity – with a similar effect to the insulin-sensitising drug metformin.[10]

- **Coenzyme Q10:** May play a role in regulating blood glucose, insulin, hormone and blood lipid levels (in some studies this is combined with vitamin E).[11]

- **Cinnamon:** May help with menstrual regularity and insulin resistance in women. Again, the evidence is not concrete, but if you enjoy it, a cheaper alternative could be to add 1–2 teaspoons of cinnamon to the diet per day. [12]

Endometriosis

Despite the fact that endometriosis affects as many as one in ten women, it takes on average eight years to get a diagnosis.[13]

Endometriosis is a condition where patches of endometrial-like tissue (that normally lines the inside of the uterus/womb) grow in other parts of the body, including the pelvic cavity, on the ovaries, bowel or bladder, and sometimes (but very rarely) on the liver and lungs. As this tissue is similar to that found in the uterus, it still responds to the hormonal fluctuations of the menstrual cycle, and so each month the tissue builds up, breaks down and causes bleeding. This causes inflammation and irritation to the surrounding tissue, leading to pain and often the formation of scar tissue.

Symptoms vary, and also depend on where the endometrial tissue is deposited, but the most common are:

- **painful or heavy periods**
- **abdominal (tummy) and pelvic pain**
- **difficulty getting pregnant**
- **pain during sex**
- **pain when opening your bowels or going for a wee**
- **fatigue**

Some women do not have any symptoms and the severity of disease doesn't always correlate well with the severity of symptoms.

What causes endometriosis?

Unfortunately, the exact cause is unknown, but there are several theories and many possible factors including genetic, immunological, hormonal and lifestyle. If your mum or sister has it, your risk of having it is higher.[14]

How is it diagnosed?

Currently, the only definitive way to diagnose endometriosis is via laparoscopic, or keyhole, surgery to see inside the pelvic cavity. As this is quite invasive, it is one of the reasons why there is a delay from onset of symptoms to diagnosis.

How is it treated?

- **Medication:** Including pain relief, such as anti-inflammatory meds such as NSAIDs, and hormone treatment, such as the pill, the hormonal coil or synthetic hormones (GnRH analogues).
- **Surgery to remove the tissue:** In very severe cases a hysterectomy (removal of the womb) may be required.

Nutrition

- **Omega-3 fatty acids:** Diets rich in omega-3 fatty acids have been associated with a reduced likelihood of developing endometriosis, likely due to their anti-inflammatory effects.[15] Trans fatty acids, found in some processed and deep-fried foods, have the opposite effect and increase the risk of endometriosis.[16]
- **Red and processed meat:** How red meat affects endometriosis is not fully understood, but observational evidence suggests that more than two servings per day increases risk compared to those who ate one or fewer servings per week.[17]
- **Antioxidants,** such as vitamins C and E, and polyphenols, such as those found in black and green tea, turmeric, dark berries and grapes, may also be beneficial in improving symptoms of endometriosis.[18]
- **Dairy:** Studies on dairy and endometriosis are inconclusive. However, most have found no link between the two, and the most recent review of the evidence found that there was a reduced risk of endometriosis with more than three servings of dairy per day.[19] This was especially true for full-fat dairy products.
- **Gluten:** There is no strong evidence to cut out gluten, but some women have reported improvement in symptoms when on a gluten-free diet.[20] Note: this requires a huge dietary overhaul and should be done under the guidance of a dietitian.

Appendix 2:
Glossary of Nutrients

Protein

Carbohydrate

Fat

Vitamin A

B Vitamins

Choline

Vitamin C

Vitamin D

Vitamin E

Vitamin K

Iron

Iodine

Calcium

Zinc

Magnesium

Phosphorus

Potassium

Selenium

Sodium

Chloride

Nutrient	Functions	Recommended Intake	Sources	Important Notes
PROTEIN	• Growth and repair • Maintains body tissues e.g. muscle, bones and skin • Creates enzymes and certain hormones • Needed for many biochemical functions e.g. in our immune system, in our blood, transporting nutrients, etc. • Provides energy (4kcals per gram)	0.75g per kg of body weight per day Athletes and those who train regularly have higher requirements: 1.4–2g of protein per kg of body weight, consumed as 20–40g of protein every 3–4 hours[1]	Animal-based: • meat • poultry • seafood • eggs • dairy Plant-based: • pulses (beans, peas, lentils and chickpeas) • soya-based products e.g. soya milk, tofu and tempeh • seitan and wheat protein • mycoprotein e.g. Quorn • pea protein • nuts and seeds • plant-based protein powders	Top tip: Vegans and vegetarians should consume a variety of protein sources across the day to meet their amino acid needs. What about supplements? Protein supplements are not necessary, but can be convenient and helpful for some people. Always make sure to stick with a high-quality and batch-tested brand.
CARBS Comes in two main forms: simple sugars and complex carbohydrates (including fibre)	• The most efficient source of energy for the body and provides 4kcals per gram • Comes in two main forms: simple sugars and complex carbohydrates (including fibre) • Fibre is important for gut health, regulating bowel movements and stabilising blood glucose. A diet rich in fibre is also linked with a reduced risk of bowel cancer, heart disease, stroke and type 2 diabetes.	Carbohydrate: 50 per cent of daily food energy Free sugars (sugar that is added to foods by the manufacturer, cook or consumer, plus sugars naturally present in honey, syrups and unsweetened fruit juices): no more than 5 per cent of daily food energy Fibre: 30g per day for adults	Starchy carbohydrates: • bread, pitta and wraps • pasta • noodles • rice • cereal • oats • barley • rye • buckwheat • quinoa • couscous • potato Free sugar: • table sugar • sweets • chocolate • cake • sweetened drinks	Are unrefined or natural sugars better? 'Unrefined' or 'natural' sugars like honey, agave nectar, rice syrup and coconut sugar are still free sugars (like table sugar) as they have a very similar impact in the body. Top tip: Consuming a variety of plant-based food (such as 30 different plants each week) provides a variety of fibre for our gut and overall health.

Nutrient	Functions	Recommended Intake	Sources	Important Notes
CARBS (cont...)	• 'Soluble fibre' can also 'mop up' LDL (bad) cholesterol in the body • Free sugar: Sugar that is 'added to foods by the manufacturer, cook or consumer, plus sugars naturally present in honey, syrups and unsweetened fruit juices'.		• honey and syrups • juices Fibre: • whole grains • fruit and vegetables • beans and pulses • nuts and seeds	
FAT Fats can be divided into saturated and unsaturated types. • Unsaturated fats can be monounsaturated (MUFA) or polyunsaturated (PUFA) • Essential fatty acids (omega-3 and -6) are a type of polyunsaturated fat, and are called 'essential' fatty acids as the body cannot make enough.- • ALA (alpha-linoleic acid), EPA (eicosapentaenoic acid) and DHA (docosahexaenoic acid) are the main long-chain omega-3 fatty acids	• Provides energy: 9kcals per gram • Needed to absorb fat-soluble vitamins A, D, E and K • Used to produce certain hormones • Forms part of cell membranes • Unsaturated fats help to regulate cholesterol levels • Omega-3s have anti-inflammatory properties and play a role in healthy brain and nervous system development of the foetus	Total fat: no more than 35 per cent of daily food energy Saturated fat: no more than 10 per cent of daily food energy Trans fat: no more than 2 per cent of daily food energy MUFA: 12 per cent of daily food energy PUFA (EPA and DHA): 0.45g per day PUFA (ALA): at least 0.2 per cent of daily food energy PUFA (linoleic acid – omega-6): at least 1 per cent of daily food energy	**Saturated fat:** • coconut oil • butter • lard • visible fat on meat • cakes • biscuits • pies and pastries • dairy **Trans fat:** Products containing 'partially hydrogenated vegetable oil' and certain fried foods and takeaways. *(Due to changes by the food industry, the average trans fat intake in the UK is well within the recommended limit.)*[2] MUFA: • olive oil • rapeseed oil • sunflower oil • nuts and seeds Omega-3: DHA and EPA: • salmon • mackerel • kippers	**Top tip:** As oily fish is the best source of omega-3, vegans and vegetarians are often recommended to consider supplementing this nutrient. Omega-3 is found in seaweed, but a high intake of seaweed can provide too much iodine. Some plant-based omega-3 (ALA) is converted into EPA and DHA, but only in small amounts.

Nutrient	Functions	Recommended Intake	Sources	Important Notes
FAT (cont..)			• sardines • herring • trout • crab • seaweed Omega-3: ALA: • rapeseed oil • soya bean oil • flax and chia seeds • walnuts • soya products e.g. edamame beans, tofu and tempeh PUFA: omega-6: • meat • eggs • sunflower oil • corn oil • safflower oil	
Vitamin A Two forms of vitamin A are available in the human diet: preformed vitamin A (retinol) and provitamin A carotenoids (beta carotene)	• Supports vision in low light • Maintains skin and membrane health (e.g. the lining of the nose) • Supports the immune system • Cell communication • Supports fertility and reproductive health	Females: 600mcg per day Pregnancy: 700mcg per day Breastfeeding: 950mcg per day Males: 700mcgs per day	Retinol: • offal e.g. liver and kidney • oily fish and fish liver oil • dairy • eggs • fortified spreads Beta carotene: • sweet potato • red pepper • carrot • green leafy vegetables e.g. spinach • tomato • mango • apricot • papaya • cantaloupe melon	Consuming excess vitamin A in the form of retinol can lead to: stomach pain, nausea, vomiting, irritability, headaches, skin issues and liver damage. Having more than 1.5mg (1,500mcg) per day consistently may worsen bone health and increase fracture risk. We are advised to eat liver or liver pâté no more than once per week to avoid consuming too much vitamin A. A high intake of vitamin A can harm an unborn baby, so pregnant women or those planning a pregnancy are advised to avoid supplements containing vitamin A, liver and liver-containing products like pâté.

Nutrient	Functions	Recommended Intake	Sources	Important Notes
B Vitamins Thiamin (B1) Riboflavin (B2) Niacin (B3) Pantothenic acid (B5) Vitamin B6 Biotin (B7) Folate (B9) Vitamin B12	Thiamin (B1): • Involved in breaking down and releasing energy from food • Cell growth and function • Needed for a healthy nervous system Riboflavin (B2): • Involved in releasing energy from food • Eye, skin and nervous system health • Supports cell growth and function Niacin (B3): • Involved in releasing energy from food • Skin and nervous system health • Supports cell function and communication Pantothenic acid (B5): • Involved in releasing energy Vitamin B6: • Using and storing energy from food • Involved in many enzyme reactions and in creating neurotransmitters (chemical messengers in the brain) • Forms haemoglobin (a protein that carries oxygen around the body) • Involved in immune function	Thiamin (B1): • Females: 0.8mg per day • Pregnancy: 0.9mg per day • Breastfeeding: 1mg per day • Males: 1mg per day or 0.9mg per day if 50 or over Riboflavin (B2): • Females: 1.1mg per day • Pregnancy: 1.4mg per day • Breastfeeding: 1.6mg per day • Males: 1.3mg per day Niacin (B3): • Females: 13mg per day, 12mg per day if 50 or over • Breastfeeding: 15mg per day • Males: 17mg per day or 16mg if 50 or over Pantothenic acid (B5): • Adults: 3–7mg per day is estimated to be adequate Vitamin B6: • Females: 1.2mg per day • Males: 1.4mg per day Biotin (B7): • Adults: 10–200mcg per day is considered safe and adequate	Thiamin (B1): • certain fortified cereals • whole grains • nuts and seeds • peas • pork • liver Riboflavin (B2): • dairy • eggs • mushrooms • fortified drinks and breakfast cereals • whole grains • meat and liver • seafood Niacin (B3): • red meat and liver • poultry • fish • eggs • whole grains • peanuts Pantothenic acid (B5): • certain fortified cereals • nuts • sunflower seeds • whole grains • dairy • meat • liver • eggs • avocado • mushrooms Vitamin B6: • certain fortified cereals • oats • meat • liver • tuna	Folic acid in pregnancy: **The UK government advise all women who could become pregnant to take 400mcg of folic acid per day prior to conception and until the twelfth week of pregnancy. Based on their medical and pregnancy history, some women are advised to take a higher dose of 5mg per day.[3] Folic acid is the synthetic form of folate found in most supplements and fortified foods. Women who carry a specific genetic mutation may be recommended to take an 'activated' or 'methylated' form of folate called 5methyltetrahydro-folate (5MTHF). Top tip: The best sources of vitamin B12 are animal products, so this is an important nutrient for vegans to supplement.

Nutrient	Functions	Recommended Intake	Sources	Important Notes
B Vitamins (cont...)	Biotin (B7): • Creates fatty acids • Obtains energy from food • Genetic function and cell signalling • Supports keratin, a protein found in our skin, hair and nails Folate (B9): • Creates healthy red blood cells • Involved in DNA production and cell division • Reduces the risk of neural tube defects in unborn babies, such as spina bifida Vitamin B12: • Keeps nerve and red blood cells healthy, including producing the fatty layer that covers nerves (myelin) • Releases energy from food • DNA formation	Folate (B9): • Adults: 200mcg per day • Pregnancy: 300mcgper day** • Breastfeeding: 260mcg per day Vitamin B12: • Adults: 1.5mcg per day • Breastfeeding: 2mcg per day	• nuts • seeds • dairy • avocado Biotin (B7): • nuts • seeds • dairy • meat • liver • salmon • gut bacteria can also create biotin Folate (B9): • fortified cereals • green vegetables like kale, cabbage, broccoli, Brussels sprouts, lettuce and spinach • beans and peas Vitamin B12: • meat • seafood • dairy products • eggs • turkey • fortified products including: nutritional yeast, certain cereals and drinks	

Nutrient	Functions	Recommended Intake	Sources	Important Notes
Choline	• Involved in brain health and function, including creation of an important chemical messenger in the brain called acetylcholine • Cell signalling, cell membranes and lipid transport • Needed for healthy brain development during pregnancy	Women: 425mg per day Pregnant women: 450mg per day Breastfeeding women: 550mg per day Men: 550mg per day	• meat • liver • eggs • potatoes • whole grains • beans, especially soya beans *Our bodies can create some choline in the liver, but not enough to meet our requirements, so it is an essential nutrient to include in our diet.*	Top tip: Animal-based foods contain higher levels of choline, so vegans may need to pay extra attention to ensure they consume enough.
Vitamin C	• Maintains healthy tissues e.g. blood vessels, skin, bone and cartilage • Important for wound healing • Antioxidant properties • Improves iron absorption from plant-based foods (i.e. haem iron) • Important for a healthy immune system	Adults: 40mg per day In the third trimester of pregnancy: 50mg per day Breastfeeding women: 70mg per day	• orange • lemon • kiwi • mango • blackcurrant • papaya • melon • strawberry • peppers • green leafy vegetables e.g. broccoli, Brussels sprouts, cabbage and kale • potato and sweet potato • liver	Should I supplement? Most people can easily meet their vitamin C requirements by consuming a variety of fruit and vegetables each day. Taking large amounts (more than 1,000mg per day) of vitamin C through supplements can lead to diarrhoea, stomach pain and a higher risk of kidney stones.
Vitamin D	• Regulates calcium and phosphate levels, which has a knock-on important role in bone, teeth and muscle health • Involved in our immune response and glucose metabolism • Plays a role in cell growth and differentiation	Adults: 10mcg per day	• oily fish and cod liver oil • egg yolks • liver • fortified drinks, spreads and cereals • mushrooms grown in UV light • sunlight	Should I supplement? As it is difficult to obtain enough vitamin D from our diet, the UK government recommends that children over four and adults take a 10mcg vitamin D supplement during the autumn and winter. This is recommended year-round for those who don't get much sunlight on their skin and for those who have dark skin.

Nutrient	Functions	Recommended Intake	Sources	Important Notes
Vitamin E	• Antioxidant i.e. helps to balance free radical levels in the body • Eye and skin health • Involved in our immune system • Plays a role in metabolic processes such as cell signalling • Involved in blood vessel dilation and reducing blood clotting	Women: 3mg per day Pregnancy: 3.8–6.2mg per day Breastfeeding: 3.8–6.2mg per day Men: 4mg per day	• rapeseed oil • olive oil • sunflower oil • corn oil • soya bean oil • safflower oil • nuts e.g. peanuts, almonds and hazelnuts • seeds e.g. sunflower seeds • wheatgerm and whole grains	A very high intake of vitamin E from supplements may be harmful. The NHS advises that up to 540mg of vitamin E from supplements is unlikely to cause harm.[4]
Vitamin K	• Blood clotting and wound healing • Supports bone, cartilage and muscle health	Adults: 1mcg per kg of body weight per day	• green leafy vegetables (like spinach, kale, broccoli, collard and turnip greens) • soya beans and (fermented soya beans) • soya bean oil • olive oil • rapeseed oil • whole grains • pine and cashew nuts • blueberries and grapes	Most healthy people should be able to reach their recommended daily intake through diet. Our gut bacteria can also make vitamin K for the body to use. Caution: Vitamin K is also involved in blood clotting and so foods that are very high in vitamin K can affect the action of blood, thinning medications such as warfarin, making them less efficient. You don't need to avoid them but you should try to maintain a regular and relatively constant amount without big changes. Those taking warfarin should not take vitamin K supplements.

Nutrient	Functions	Recommended Intake	Sources	Important Notes
Iron There are two main forms of iron: haem and non-haem	• Creates proteins that carry oxygen around the body (haemoglobin and myoglobin) • Needed for growth and brain development in babies and children • Involved in the creation of certain hormones and a healthy immune system	Women (from 11–50 years old): 14.8mg per day Women over 50: 8.7mg per day Men: 8.7mg per day	Haem iron: • red meat • liver Non-haem iron: • fortified cereals • eggs • beans, lentils and chickpeas • tofu • green leafy vegetables like spinach and chard • nuts • seeds • spirulina • dried fruit e.g. apricots, figs, raisins	Haem iron is found in animal-based products. Non-haem iron is found mostly in plant-based products and is more difficult for the body to access and use. See page 26 for tips on how to increase absorption.
Iodine	• Needed to create thyroid hormones which play an essential role in our metabolism • Involved in the brain and bone development of a foetus and baby • Supports fertility	Adults: 140mcg per day (Note: the European Food Safety Authority (EFSA) recommends higher intakes of 200mcg for pregnant and breastfeeding women)	• milk • yogurt • haddock and cod • seaweed • scampi and oysters • eggs • certain fortified drinks • iodised salt	Seafood, milk and yogurt are the main sources of iodine in the UK diet, therefore vegans may benefit from supplements in the form of potassium iodate or potassium iodide (the dose should not be above the daily recommended intake). There is a possible risk of consuming too much iodine from supplements and types of seaweed.

Nutrient	Functions	Recommended Intake	Sources	Important Notes
Calcium	• For healthy bones and teeth • Muscle, nerve and blood vessel function • Involved in hormone secretion	Adults : 700mg per day Breastfeeding women: 1250mg per day Post-menopausal women and men over 55 years of age: 1200mg/day Those with coeliac disease/osteoporosis/ inflammatory bowel disease (IBD): 1000mg/day[5]	• dairy products • certain fortified drinks, yogurts and cereals • green leafy vegetables like kale, pak choi and okra • tahini • calcium-set tofu • dried fig • nuts and seeds • fortified flour and bread • tinned fish with bones like sardines and pilchards	Vitamin D and magnesium are needed for calcium absorption. A high intake of calcium from supplements may increase the risk of hardening the arteries over time.[6]
Zinc	• Wound healing • Immune system function • Making DNA and proteins • Growth of babies and children • Involved in our senses of taste and smell	Women: 7mg per day Pregnant women: 13mg per day Breastfeeding women: 9.5mg per day Men: 9.5mg per day	• meat • dairy, especially cheese • shellfish • beans and chickpeas • nuts • seeds • whole grains • beans and lentils	Top tip: Leavened bread and sprouted beans, chickpeas and lentils may help to increase zinc absorption.
Magnesium	• Healthy muscle and nerve function • Bone health related to calcium absorption, vitamin D and parathyroid function • DNA and protein creation • Regulating blood pressure and blood glucose • Converting food to energy • Regulating certain hormones and neurotransmitters (chemical messengers)	Women: 270mg per day Pregnant or breastfeeding women: 320mg per day Men: 300mg per day	• seeds, especially pumpkin • nuts • spinach • soya beans • black beans • whole grains • dark chocolate	Magnesium supplements can cause diarrhoea (especially at doses >400mg) and also interact or interfere with some medicines and compete for absorption with other minerals like iron and zinc.

Nutrient	Functions	Recommended Intake	Sources	Important Notes
Phosphorus	• Needed for our bones, teeth, DNA and cell membranes • Combines with calcium in the bones and in teeth • Converts energy from food • Enzyme function • pH balance	Adults: 550mg per day Pregnant or breastfeeding women: 990mg per day	• dairy products • meat • fish • tofu • eggs • beans and pulses • whole grains • potatoes (with skin) • nuts • seeds	
Potassium	• Needed for normal cell function and maintaining fluid balance • Heart and kidney function • Muscle contraction and nerve transmission	Adults: 3,500mg per day	• banana • dried fruit • tomatoes • potatoes • avocado • beetroot • beans and pulses • nuts • seeds • dairy • meat • fish	
Selenium	• Supports a healthy immune system • Involved in thyroid function • Involved in DNA production • Supports fertility • Antioxidant properties	Women: 60mcg per day Pregnant or breastfeeding women: 75mcg per day Men: 75mcg per day	• nuts, especially Brazil nuts • seeds • meat • fish • eggs • beans and pulses	Selenium content varies between different regions due to differences in the soil. The best sources of selenium are animal-based foods, with the exception of Brazil nuts. In fact, in some cases just one Brazil nut can contain our daily selenium requirements.

Nutrient	Functions	Recommended Intake	Sources	Important Notes
Sodium	• Balances fluid and pH levels • Regulates blood pressure • Transports and absorbs nutrients • Muscle contraction and relaxation • Nerve signalling	Adults: 1600mg per day (no more than 2.4g per day) Salt: no more than 6g per day	• salt • soy sauce • stock cubes • gravy • crisps • salted nuts • pickled food • processed meat like bacon and salami • cheese • many takeaways and ready meals	Salt is a combination of sodium and chloride. A high intake of salt is linked with increased blood pressure, which may increase the risk of heart disease, as well as a higher risk of stomach cancer and kidney stones. The average UK intake of salt is significantly above the recommended limit of 6g per day.[7]
Chloride	• Balances fluid and pH levels • Maintains blood pressure • Movement of nutrients in and out of cells • Nerve and red blood cell function • Muscle and heart contraction • Production of stomach acid – vital for digestion	Adults: 2,500mg per day	• Mainly found in salt and salty foods (listed above) • Found in smaller amounts in meat, fish and plant-based products	

Note: RNI = reference nutrient intake: this is the amount of a nutrient that is needed to meet the needs of nearly all a group (97.5 per cent). UK adult RNIs and nutrition requirements from the Committee on the Medical Aspects of Food Policy (COMA) and the Scientific Advisory Committee on Nutrition (SACN) are provided here. Please note that recommended intakes are based on population recommendations for adults – please seek individual advice where needed.[8]

References

Introduction

[1] Beery, A. K. and Zucker, I., 2011. Sex bias in neuroscience and biomedical research. *Neuroscience & Biobehavioral Reviews*, 35(3), pp. 565–72. Available at https://www.sciencedirect.com/science/article/abs/pii/S0149763410001156.

[2] Ibid.

[3] Zucker, I. and Prendergast, B. J., 2020. Sex differences in pharmacokinetics predict adverse drug reactions in women. *Biology of Sex Differences*, 11, pp. 1–14. Available at https://www.ncbi.nlm.nih.gov/pmc/articles/PMC7275616/.

[4] United States General Accounting Office, 2001. Drug Safety: Most Drugs withdrawn in recent years had greater health risks. Available at https://books.google.co.uk/books?hl=en&lr=&id=aj__g6FJs7YC&oi=fnd&pg=PA7&ots=gB-UOdGegC&sig=6L1cgqrqoeVAEzP2jqXTYshXpS4&redir_esc=y#v=onepage&q&f=false; Liu, K. A. and Dipietro Mager, N. A., 2016. Women's involvement in clinical trials: Historical perspective and future implications. Pharmacy Practice (Granada), 14(1), p. 708. Available at https://www.ncbi.nlm.nih.gov/pmc/articles/PMC4800017/#ref27.

[5] Soldin, O. P. and Mattison, D. R., 2009. Sex differences in pharmacokinetics and pharmacodynamics. *Clinical Pharmacokinetics*, 48(3), pp. 143–57. Available at https://www.ncbi.nlm.nih.gov/pmc/articles/PMC3644551/; Anderson, G. D., 2008. Gender differences in pharmacological response. International Review of Neurobiology, 83, pp. 1–10. Available at https://www.sciencedirect.com/science/article/abs/pii/S0074774208000019.

[6] UK Clinical Research Collaboration, 2015. UK health research analysis 2014. Available at https://www.ukcrc.org/wp-content/uploads/2015/08/UKCRCHealthResearchAnalysis2014-WEB.pdf; Public Health England, 26 Jun. 2018. Survey reveals women experience severe reproductive health issues. Available at https://www.gov.uk/government/news/survey-reveals-women-experience-severe-reproductive-health-issues.

[7] Bougie, O., Yap, M. I., Sikora, L., Flaxman, T. and Singh, S., 2019. Influence of race/ethnicity on prevalence and presentation of endometriosis: A systematic review and meta-analysis. BJOG: *An International Journal of Obstetrics & Gynaecology*, 126(9), pp. 1104–15. Available at https://obgyn.onlinelibrary.wiley.com/doi/abs/10.1111/1471-0528.15692.

[8] World Health Organization, 11 Jun. 2021. Cardiovascular diseases. Available at https://www.who.int/news-room/fact-sheets/detail/cardiovascular-diseases-(cvds).

[9] Miller, D. I., Nolla, K. M., Eagly, A. H. and Uttal, D. H., 2018. The development of children's gender-science stereotypes: A meta-analysis of 5 decades of US draw-a-scientist studies. *Child Development*, 89(6), pp. 1943–55. Available at https://srcd.onlinelibrary.wiley.com/doi/full/10.1111/cdev.13039.

[10] Caldwell, E. F. and Wilbraham, S. J., 2018. Hairdressing in space: Depiction of gender in science books for children. *Journal of Science & Popular Culture*, 1(2), pp. 101–18. Available at https://www.ingentaconnect.com/contentone/intellect/jspc/2018/00000001/00000002/art00002.

[11] https://www.jci.org/articles/view/142029

[12] https://www.liebertpub.com/doi/10.1089/trgh.2017.0004

[13] https://pubmed.ncbi.nlm.nih.gov/21294024/

CH 01 - Nutrition

[1] Barroso, F., Allard, S., Kahan, B. C., Connolly, C., Smethurst, H., Choo, L., Khan, K. and Stanworth, S., 2011. Prevalence of maternal anaemia and its predictors: A multi-centre study. *European Journal of Obstetrics & Gynecology and Reproductive Biology*, 159(1), pp. 99–105. Available at https://pubmed.ncbi.nlm.nih.gov/21890259/; Stevens, G. A., Finucane, M. M., De-Regil, L. M., Paciorek, C. J., Flaxman, S. R., Branca, F., Peña-Rosas, J. P., Bhutta, Z. A., Ezzati, M. and Nutrition Impact Model Study Group, 2013. Global, regional, and national trends in haemoglobin concentration and prevalence of total and severe anaemia in children and pregnant and non-pregnant women for 1995–2011: A systematic analysis of population-representative data. *The Lancet Global Health*, 1(1), pp. e16–25. Available at https://www.ncbi.nlm.nih.gov/pmc/articles/PMC4547326/.

[2] Benton, M. J., Hutchins, A. M. and Dawes, J. J., 2020. Effect of menstrual cycle on resting metabolism: A systematic review and meta-analysis. *PloS One*, 15(7), p. e0236025. Available at https://journals.plos.org/plosone/article?id=10.1371/journal.pone.0236025.

[3] Dye, L. and Blundell, J. E., 1997. Menstrual cycle and appetite control: Implications for weight regulation. *Human Reproduction*, 12(6), pp. 1142–51. Available at https://pubmed.ncbi.nlm.nih.gov/9221991/; Davidsen, L., Vistisen, B. and Astrup, A., 2007. Impact of the menstrual cycle on determinants of energy balance: A putative role in weight loss attempts. *International Journal of Obesity*, 31(12), pp. 1777–85. Available at https://pubmed.ncbi.nlm.nih.gov/17684511/.

[4] Davidsen, L., Vistisen, B. and Astrup, A., 2007. Impact of the menstrual cycle on determinants of energy balance: A putative role in weight loss attempts. *International Journal of Obesity*, 31(12), pp. 1777–85. Available at https://pubmed.ncbi.nlm.nih.gov/17684511/; Gorczyca, A. M., Sjaarda, L. A., Mitchell, E. M., Perkins, N. J., Schliep, K. C., Wactawski-Wende, J. and Mumford, S. L., 2016. Changes in macronutrient, micronutrient, and food group intakes throughout the menstrual cycle in healthy, premenopausal women. *European Journal of Nutrition*, 55(3), pp. 1181–8. Available at https://pubmed.ncbi.nlm.nih.gov/26043860/.

[5] Hill, A. J. and Heaton-Brown, L., 1994. The experience of food craving: A prospective investigation in healthy women. *Journal of Psychosomatic Research*, 38(8), pp. 801–14. Available at https://pubmed.ncbi.nlm.nih.gov/7722960/; Weingarten, H. P. and Elston, D., 1991. Food cravings in a college population. *Appetite*, 17(3), pp. 167–75. Available at https://pubmed.ncbi.nlm.nih.gov/1799279/.

[6] Hallam, J., Boswell, R. G., DeVito, E. E. and Kober, H., 2016. Gender-related differences in food craving and obesity. *Yale Journal of Biology and Medicine*, 89(2), pp. 161–73. Available at https://pubmed.ncbi.nlm.nih.gov/27354843/.

[7] Valdes, C. T. and Elkind-Hirsch, K. E., 1991. Intravenous glucose tolerance test-derived insulin sensitivity changes during the menstrual cycle. *Journal of Clinical Endocrinology & Metabolism*, 72(3), pp. 642–6. Available at https://pubmed.ncbi.nlm.nih.gov/1997519/; Pulido, J. M. E. and Salazar, M. A., 1999. Changes in insulin sensitivity, secretion and glucose effectiveness during menstrual cycle. *Archives of Medical Research*, 30(1), pp. 19–22. Available at https://pubmed.ncbi.nlm.nih.gov/10071420/.

[8] Hallam, J., Boswell, R. G., DeVito, E. E. and Kober, H., 2016. Gender-related differences in food craving and obesity. *Yale Journal of Biology and Medicine*, 89(2), pp. 161–73. Available at https://pubmed.ncbi.nlm.nih.gov/27354843/.

[9] Ibid.

[10] Davidsen, L., Vistisen, B. and Astrup, A., 2007. Impact of the menstrual cycle on determinants of energy balance: A putative role in weight loss attempts. *International Journal of Obesity*, 31(12), pp. 1777–85. Available at https://pubmed.ncbi.nlm.nih.gov/17684511/.

[11] Ibid.

[12] Gallo, M. F., Lopez, L. M., Grimes, D. A., Carayon, F., Schulz, K. F. and Helmerhorst, F. M., 2014. Combination contraceptives: effects on weight. *Cochrane Database of Systematic Reviews*, (1). Available at https://www.cochranelibrary.com/cdsr/doi/10.1002/14651858.CD003987.pub5/full.

[13] Houghton, S. C., Manson, J. E., Whitcomb, B. W., Hankinson, S. E., Troy, L. M., Bigelow, C. and Bertone-Johnson, E. R., 2018. Carbohydrate and fiber intake and the risk of premenstrual syndrome. *European Journal of Clinical Nutrition*, 72(6), pp. 861–70. Available at https://pubmed.ncbi.nlm.nih.gov/29379144/.

[14] Quaranta, S., Buscaglia, M. A., Meroni, M. G., Colombo, E. and Cella, S., 2007. Pilot study of the efficacy and safety of a modified-release magnesium 250mg tablet (Sincromag®) for the treatment of premenstrual syndrome. *Clinical Drug Investigation*, 27(1), pp. 51–8. Available at https://pubmed.ncbi.nlm.nih.gov/17177579/; Walker, A. F., De Souza, M. C., Vickers, M. F., Abeyasekera, S., Collins, M. L. and Trinca, L. A., 1998. Magnesium supplementation alleviates premenstrual symptoms of fluid retention. *Journal of Women's Health*, 7(9), pp. 1157–65. Available at https://pubmed.ncbi.nlm.nih.gov/9861593/.

[15] Fathizadeh, N., Ebrahimi, E., Valiani, M., Tavakoli, N. and Yar, M. H., 2010. Evaluating the effect of magnesium and magnesium plus vitamin B6 supplement on the severity of premenstrual syndrome. *Iranian Journal of Nursing and Midwifery Research*, 15(Suppl1), pp. 401–5. Available at https://pubmed.ncbi.nlm.nih.gov/22069417/.

[16] Chocano-Bedoya, P. O., Manson, J. E., Hankinson, S. E., Johnson, S. R., Chasan-Taber, L., Ronnenberg, A. G., Bigelow, C. and Bertone-Johnson, E. R., 2013. Intake of selected minerals and risk of premenstrual syndrome. *American Journal of Epidemiology*, 177(10), pp. 1118–27. Available at https://www.ncbi.nlm.nih.gov/pmc/articles/PMC3649635/.

[17] Abdi, F., Ozgoli, G. and Rahnemaie, F. S., 2019. A systematic review of the role of vitamin D and calcium in premenstrual syndrome. *Obstetrics & Gynecology Science*, 62(2), pp. 73–86. Available at https://www.ncbi.nlm.nih.gov/pmc/articles/PMC6422848/.

[18] Shobeiri, F., Araste, F. E., Ebrahimi, R., Jenabi, E. and Nazari, M., 2017. Effect of calcium on premenstrual syndrome: A double-blind randomized clinical trial. *Obstetrics & Gynecology Science*, 60(1), pp. 100–5. Available at https://www.ncbi.nlm.nih.gov/pmc/articles/PMC5313351/.

[19] Chocano-Bedoya, P. O., Manson, J. E., Hankinson, S. E., Willett, W. C., Johnson, S. R., Chasan-Taber, L., Ronnenberg, A. G., Bigelow, C. and Bertone-Johnson, E. R., 2011. Dietary B vitamin intake and incident premenstrual syndrome. *American Journal of Clinical Nutrition*, 93(5), pp. 1080–6. Available at https://pubmed.ncbi.nlm.nih.gov/21346091/.

[20] Wyatt, K. M., Dimmock, P. W., Jones, P. W. and O'Brien, P. S., 1999. Efficacy of vitamin B-6 in the treatment of premenstrual syndrome: Systematic review. *BMJ*, 318(7195), pp. 1375–81. Available at https://pubmed.ncbi.nlm.nih.gov/10334745/; BMJ Best Practice, 1 Nov. 2019. Premenstrual syndrome and dysphoric disorder. Available at https://bestpractice.bmj.com/topics/en-gb/419#referencePop59.

[21] van Die, M. D., Burger, H. G., Teede, H. J. and Bone, K. M., 2013. Vitex agnus-castus extracts for female reproductive disorders: A systematic review of clinical trials. *Planta Medica*, 79(07), pp. 562–75. Available at https://pubmed.ncbi.nlm.nih.gov/23136064/.

[22] Huntley, A. L. and Ernst, E., 2004. Soy for the treatment of perimenopausal symptoms – a systematic review. *Maturitas*, 47(1), pp. 1–9. Available at https://pubmed.ncbi.nlm.nih.gov/14706760/; Kim, H. W., Kwon, M. K., Kim, N. S. and Reame, N. E., 2006. Intake of dietary soy isoflavones in relation to perimenstrual symptoms of Korean women living in the USA. *Nursing & Health Sciences*, 8(2), pp. 108–13. Available at https://pubmed.ncbi.nlm.nih.gov/16764563/. https://obgyn.onlinelibrary.wiley.com/doi/epdf/10.1111/jog.15217

[23] Vander Borght, M. and Wyns, C., 2018. Fertility and infertility: Definition and epidemiology. *Clinical Biochemistry*, 62, pp. 2–10. Available at https://pubmed.ncbi.nlm.nih.gov/29555319/.

[24] Salas-Huetos, A., Babio, N., Carrell, D. T., Bulló, M. and Salas-Salvadó, J., 2019. Adherence to the Mediterranean diet is positively associated with sperm motility: A cross-sectional analysis. *Scientific Reports*, 9(1), pp. 1–8. Available at https://www.nature.com/articles/s41598-019-39826-7; Toledo, E., Lopez-del Burgo, C., Ruiz-Zambrana, A., Donazar, M., Navarro-Blasco, Í., Martínez-González, M.A. and de Irala, J., 2011. Dietary patterns and difficulty conceiving: A nested case-control study. *Fertility and Sterility*, 96(5), pp. 1149–53. Available at https://pubmed.ncbi.nlm.nih.gov/21943725/; Karayiannis, D., Kontogianni, M. D., Mendorou, C., Mastrominas, M. and Yiannakouris, N., 2018. Adherence to the Mediterranean diet and IVF success rate among non-obese women attempting fertility. *Human Reproduction*, 33(3), pp. 494–502. Available at https://pubmed.ncbi.nlm.nih.gov/29390148/; Vujkovic, M., de Vries, J. H., Lindemans, J., Macklon, N. S., van der Spek, P. J., Steegers, E. A. and Steegers-Theunissen, R. P., 2010. The preconception Mediterranean dietary pattern in couples undergoing in vitro fertilization/intracytoplasmic sperm injection treatment increases the chance of pregnancy. *Fertility and Sterility*, 94(6), pp. 2096–101. Available at https://pubmed.ncbi.nlm.nih.gov/20189169/.

[25] Eslamian, G., Amirjannati, N., Rashidkhani, B., Sadeghi, M. R., Baghestani, A. R. and Hekmatdoost, A., 2015. Dietary fatty acid intakes and asthenozoospermia: A case-control study. *Fertility and Sterility*, 103(1), pp. 190–8. Available at https://pubmed.ncbi.nlm.nih.gov/25456794/; Chiu, Y. H., Karmon, A. E., Gaskins, A. J., Arvizu, M., Williams, P. L., Souter, I., Rueda, B. R., Hauser, R., Chavarro, J.E. and EARTH Study Team, 2018. Serum omega-3 fatty acids and treatment outcomes among women undergoing assisted reproduction. *Human Reproduction*, 33(1), pp. 156–65. Available at https://pubmed.ncbi.nlm.nih.gov/29136189/; Esmaeili, V., Shahverdi, A. H., Moghadasian, M. H. and Alizadeh, A., 2015. Dietary fatty acids affect semen quality: A review. *Andrology*, 3(3), pp. 450–61. Available at https://pubmed.ncbi.nlm.nih.gov/25951427/; Chavarro, J. E., Rich-Edwards, J. W., Rosner, B. A. and Willett, W. C., 2007. Dietary fatty acid intakes and the risk of ovulatory infertility. *American Journal of Clinical Nutrition*, 85(1), pp. 231–7. Available at https://pubmed.ncbi.nlm.nih.gov/17209201/.

[26] Chavarro, J. E., Rich-Edwards, J. W., Rosner, B. A. and Willett, W. C., 2008. Protein intake and ovulatory infertility. *American Journal of Obstetrics and Gynecology*, 198(2), pp. 210–e1. Available at https://pubmed.ncbi.nlm.nih.gov/18226626/.

[27] Chavarro, J. E., Rich-Edwards, J. W., Rosner, B. A. and Willett, W. C., 2007. Diet and lifestyle in the prevention of ovulatory disorder infertility. *Obstetrics & Gynecology*, 110(5), pp. 1050–8. Available at https://pubmed.ncbi.nlm.nih.gov/17978119/.

[28] Nehra, D., Le, H. D., Fallon, E. M., Carlson, S. J., Woods, D., White, Y. A., Pan, A. H., Guo, L., Rodig, S. J., Tilly, J. L. and Rueda, B. R., 2012. Prolonging the female reproductive lifespan and improving egg quality with dietary omega-3 fatty acids. *Aging Cell*, 11(6), pp. 1046–54. Available at https://pubmed.ncbi.nlm.nih.gov/22978268/.

[29] Agarwal, A., Gupta, S. and Sikka, S., 2006. The role of free radicals and antioxidants in reproduction. *Current Opinion in Obstetrics and Gynecology*, 18(3), pp. 325–32. Available at https://pubmed.ncbi.nlm.nih.gov/16735834/.

[30] Salas-Huetos, A., Rosique-Esteban, N., Becerra-Tomás, N., Vizmanos, B., Bulló, M. and Salas-Salvadó, J., 2018. The effect of nutrients and dietary supplements on sperm quality parameters: A systematic review and meta-analysis of randomized clinical trials. *Advances in Nutrition*, 9(6), pp. 833–48. Available at https://pubmed.ncbi.nlm.nih.gov/30462179/; Grieger, J. A., Grzeskowiak, L. E., Wilson, R. L., Bianco-Miotto, T., Leemaqz, S. Y., Jankovic-Karasoulos, T., Perkins, A. V., Norman, R. J., Dekker, G. A. and Roberts, C. T., 2019. Maternal selenium, copper and zinc concentrations in early pregnancy, and the association with fertility. *Nutrients*, 11(7), p. 1609. Available at https://www.ncbi.nlm.nih.gov/pmc/articles/PMC6683068/; Ahmadi, S., Bashiri, R., Ghadiri-Anari, A. and Nadjarzadeh, A., 2016. Antioxidant supplements and semen parameters: An evidence-based review. *International Journal of Reproductive BioMedicine*, 14(12), pp. 729–36. Available at https://www.ncbi.nlm.nih.gov/pmc/articles/PMC5203687/.

[31] Showell, M. G., Mackenzie-Proctor, R., Jordan, V. and Hart, R. J., 2020. Antioxidants for female subfertility. *Cochrane Database of Systematic Reviews*, (8). Available at https://www.cochranelibrary.com/cdsr/doi/10.1002/14651858.CD007807.pub3/full; Gaskins, A. J. and Chavarro, J. E., 2018. Diet and fertility: A review. *American Journal of Obstetrics and Gynecology*, 218(4), pp. 379–89. Available at https://www.sciencedirect.com/science/article/abs/pii/S0002937817309456.

[32] Florou, P., Anagnostis, P., Theocharis, P., Chourdakis, M. and Goulis, D. G., 2020. Does coenzyme Q 10 supplementation improve fertility outcomes in women undergoing assisted reproductive technology procedures? A systematic review and meta-analysis of randomized-controlled trials. *Journal of Assisted Reproduction and Genetics*, 37(10), pp. 2377–87. Available at https://pubmed.ncbi.nlm.nih.gov/32767206/; Salvio, G., Cutini, M., Ciarloni, A., Giovannini, L., Perrone, M. and Balercia, G., 2021. Coenzyme Q10 and male infertility: A systematic review. *Antioxidants*, 10(6), p. 874. Available at https://www.ncbi.nlm.nih.gov/pmc/articles/PMC8226917/.

[33] Chen, J. H., Lin, X., Bu, C. and Zhang, X., 2018. Role of advanced glycation end products in mobility and considerations in possible dietary and nutritional intervention strategies. *Nutrition & Metabolism*, 15(1), pp. 1–18. Available at https://www.ncbi.nlm.nih.gov/pmc/articles/PMC6180645/.

[34] Ibid.

[35] Chavarro, J. E., Rich-Edwards, J. W., Rosner, B. A. and Willett, W. C., 2007. Diet and lifestyle in the prevention of ovulatory disorder infertility. *Obstetrics & Gynecology*, 110(5), pp. 1050–8. Available at https://pubmed.ncbi.nlm.nih.gov/17978119/; Hahn, K. A., Wesselink, A. K., Wise, L. A., Mikkelsen, E. M., Cueto, H. T., Tucker, K. L., Vinceti, M., Rothman, K. J., Sorensen, H. T. and Hatch, E. E., 2019. Iron consumption is not consistently associated with fecundability among North American and Danish pregnancy planners. *Journal of Nutrition*, 149(9), pp. 1585–95. Available at https://academic.oup.com/jn/article/149/9/1585/5510077.

[36] Geerligs, P. P., Brabin, B. J. and Omari, A. A. A., 2003. Food prepared in iron cooking pots as an intervention for reducing iron deficiency anaemia in developing countries: A systematic review. *Journal of Human Nutrition and Dietetics*, 16(4), pp. 275–81. Available at https://pubmed.ncbi.nlm.nih.gov/12859709/.

[37] The British Dietetic Association, May 2019. Iodine: Food fact sheet. Available at https://www.bda.uk.com/resource/iodine.html; Fallon, N. and Dillon, S. A., 2020. Low intakes of iodine and selenium amongst vegan and vegetarian women highlight a potential nutritional vulnerability. *Frontiers in Nutrition*, 7, p. 72. Available at https://www.ncbi.nlm.nih.gov/pmc/articles/PMC7251157/.

[38] The British Dietetic Association, 10 May 2021. A clinical update on diet and fertility. Available at https://www.bda.uk.com/resource/a-clinical-update-on-diet-and-fertility.html.

[39] Chu, J., Gallos, I., Tobias, A., Tan, B., Eapen, A. and Coomarasamy, A., 2018. Vitamin D and assisted reproductive treatment outcome: A systematic review and meta-analysis. *Human Reproduction*, 33(1), pp. 65–80. Available at https://academic.oup.com/humrep/article/33/1/65/4582928?login=true.

[40] British Nutrition Foundation, Aug. 2019. Nutrition requirements. Available at https://archive.nutrition.org.uk/attachments/article/907/Nutrition%20Requirements_Revised%20August%202019.pdf.

[41] Ibid.

[42] European Food Safety Authority (EFSA), 23 Sep. 2019. Dietary reference values for nutrients: Summary report. Available at https://efsa.onlinelibrary.wiley.com/doi/pdf/10.2903/sp.efsa.2017.e15121.

[43] NHS, 4 Dec. 2018. Fish and shellfish. Available at https://www.nhs.uk/live-well/eat-well/fish-and-shellfish-nutrition/#:~:text=You%20can%20give%20boys%20up,baby%20during%20a%20future%20pregnancy

[44] The British Dietetic Association, May 2019. Iodine: Food fact sheet. Available at https://www.bda.uk.com/resource/iodine.html.

[45] American Society of Hematology, n.d. Anemia and pregnancy. Available at https://www.hematology.org/education/patients/anemia/pregnancy.

[46] Rahmati, S., Azami, M., Badfar, G., Parizad, N. and Sayehmiri, K., 2020. The relationship between maternal anemia during pregnancy with preterm birth: A systematic review and meta-analysis. *Journal of Maternal-Fetal & Neonatal Medicine*, 33(15), pp. 2679–89. Available at https://pubmed.ncbi.nlm.nih.gov/30522368/; Rahmati, S., Delpishe, A., Azami, M., Ahmadi, M. R. H. and Sayehmiri, K., 2017. Maternal anemia during pregnancy and infant low birth weight: A systematic review and meta-analysis. *International Journal of Reproductive Biomedicine*, 15(3), pp. 125–34. Available at https://www.ncbi.nlm.nih.gov/pmc/articles/PMC5447828/.

[47] The British Dietetic Association, 1 Feb. 2021. Pregnancy and diet: Food fact sheet. Available at https://www.bda.uk.com/resource/pregnancy-diet.html.

[48] Räikkönen, K., Martikainen, S., Pesonen, A. K., Lahti, J., Heinonen, K., Pyhälä, R., Lahti, M., Tuovinen, S., Wehkalampi, K., Sammallahti, S. and Kuula, L., 2017. Maternal licorice consumption during pregnancy and pubertal, cognitive, and psychiatric outcomes in children. *American Journal of Epidemiology*, 185(5), pp. 317–28. Available at https://academic.oup.com/aje/article/185/5/317/2967089.

[49] Grosso, G., Godos, J., Galvano, F. and Giovannucci, E. L., 2017. Coffee, caffeine, and health outcomes: An umbrella review. *Annual Review of Nutrition*, 37, pp. 131–56. Available at https://pubmed.ncbi.nlm.nih.gov/28826374/.

[50] NHS, 30 Sep. 2019. Severe vomiting in pregnancy. Available at https://www.nhs.uk/pregnancy/related-conditions/complications/severe-vomiting/.

[51] Bustos, M., Venkataramanan, R. and Caritis, S., 2017. Nausea and vomiting of pregnancy –What's new? *Autonomic Neuroscience*, 202, pp. 62–72. Available at https://www.ncbi.nlm.nih.gov/pmc/articles/PMC5107351/.

[52] Thomson, M., Corbin, R. and Leung, L., 2014. Effects of ginger for nausea and vomiting in early pregnancy: A meta-analysis. *Journal of the American Board of Family Medicine*, 27(1), pp. 115–22. Available at https://pubmed.ncbi.nlm.nih.gov/24390893/.

[53] Vazquez, J. C., 2015. Heartburn in pregnancy. *BMJ Clinical Evidence*, p. 1411. Available at https://www.ncbi.nlm.nih.gov/pmc/articles/PMC4562453/.

[54] European Food Safety Authority (EFSA), 25 Mar. 2010. Specific opinion on dietary reference values for water. Available at https://www.efsa.europa.eu/en/efsajournal/pub/1459.

[55] British Nutrition Foundation, Nov. 2016. Breastfeeding – an introduction. Available at https://www.nutrition.org.uk/life-stages/baby/breastfeeding/breastfeeding-an-introduction/?level=Consumer.

[56] NHS, 15 Oct. 2021. Alcohol units. Available at https://www.nhs.uk/live-well/alcohol-support/calculating-alcohol-units/.

[57] Polotsky, H. N. and Polotsky, A. J., 2010. Metabolic implications of menopause. *Seminars in Reproductive Medicine*, 28(5), pp. 426–34. Available at https://pubmed.ncbi.nlm.nih.gov/20865657/.

[58] Toth, M. J., Tchernof, A., Sites, C. K. and Poehlman, E. T., 2000. Menopause-related changes in body fat distribution. *Annals of the New York Academy of Sciences*, 904(1), pp. 502–6. Available at https://pubmed.ncbi.nlm.nih.gov/10865795/#:~:text=Postmenopausal%20women%20had%2036%25%20more,%3C%200.05)%20than%20premenopausal%20women.

[59] Polotsky, H. N. and Polotsky, A. J., 2010. Metabolic implications of menopause. *Seminars in Reproductive Medicine*, 28(5), pp. 426–34. Available at https://pubmed.ncbi.nlm.nih.gov/20865657/.

[60] Li, Q., Wang, X., Ni, Y., Hao, H., Liu, Z., Wen, S., Shao, X., Wu, X., Yu, W. and Hu, W., 2019. Epidemiological characteristics and risk factors of T2DM in Chinese premenopausal and postmenopausal women. *Lipids in Health and Disease*, 18(1), pp. 1–8. Available at https://lipidworld.biomedcentral.com/articles/10.1186/s12944-019-1091-7.

[61] Millett, E. R., Peters, S. A. and Woodward, M., 2018. Sex differences in risk factors for myocardial infarction: Cohort study of UK Biobank participants. *BMJ*, 363. Available at https://www.bmj.com/content/363/bmj.k4247.

[62] Aune, D., Keum, N., Giovannucci, E., Fadnes, L. T., Boffetta, P., Greenwood, D. C., Tonstad, S., Vatten, L. J., Riboli, E. and Norat, T., 2016. Whole grain consumption and risk of cardiovascular disease, cancer, and all cause and cause specific mortality: Systematic review and dose-response meta-analysis of prospective studies. *BMJ*, 353, p. i2716. Available at https://pubmed.ncbi.nlm.nih.gov/27301975/.

[63] McRae, M. P., 2017. Dietary fiber is beneficial for the prevention of cardiovascular disease: An umbrella review of meta-analyses. *Journal of Chiropractic Medicine*, 16(4), pp. 289–99. Available at https://pubmed.ncbi.nlm.nih.gov/29276461/.

[64] Gunness, P. and Gidley, M. J., 2010. Mechanisms underlying the cholesterol-lowering properties of soluble dietary fibre polysaccharides. *Food & Function*, 1(2), pp. 149–55. Available at https://pubmed.ncbi.nlm.nih.gov/21776465/.

[65] Blanco Mejia, S., Messina, M., Li, S. S., Viguiliouk, E., Chiavaroli, L., Khan, T. A., Srichaikul, K., Mirrahimi, A., Sievenpiper, J. L., Kris-Etherton, P. and Jenkins, D. J., 2019. A meta-analysis of 46 studies identified by the FDA demonstrates that soy protein decreases circulating LDL and total cholesterol concentrations in adults. *Journal of Nutrition*, 149(6), pp. 968–81. Available at https://www.ncbi.nlm.nih.gov/pmc/articles/PMC6543199/.

[66] Del Gobbo, L. C., Falk, M. C., Feldman, R., Lewis, K. and Mozaffarian, D., 2015. Effects of tree nuts on blood lipids, apolipoproteins, and blood pressure: Systematic review, meta-analysis, and dose-response of 61 controlled intervention trials. *American Journal of Clinical Nutrition*, 102(6), pp. 1347–56. Available at https://pubmed.ncbi.nlm.nih.gov/26561616/.

[67] He, F. J., Li, J. and MacGregor, G. A., 2013. Effect of longer-term modest salt reduction on blood pressure. *Cochrane Database of Systematic Reviews*, (4). Available at https://pubmed.ncbi.nlm.nih.gov/23633321/; Cogswell, M. E., Mugavero, K., Bowman, B. A. and Frieden, T. R., 2016. Dietary sodium and cardiovascular disease risk – measurement matters. *New England Journal of Medicine*, 375(6), pp. 580–6. Available at https://www.ncbi.nlm.nih.gov/pmc/articles/PMC5381724/.

[68] Musa-Veloso, K., Poon, T. H., Elliot, J. A. and Chung, C., 2011. A comparison of the LDL-cholesterol lowering efficacy of plant stanols and plant sterols over a continuous dose range:

Results of a meta-analysis of randomized, placebo-controlled trials. *Prostaglandins, Leukotrienes and Essential Fatty Acids*, 85(1), pp .9–28. Available at https://pubmed.ncbi.nlm.nih.gov/21345662/.

[69] Heart UK, n.d. Six cholesterol-lowering foods. Available at https://www.heartuk.org.uk/healthy-living/cholesterol-lowering-foods.

[70] The British Dietetic Association, Jul. 2017. Calcium: Food fact sheet. Available at https://www.bda.uk.com/uploads/assets/b1f5f83d-fdd0-41be-b7ef16c174fdcbc8/Calcium2017-food-fact-sheet.pdf.

[71] The British Dietetic Association, 8 Jun. 2021. Calcium: Food fact sheet. Available at https://www.bda.uk.com/resource/calcium.html.

[72] Rizzoli, R., Stevenson, J. C., Bauer, J. M., van Loon, L. J., Walrand, S., Kanis, J. A., Cooper, C., Brandi, M. L., Diez-Perez, A. and Reginster, J. Y., 2014. The role of dietary protein and vitamin D in maintaining musculoskeletal health in postmenopausal women: A consensus statement from the European Society for Clinical and Economic Aspects of Osteoporosis and Osteoarthritis (ESCEO). Maturitas, 79(1), pp. 122–32. Available at https://pubmed.ncbi.nlm.nih.gov/25082206/.

[73] Palermo, A., Tuccinardi, D., D'Onofrio, L., Watanabe, M., Maggi, D., Maurizi, A. R., Greto, V., Buzzetti, R., Napoli, N., Pozzilli, P. and Manfrini, S., 2017. Vitamin K and osteoporosis: Myth or reality? Metabolism, 70, pp. 57–71. Available at https://www.researchgate.net/publication/313357045_Vitamin_K_and_Osteoporosis_Myth_or_Reality.

[74] Movassagh, E. Z. and Vatanparast, H., 2017. Current evidence on the association of dietary patterns and bone health: A scoping review. Advances in Nutrition, 8(1), pp. 1–16. Available at https://academic.oup.com/advances/article/8/1/1/4566585#110893649.

[75] Bansal, R. and Aggarwal, N., 2019. Menopausal hot flashes: A concise review. Journal of Mid-life Health, 10(1), p. 6. Available at https://www.ncbi.nlm.nih.gov/pmc/articles/PMC6459071/.

[76] Freedman, R. R., 2005. Hot flashes: Behavioral treatments, mechanisms, and relation to sleep. The American Journal of Medicine, 118(12), pp. 124–30. Available at https://pubmed.ncbi.nlm.nih.gov/16414337/.

[77] Kandiah, J. and Amend, V., 2010. An exploratory study on perceived relationship of alcohol, caffeine, and physical activity on hot flashes in menopausal women. Health, 2(9), p. 989. Available at https://www.scirp.org/journal/paperinformation.aspx?paperid=2617; Pimenta, F., Leal, I., Maroco, J. and Ramos, C., 2011. Perceived control, lifestyle, health, socio-demographic factors and menopause: Impact on hot flashes and night sweats. Maturitas, 69(4), pp. 338–42. Available at https://pubmed.ncbi.nlm.nih.gov/21680119/.

[78] Hunter, M. S., Gupta, P., Chedraui, P., Blümel, J. E., Tserotas, K., Aguirre, W., Palacios, S. and Sturdee, D. W., 2012. The international menopause study of climate, altitude, temperature (IMS-CAT) and vasomotor symptoms. Climacteric, 16(1), pp. 8–16. Available at https://pubmed.ncbi.nlm.nih.gov/22946508/.

[79] Bacciottini, L., Falchetti, A., Pampaloni, B., Bartolini, E., Carossino, A. M. and Brandi, M.L., 2007. Phytoestrogens: Food or drug? Clinical Cases in Mineral and Bone Metabolism, 4(2), pp. 123–30. Available at https://www.ncbi.nlm.nih.gov/pmc/articles/PMC2781234/; Taku, K., Melby, M. K., Kronenberg, F., Kurzer, M. S. and Messina, M., 2012. Extracted or synthesized soybean isoflavones reduce menopausal hot flash frequency and severity: Systematic review and meta-analysis of randomized controlled trials. Menopause, 19(7), pp. 776–90. Available at https://pubmed.ncbi.nlm.nih.gov/22433977/.

[80] National Institute for Health and Care Excellence, 5 Dec. 2019. Menopause: Diagnosis and Management. Available at https://www.nice.org.uk/guidance/ng23/chapter/Recommendations#long-term-benefits-and-risks-of-hormone-replacement-therapy.

[81] Hickey, M., Elliott, J. and Davison, S. L., 2012. Hormone replacement therapy. BMJ, 344. Available at https://www.bmj.com/content/344/bmj.e763/rapid-responses.

[82] Collaborative Group on Epidemiological Studies of Ovarian Cancer, 2015. Menopausal hormone use and ovarian cancer risk: Individual participant meta-analysis of 52 epidemiological studies. The Lancet, 385(9980), pp. 1835–42. Available at https://www.thelancet.com/journals/lancet/article/PIIS0140-6736(14)61687-1/fulltext.

[83] Grady, D., Gebretsadik, T., Kerlikowske, K., Ernster, V. and Petitti, D., 1995. Hormone replacement therapy and endometrial cancer risk: A meta-analysis. Obstetrics & Gynecology, 85(2), pp. 304–13. Available at https://pubmed.ncbi.nlm.nih.gov/7824251/.

[84] National Institute for Health and Care Excellence, 5 Dec. 2019. Menopause: Diagnosis and Management. Available at https://www.nice.org.uk/guidance/ng23/chapter/Recommendations#long-term-benefits-and-risks-of-hormone-replacement-therapy.

[85] Vinogradova, Y., Dening, T., Hippisley-Cox, J., Taylor, L., Moore, M. and Coupland, C., 2021. Use of menopausal hormone therapy and risk of dementia: Nested case-control studies using QResearch and CPRD databases. BMJ, 374. Available at https://www.bmj.com/content/374/bmj.n2182.

[86] National Institute for Health and Care Excellence, 5 Dec. 2019. Menopause: Diagnosis and Management. Available at https://www.nice.org.uk/guidance/ng23/chapter/Recommendations#long-term-benefits-and-risks-of-hormone-replacement-therapy.

[87] Archer, D. F., 2012. Postmenopausal skin and estrogen. *Gynecological Endocrinology*, 28(sup2), pp. 2–6. Available at https://pubmed.ncbi.nlm.nih.gov/22849791/.

[88] Mørch, L. S., Lidegaard, Ø., Keiding, N., Løkkegaard, E. and Kjær, S. K., 2016. The influence of hormone therapies on colon and rectal cancer. *European Journal of Epidemiology*, 31(5), pp. 481–9. Available at https://pubmed.ncbi.nlm.nih.gov/26758900/.

[89] National Institute for Health and Care Excellence, 5 Dec. 2019. Menopause: Diagnosis and Management. Available at https://www.nice.org.uk/guidance/ng23/chapter/Recommendations#long-term-benefits-and-risks-of-hormone-replacement-therapy.

[90] Ibid.

[91] Ibid.

CH 02 - Movement

[1] Longman, J., 23 Jun. 1996. How the women won. *New York Times Magazine*. Available at https://www.nytimes.com/1996/06/23/magazine/how-the-women-won.html.

[2] International Olympic Committee, 3 Nov. 2019. In Amsterdam in 1928… Available at https://olympics.com/en/news/in-amsterdam-in-1928-lina-radke-was-the-first-female-olympic-800m-champion-but.

[3] Kathrineswitzer.com, n.d. The real story. Available at https://kathrineswitzer.com/1967-boston-marathon-the-real-story/.

[4] International Olympic Committee, 14 Aug. 2021. The women that wowed. Available at https://olympics.com/en/news/the-women-that-wowed-at-tokyo-2020; Cowley, E. S., Olenick, A. A., McNulty, K. L. and Ross, E. Z., 2021. 'Invisible sportswomen': The sex data gap in sport and exercise science research. *Women in Sport and Physical Activity Journal*, 29(2), pp. 146–51. Available at https://www.researchgate.net/publication/354739161_Invisible_Sportswomen_The_Sex_Data_Gap_in_Sport_and_Exercise_Science_Research.

[5] Cowley, E. S., Olenick, A. A., McNulty, K. L. and Ross, E. Z., 2021. 'Invisible sportswomen': The sex data gap in sport and exercise science research. *Women in Sport and Physical Activity Journal*, 29(2), pp. 146–51. Available at https://journals.humankinetics.com/view/journals/wspaj/29/2/article-p146.xml.

[6] Craft, B. B., Carroll, H. A. and Lustyk, M. K. B., 2014. Gender differences in exercise habits and quality of life reports: Assessing the moderating effects of reasons for exercise. *International Journal of Liberal Arts and Social Science*, 2(5), pp. 65–76. Available at https://www.ncbi.nlm.nih.gov/pmc/articles/PMC5033515/.

[7] Devries, M. C., Hamadeh, M. J., Phillips, S. M. and Tarnopolsky, M. A., 2006. Menstrual cycle phase and sex influence muscle glycogen utilization and glucose turnover during moderate-intensity endurance exercise. *American Journal of Physiology-Regulatory, Integrative and Comparative Physiology*, 291(4), pp. R1120–8. Available at https://pubmed.ncbi.nlm.nih.gov/16690766/; Willett, H. N., Koltun, K. J. and Hackney, A. C., 2021. Influence of menstrual cycle estradiol-□-17 fluctuations on energy substrate utilization-oxidation during aerobic, endurance exercise. *International Journal of Environmental Research and Public Health*, 18(13), p. 7209. Available at https://pubmed.ncbi.nlm.nih.gov/34281146/.

[8] Tiller, N. B., Elliott-Sale, K. J., Knechtle, B., Wilson, P. B., Roberts, J. D. and Millet, G. Y., 2021. Do sex differences in physiology confer a female advantage in ultra-endurance sport? *Sports Medicine*, 51(5), pp. 895–915. Available at https://pubmed.ncbi.nlm.nih.gov/33502701/; Lariviere, F., Moussalli, R. and Garrel, D. R., 1994. Increased leucine flux and leucine oxidation during the luteal phase of the menstrual cycle in women. *American Journal of Physiology-Endocrinology and Metabolism*, 267(3), pp. E422–8. Available at https://pubmed.ncbi.nlm.nih.gov/7943222/; Sawai, A., Tsuzuki, K., Yamauchi, M., Kimura, N., Tsushima, T., Sugiyama, K., Ota, Y., Sawai, S. and Tochikubo, O., 2020. The effects of estrogen and progesterone on plasma amino acids levels: Evidence from change plasma amino acids levels during the menstrual cycle in women. *Biological Rhythm Research*, 51(1), pp. 151–64. Available at https://www.tandfonline.com/doi/abs/10.1080/09291016.2018.1526496.

[9] Hallam, J., Boswell, R. G., DeVito, E. E. and Kober, H., 2016. Gender-related differences in food craving and obesity. *Yale Journal of Biology and Medicine*, 89(2), pp. 161–73. Available at https://pubmed.ncbi.nlm.nih.gov/27354843/.

[10] Kirchengast, S. and Huber, J., 2001. Body composition characteristics and body fat distribution in lean women with polycystic ovary syndrome. *Human Reproduction*, 16(6), pp. 1255-60. Available at https://academic.oup.com/humrep/article/16/6/1255/619529.

[11] Bean, A., 2017. *The Complete Guide to Sports Nutrition*. Bloomsbury [8th edition].

[12] Nedungadi, T. P. and Clegg, D. J., 2009. Sexual dimorphism in body fat distribution and risk for cardiovascular diseases. *Journal of Cardiovascular Translational Research*, 2(3), pp. 321–7. Available at https://www.researchgate.net/profile/Thekkethil-Nedungadi/publication/44684678_Sexual_Dimorphism_in_Body_Fat_Distribution_and_Risk_for_Cardiovascular_Diseases/links/004635314b9e75e32b000000/Sexual-Dimorphism-in-Body-Fat-Distribution-and-Risk-for-Cardiovascular-Diseases.pdf

[13] Gehlsen, G. and Albohm, M., 1980. Evaluation of sports bras. *The Physician and Sportsmedicine*, 8(10), pp. 88–97. Available at https://www.tandfonline.com/doi/abs/10.1080/00913847.1980.11948653.

[14] Brown, N., White, J., Brasher, A. and Scurr, J., 2014. The experience of breast pain (mastalgia) in female runners of the 2012 London Marathon and its effect on exercise behaviour. *British Journal of Sports Medicine*, 48(4), pp. 320–5. Available at https://pubmed.ncbi.nlm.nih.gov/23603819/.

[15] Scurr, J. C., White, J. L. and Hedger, W., 2011. Supported and unsupported breast displacement in three dimensions across treadmill activity levels. *Journal of Sports Sciences*, 29(1), pp. 55–61. Available at https://pubmed.ncbi.nlm.nih.gov/21077006/; Bridgman, C., Scurr, J., White, J., Hedger, W. and Galbraith, H., 2010. Three-dimensional kinematics of the breast during a two-step star jump. *Journal of Applied Biomechanics*, 26(4), pp. 465–72. Available at https://www.researchgate.net/publication/49765482_Three-Dimensional_Kinematics_of_the_Breast_During_a_Two-Step_Star_Jump.

[16] McGhee, D. E. and Steele, J. R., 2020. Biomechanics of breast support for active women. *Exercise and Sport Sciences Reviews*, 48(3), pp. 99–109. Available at https://pubmed.ncbi.nlm.nih.gov/32271181/.

[17] McGhee, D. E. and Steele, J. R., 2020. Biomechanics of breast support for active women. *Exercise and Sport Sciences Reviews*, 48(3), pp. 99–109. Available at https://journals.lww.com/acsm-essr/fulltext/2020/07000/biomechanics_of_breast_support_for_active_women.1.aspx.

[18] McGhee, D. E. and Steele, J. R., 2010. Breast elevation and compression decrease exercise-induced breast discomfort. *Medicine and Science in Sports and Exercise*, 42(7), pp. 1333–8. Available at https://pubmed.ncbi.nlm.nih.gov/20019639/.

[19] McGhee, D. E. and Steele, J. R., 2020. Biomechanics of breast support for active women. *Exercise and Sport Sciences Reviews*, 48(3), pp. 99–109. Available at https://pubmed.ncbi.nlm.nih.gov/32271181/; Coltman, C. E., McGhee, D. E. and Steele, J. R., 2015. Bra strap orientations and designs to minimise bra strap discomfort and pressure during sport and exercise in women with large breasts. *Sports Medicine – Open*, 1(21), pp. 1–8. Available at https://sportsmedicine-open.springeropen.com/articles/10.1186/s40798-015-0014-z.

[20] Anthony, K., 29 Sep. 2018. Breast asymmetry. *Healthline*. Available at https://www.healthline.com/health/breast-asymmetry.

[21] Parthasarathi, V., Raaja Priya, T., Sivaranjani, S. and Dhivya, A., 2016. Design and development of sports intimate apparel – a review. *Smart Moves Journal Ijosthe*, 3(1). Available at https://ijosthe.com/index.php/ojssports/article/view/52.

[22] Norris, M., Blackmore, T., Horler, B. and Wakefield-Scurr, J., 2021. How the characteristics of sports bras affect their performance. *Ergonomics*, 64(3), pp. 410–25. Available at https://pubmed.ncbi.nlm.nih.gov/32981459/.

[23] Cancer Research UK, n.d. Breast cancer statistics. Available at https://www.cancerresearchuk.org/health-professional/cancer-statistics/statistics-by-cancer-type/breast-cancer#:~:text=A%20person's%20risk%20of%20developing,in%20the%20UK%20are%20preventable.

[24] Janssen, I., Heymsfield, S. B., Wang, Z. and Ross, R., 2000. Skeletal muscle mass and distribution in 468 men and women aged 18–88 yr. *Journal of Applied Physiology*, 89(1), pp. 81–8. Available at https://journals.physiology.org/doi/full/10.1152/jappl.2000.89.1.81.

[25] Staron, R. S., Hagerman, F. C., Hikida, R. S., Murray, T. F., Hostler, D. P., Crill, M. T., Ragg, K. E. and Toma, K., 2000. Fiber type composition of the vastus lateralis muscle of young men and women. *Journal of Histochemistry & Cytochemistry*, 48(5), pp. 623–9. Available at https://journals.sagepub.com/doi/10.1177/002215540004800506?url_ver=Z39.88-2003&rfr_id=ori%3Arid%3Acrossref.org&rfr_dat=cr_pub++0pubmed&.

[26] Tarnopolsky, M. A., 2008. Sex differences in exercise metabolism and the role of 17-beta estradiol. *Medicine and Science in Sports and Exercise*, 40(4), pp. 648–54. Available at https://pubmed.ncbi.nlm.nih.gov/18317381/; Hunter, S. K., 2014. Sex differences in human fatigability: Mechanisms and insight to physiological responses. *Acta Physiologica*, 210(4), pp. 768–89. Available at https://www.ncbi.nlm.nih.gov/pmc/articles/PMC4111134/; Hicks, A. L., Kent-Braun, J. and Ditor, D. S., 2001. Sex differences in human skeletal muscle fatigue. *Exercise and Sport Sciences Reviews*, 29(3), pp. 109–12. Available at https://pubmed.ncbi.nlm.nih.gov/11474957/.

27 Smith, G. I. and Mittendorfer, B., 2012. Similar muscle protein synthesis rates in young men and women: Men aren't from Mars and women aren't from Venus. *Journal of Applied Physiology*, 112(11), pp. 1803–4. Available at https://journals.physiology.org/doi/full/10.1152/japplphysiol.00354.2012.

28 Alway, S. E., Grumbt, W. H., Gonyea, W. J. and Stray-Gundersen, J., 1989. Contrasts in muscle and myofibers of elite male and female bodybuilders. *Journal of Applied Physiology*, 67(1), pp. 24–31. Available at https://journals.physiology.org/doi/pdf/10.1152/jappl.1989.67.1.24.

29 Miller, A. E. J., MacDougall, J. D., Tarnopolsky, M. A. and Sale, D. G., 1993. Gender differences in strength and muscle fiber characteristics. European *Journal of Applied Physiology and Occupational Physiology*, 66(3), pp. 254–62. Available at https://pubmed.ncbi.nlm.nih.gov/8477683/.

30 Hilton, E. N. and Lundberg, T. R., 2021. Transgender women in the female category of sport: Perspectives on testosterone suppression and performance advantage. *Sports Medicine*, 51(2), pp. 199–214. Available at https://link.springer.com/article/10.1007/s40279-020-01389-3.

31 Dworkin, S. L., 2001. 'Holding back': Negotiating a glass ceiling on women's muscular strength. *Sociological Perspectives*, 44(3), pp. 333–50. Available at https://www.jstor.org/stable/10.1525/sop.2001.44.3.333.

32 Larry Kenney, W., Wilmore, J. H. and Costill, D. L., 2011. *Physiology of Sport and Exercise*. Human Kinetics Publishers [5th edition].

33 Abrams, S. A., 2003. Normal acquisition and loss of bone mass. *Hormone Research in Paediatrics*, 60(Suppl. 3), pp.71–6. Available at https://pubmed.ncbi.nlm.nih.gov/14671401/.

34 Reeve, J., Walton, J., Russell, L. J., Lunt, M., Wolman, R., Abraham, R. A., Justice, J., Nicholls, A., Wardley-Smith, B., Green, J. R. and Mitchell, A., 1999. Determinants of the first decade of bone loss after menopause at spine, hip and radius. *QJM*, 92(5), pp. 261–73. Available at https://academic.oup.com/qjmed/article/92/5/261/1592959.

35 Alswat, K. A., 2017. Gender disparities in osteoporosis. *Journal of Clinical Medicine Research*, 9(5), pp. 382–7. Available at https://www.ncbi.nlm.nih.gov/pmc/articles/PMC5380170/#:~:text=Women%20start%20losing%20bone%20at,years%20earlier%20compared%20with%20men.

36 Weaver, C. M., Gordon, C. M., Janz, K. F., Kalkwarf, H. J., Lappe, J. M., Lewis, R., O'Karma, M., Wallace, T. C. and Zemel, B. S., 2016. The National Osteoporosis Foundation's position statement on peak bone mass development and lifestyle factors: A systematic review and implementation recommendations. *Osteoporosis International*, 27(4), pp. 1281–386. Available at https://www.ncbi.nlm.nih.gov/pmc/articles/PMC4791473/.

37 Ibid.

38 Lewis, A., 22 Jan. 2015. Curse or myth – do periods affect performance? BBC Sport. Available at https://www.bbc.co.uk/sport/tennis/30926244.

39 BBC Sport, 22 Jan. 2015. Paula Radcliffe: Sport has not learned about periods. Available at https://www.bbc.co.uk/sport/athletics/30927245.

40 McNulty, K. L., Elliott-Sale, K. J., Dolan, E., Swinton, P. A., Ansdell, P., Goodall, S., Thomas, K. and Hicks, K. M., 2020. The effects of menstrual cycle phase on exercise performance in eumenorrheic women: A systematic review and meta-analysis. *Sports Medicine*, 50(10), pp. 1813–27. Available at https://pubmed.ncbi.nlm.nih.gov/32661839/.

41 Bharati, M., 2016. Comparing the effects of yoga & oral calcium administration in alleviating symptoms of premenstrual syndrome in medical undergraduates. *Journal of Caring Sciences*, 5(3), pp. 179–85. Available at https://pubmed.ncbi.nlm.nih.gov/27752483/; El-Lithy, A., El-Mazny, A., Sabbour, A. and El-Deeb, A., 2015. Effect of aerobic exercise on premenstrual symptoms, haematological and hormonal parameters in young women. *Journal of Obstetrics and Gynaecology*, 35(4), pp. 389–92. Available at https://pubmed.ncbi.nlm.nih.gov/25279689/; Petersen, A. M. W. and Pedersen, B. K., 2005. The anti-inflammatory effect of exercise. *Journal of Applied Physiology*, 98(4), pp. 1154–62. Available at https://pubmed.ncbi.nlm.nih.gov/15772055/; Tsai, S. Y., 2016. Effect of yoga exercise on premenstrual symptoms among female employees in Taiwan. International *Journal of Environmental Research and Public Health*, 13(7), p. 721. Available at https://www.ncbi.nlm.nih.gov/pmc/articles/PMC4962262/; Vaghela, N., Mishra, D., Sheth, M. and Dani, V. B., 2019. To compare the effects of aerobic exercise and yoga on Premenstrual syndrome. *Journal of Education and Health Promotion*, 8, p. 199. Available at https://pubmed.ncbi.nlm.nih.gov/31867375/.

42 Ansdell, P., Brownstein, C. G., Škarabot, J., Hicks, K. M., Simoes, D. C., Thomas, K., Howatson, G., Hunter, S. K. and Goodall, S., 2019. Menstrual cycle-associated modulations in neuromuscular function and fatigability of the knee extensors in eumenorrheic women. *Journal of Applied Physiology*, 126(6), pp. 1701–12. Available at https://pubmed.ncbi.nlm.nih.gov/30844334/; Baltgalvis, K. A., Greising, S. M., Warren, G. L. and Lowe, D. A., 2010. Estrogen regulates estrogen receptors and antioxidant gene expression in mouse skeletal muscle. *PloS One*, 5(4), p. e10164. Available at https://pubmed.ncbi.nlm.nih.gov/20450008/; Lowe, D. A., Baltgalvis, K. A. and Greising, S. M., 2010. Mechanisms behind estrogens' beneficial effect on muscle strength in females. Exercise and Sport Sciences Reviews, 38(2), pp. 61–7. Available at https://www.ncbi.nlm.nih.gov/pmc/articles/PMC2873087/; Wihlbäck, A. C., Poromaa, I. S., Bixo, M., Allard, P., Mjörndal, T. and Spigset, O., 2004. Influence of menstrual cycle on platelet serotonin uptake site and serotonin2A receptor binding. *Psychoneuroendocrinology*, 29(6), pp. 757–66. Available at https://pubmed.ncbi.nlm.nih.gov/15110925/.

43 Herzberg, S. D., Motu'apuaka, M. L., Lambert, W., Fu, R., Brady, J. and Guise, J. M., 2017. The effect of menstrual cycle and contraceptives on ACL injuries and laxity: A systematic review and meta-analysis. *Orthopaedic Journal of Sports Medicine*, 5(7), p. 2325967117718781. Available at https://pubmed.ncbi.nlm.nih.gov/28795075/.

44 Bushman, B., Masterson, G. and Nelsen, J., 2006. Anaerobic power performance and the menstrual cycle: Eumenorrheic and oral contraceptive users. *Journal of Sports Medicine and Physical Fitness*, 46(1), pp. 132–7. Available at https://pubmed.ncbi.nlm.nih.gov/16596112/; Ekenros, L., Hirschberg, A. L., Heijne, A. and Fridén, C., 2013. Oral contraceptives do not affect muscle strength and hop performance in active women. *Clinical Journal of Sport Medicine*, 23(3), pp. 202–7. Available at https://pubmed.ncbi.nlm.nih.gov/22948447/; Elliott, K. J., Cable, N. T. and Reilly, T., 2005. Does oral contraceptive use affect maximum force production in women? *British Journal of Sports Medicine*, 39(1), pp. 15–19. Available at https://pubmed.ncbi.nlm.nih.gov/15618333/; Peters, C. and Burrows, M., 2006. Androgenicity of the progestin in oral contraceptives does not affect maximal leg strength. *Contraception*, 74(6), pp. 487–91. Available at https://pubmed.ncbi.nlm.nih.gov/17157107/; Sunderland, C., Tunaley, V., Horner, F., Harmer, D. and Stokes, K. A., 2011. Menstrual cycle and oral contraceptives' effects on growth hormone response to sprinting. *Applied Physiology, Nutrition, and Metabolism*, 36(4), pp. 495–502. Available at https://pubmed.ncbi.nlm.nih.gov/21848445/; Lynch, N. J., De Vito, G. and Nimmo, M. A., 2001. Low dosage monophasic oral contraceptive use and intermittent exercise performance and metabolism in humans. *European Journal of Applied Physiology*, 84(4), pp. 296–301. Available at https://pubmed.ncbi.nlm.nih.gov/11374113/.

45 Elliott-Sale, K. J., McNulty, K. L., Ansdell, P., Goodall, S., Hicks, K. M., Thomas, K., Swinton, P. A. and Dolan, E., 2020. The effects of oral contraceptives on exercise performance in women: A systematic review and meta-analysis. *Sports Medicine*, 50(10), pp. 1785–812. Available at https://pubmed.ncbi.nlm.nih.gov/32666247/.

46 De Souza, M. J., Toombs, R. J., Scheid, J. L., O'Donnell, E., West, S. L. and Williams, N. I., 2010. High prevalence of subtle and severe menstrual disturbances in exercising women: Confirmation using daily hormone measures. *Human Reproduction*, 25(2), pp. 491–503. Available at https://academic.oup.com/humrep/article/25/2/491/674505.

47 Practice Committee of the American Society for Reproductive Medicine, 2006. Current evaluation of amenorrhea. Fertility and Sterility, 86(5), pp. S148–55. Available at https://pubmed.ncbi.nlm.nih.gov/17055812/.

48 Eunice Kennedy Shriver National Institute of Child Health and Human Development, 13 Sep. 2021. Menstrual cycles as a fifth vital sign. Available at https://www.nichd.nih.gov/about/org/od/directors_corner/prev_updates/menstrual-cycles.

49 Nike, 2021. The toughest athletes. Available at https://www.instagram.com/p/CMZEIfdhFIS/?utm_source=ig_embed&ig_rid=3b7affec-8f94-487c-9356-b6efdc4ff259.

50 Thurber, C., Dugas, L. R., Ocobock, C., Carlson, B., Speakman, J. R. and Pontzer, H., 2019. Extreme events reveal an alimentary limit on sustained maximal human energy expenditure. *Science Advances*, 5(6), p. eaaw0341. Available at https://www.science.org/doi/10.1126/sciadv.aaw0341.

51 Department of Health and Social Care, 7 Sep. 2019. UK Chief Medical Officer's physical activity guidelines. Available at https://assets.publishing.service.gov.uk/government/uploads/system/uploads/attachment_data/file/832868/uk-chief-medical-officers-physical-activity-guidelines.pdf; Mottola, M. F., Davenport, M. H., Ruchat, S. M., Davies, G. A., Poitras, V. J., Gray, C. E., Garcia, A. J., Barrowman, N., Adamo, K. B., Duggan, M. and Barakat, R., 2018. 2019 Canadian guideline for physical activity throughout pregnancy. *British Journal of Sports Medicine*, 52(21), pp. 1339–46. Available at https://pubmed.ncbi.nlm.nih.gov/30337460/; World Health Organization, 25 Nov. 2020. WHO guidelines on physical activity and sedentary behaviour. Available at https://www.who.int/publications/i/item/9789240015128.

52 Ibid.

[53] Currie, S., Sinclair, M., Murphy, M. H., Madden, E., Dunwoody, L. and Liddle, D., 2013. Reducing the decline in physical activity during pregnancy: A systematic review of behaviour change interventions. *PloS One*, 8(6), p. e66385. Available at https://pubmed.ncbi.nlm.nih.gov/23799096/.

[54] Sytsma, T. T., Zimmerman, K. P., Manning, J. B., Jenkins, S. M., Nelson, N. C., Clark, M. M., Boldt, K. and Borowski, K. S., 2018. Perceived barriers to exercise in the first trimester of pregnancy. *Journal of Perinatal Education*, 27(4), pp. 198–206. Available at https://pubmed.ncbi.nlm.nih.gov/31073266/.

[55] Meah, V. L., Davies, G. A. and Davenport, M. H., 2020. Why can't I exercise during pregnancy? Time to revisit medical 'absolute' and 'relative' contraindications: Systematic review of evidence of harm and a call to action. *British Journal of Sports Medicine*, 54(23), pp. 1395–404. Available at https://pubmed.ncbi.nlm.nih.gov/32513676/.

[56] Mottola, M. F., Davenport, M. H., Ruchat, S. M., Davies, G. A., Poitras, V. J., Gray, C. E., Garcia, A. J., Barrowman, N., Adamo, K. B., Duggan, M. and Barakat, R., 2018. 2019 Canadian guideline for physical activity throughout pregnancy. *British Journal of Sports Medicine*, 52(21), pp. 1339–46. Available at https://pubmed.ncbi.nlm.nih.gov/30337460/; e-Learning for Healthcare, 10 Mar. 2020. Pregnancy and postnatal period: Being active [course]. Available at https://portal.e-lfh.org.uk/Component/Details/604251.

[57] Department of Health and Social Care, 7 Sep. 2019. UK Chief Medical Officer's physical activity guidelines: Physical activity for pregnant women. Available at https://assets.publishing.service.gov.uk/government/uploads/system/uploads/attachment_data/file/829894/5-physical-activity-for-pregnant-women.pdf.

[58] Kołomańska-Bogucka, D. and Mazur-Bialy, A. I., 2019. Physical activity and the occurrence of postnatal depression – a systematic review. *Medicina*, 55(9), p. 560. Available at https://www.ncbi.nlm.nih.gov/pmc/articles/PMC6780177/.

[59] Department of Health and Social Care, 7 Sep. 2019. UK Chief Medical Officer's physical activity guidelines: Physical activity for women after childbirth (birth to 12 months). Available at https://assets.publishing.service.gov.uk/government/uploads/system/uploads/attachment_data/file/841936/Postpartum_infographic.pdf.

[60] El-Shamy, F. F. and Abd El Fatah, E., 2017. Effect of antenatal pelvic floor muscle exercise on mode of delivery: A randomized controlled trial. *Integrative Medicine International*, 4(3–4), pp. 187–97. Available at https://www.researchgate.net/publication/324760782_Effect_of_Antenatal_Pelvic_Floor_Muscle_Exercise_on_Mode_of_Delivery_A_Randomized_Controlled_Trial; Agur, W., Steggles, P., Waterfield, M. and Freeman, R., 2008. Does antenatal pelvic floor muscle training affect the outcome of labour? A randomised controlled trial. *International Urogynecology Journal*, 19(1), pp. 85–8. Available at https://pubmed.ncbi.nlm.nih.gov/17530154/; Salvesen, K. Å. and Mørkved, S., 2004. Randomised controlled trial of pelvic floor muscle training during pregnancy. *BMJ*, 329(7462), pp. 378–80. Available at https://pubmed.ncbi.nlm.nih.gov/15253920/; Bø, K., Fleten, C. and Nystad, W., 2009. Effect of antenatal pelvic floor muscle training on labor and birth. *Obstetrics & Gynecology*, 113(6), pp. 1279–84. Available at https://pubmed.ncbi.nlm.nih.gov/19461423/.

[61] Lowenstein, L., Gruenwald, I., Gartman, I. and Vardi, Y., 2010. Can stronger pelvic muscle floor improve sexual function? *International Urogynecology Journal*, 21(5), pp. 553–6. Available at https://pubmed.ncbi.nlm.nih.gov/20087572/; Sacomori, C., Virtuoso, J. F., Kruger, A. P. and Cardoso, F. L., 2015. Pelvic floor muscle strength and sexual function in women. *Fisioterapia em Movimento*, 28, pp. 657–65. Available at https://scielo.br/j/fm/a/Zy3kbm3dtcXT6TrcyZKVFkb/abstract/?lang=en; Ferreira, C. H. J., Dwyer, P. L., Davidson, M., De Souza, A., Ugarte, J. A. and Frawley, H. C., 2015. Does pelvic floor muscle training improve female sexual function? A systematic review. *International Urogynecology Journal*, 26(12), pp. 1735–50. Available at https://pubmed.ncbi.nlm.nih.gov/26072126/.

[62] Ferreira, C. H. J., Dwyer, P. L., Davidson, M., De Souza, A., Ugarte, J. A. and Frawley, H. C., 2015. Does pelvic floor muscle training improve female sexual function? A systematic review. *International Urogynecology Journal*, 26(12), pp. 1735–50. Available at https://pubmed.ncbi.nlm.nih.gov/26072126/; Sobhgol, S. S., Priddis, H., Smith, C. A. and Dahlen, H. G., 2019. Evaluation of the effect of an antenatal pelvic floor muscle exercise programme on female sexual function during pregnancy and the first 3 months following birth: Study protocol for a pragmatic randomised controlled trial. *Trials*, 20(144), pp. 1–11. Available at https://trialsjournal.biomedcentral.com/articles/10.1186/s13063-019-3226-6.

[63] National Institute for Health and Care Excellence, 9 Dec. 2021. Pelvic floor dysfunction: Prevention and non-surgical management. Available at https://www.nice.org.uk/guidance/NG210.

[64] London Sport, n.d. Menopause, me and physical activity. *Women in Sport*. Available at https://www.womeninsport.org/wp-content/uploads/2018/06/Menopause-report-PDF-final-1-2.pdf.

[65] Women in Sport, n.d. Menopause. Available at https://www.womeninsport.org/menopause/.

[66] Shojaa, M., Von Stengel, S., Schoene, D., Kohl, M., Barone, G., Bragonzoni, L., Dallolio, L., Marini, S., Murphy, M. H., Stephenson, A. and Mänty, M., 2020. Effect of exercise training on bone mineral density in post-menopausal women: A systematic review and meta-analysis of intervention studies. Frontiers in Physiology, 11, p. 652. Available at https://www.ncbi.nlm.nih.gov/pmc/articles/PMC7325605/; Kemmler, W. and Von Stengel, S., 2014. Dose–response effect of exercise frequency on bone mineral density in post-menopausal, osteopenic women. *Scandinavian Journal of Medicine & Science in Sports*, 24(3), pp. 526–34. Available at https://onlinelibrary.wiley.com/doi/10.1111/sms.12024.

[67] Dubnov, G., Brzezinski, A. and Berry, E. M., 2003. Weight control and the management of obesity after menopause: The role of physical activity. *Maturitas*, 44(2), pp. 89–101. Available at https://pubmed.ncbi.nlm.nih.gov/12590004/; Hagner-Derengowska, M., Kaluzny, K., Kochanski, B., Hagner, W., Borkowska, A., Czamara, A. and Budzynski, J., 2015. Effects of Nordic Walking and Pilates exercise programs on blood glucose and lipid profile in overweight and obese postmenopausal women in an experimental, nonrandomized, open-label, prospective controlled trial. Menopause, 22(11), pp. 1215–23. Available at https://pubmed.ncbi.nlm.nih.gov/25803666/; Aragão, F. R., Abrantes, C. G., Gabriel, R. E., Sousa, M. F., Castelo-Branco, C. and Moreira, M. H., 2014. Effects of a 12-month multi-component exercise program on the body composition of postmenopausal women. Climacteric, 17(2), pp. 155–63. Available at https://www.tandfonline.com/doi/full/10.3109/13697137.2013.819328.

[68] Bunyaratavej, N., 2015. Effects of circuit aerobic step exercise program on musculoskeletal for prevention of falling and enhancement of postural balance in postmenopausal women. *Journal of the Medical Association of Thailand*, 98(8), pp. S88–94. Available at https://www.thaiscience.info/journals/Article/JMAT/10976918.pdf; Cruz-Díaz, D., Martínez-Amat, A., Manuel, J., Casuso, R. A., de Guevara, N. M. L. and Hita-Contreras, F., 2015. Effects of a six-week Pilates intervention on balance and fear of falling in women aged over 65 with chronic low-back pain: A randomized controlled trial. Maturitas, 82(4), pp. 371–6. Available at https://pubmed.ncbi.nlm.nih.gov/26277254/.

[69] Mazurek, K., Żmijewski, P., Kozdroń, E., Fojt, A., Czajkowska, A., Szczypiorski, P. and Mazurek, T., 2017. Cardiovascular risk reduction in sedentary postmenopausal women during organised physical activity. Kardiologia Polska (Polish Heart Journal), 75(5), pp. 476–85. Available at https://pubmed.ncbi.nlm.nih.gov/28281730/; Colpani, V., Oppermann, K. and Spritzer, P. M., 2013. Association between habitual physical activity and lower cardiovascular risk in premenopausal, perimenopausal, and postmenopausal women: A population-based study. Menopause, 20(5), pp. 525–31. Available at https://journals.lww.com/menopausejournal/Abstract/2013/05000/Association_between_habitual_physical_activity_and.9.aspx; Seals, D. R., Silverman, H. G., Reiling, M. J. and Davy, K. P., 1997. Effect of regular aerobic exercise on elevated blood pressure in postmenopausal women. *American Journal of Cardiology*, 80(1), pp. 49–55. Available at https://www.ajconline.org/article/S0002-9149(97)00282-8/pdf; Mandrup, C. M., Egelund, J., Nyberg, M., Slingsby, M. H. L., Andersen, C. B., Løgstrup, S., Bangsbo, J., Suetta, C., Stallknecht, B. and Hellsten, Y., 2017. Effects of high-intensity training on cardiovascular risk factors in premenopausal and postmenopausal women. *American Journal of Obstetrics and Gynecology*, 216(4), pp. 384e1–e11. Available at https://pubmed.ncbi.nlm.nih.gov/28024987/.

[70] Najar, J., Östling, S., Gudmundsson, P., Sundh, V., Johansson, L., Kern, S., Guo, X., Hällström, T. and Skoog, I., 2019. Cognitive and physical activity and dementia: A 44-year longitudinal population study of women. Neurology, 92(12), pp. e1322–30. Available at https://n.neurology.org/content/92/12/e1322.abstract; Erickson, K. I., Hillman, C., Stillman, C. M., Ballard, R. M., Bloodgood, B., Conroy, D. E., Macko, R., Marquez, D. X., Petruzzello, S. J. and Powell, K. E., 2019. Physical activity, cognition, and brain outcomes: A review of the 2018 physical activity guidelines. *Medicine and Science in Sports and Exercise*, 51(6), pp. 1242–51. Available at https://www.ncbi.nlm.nih.gov/pmc/articles/PMC6527141/.

[71] Kline, C. E., Irish, L. A., Krafty, R. T., Sternfeld, B., Kravitz, H. M., Buysse, D. J., Bromberger, J. T., Dugan, S. A. and Hall, M. H., 2013. Consistently high sports/exercise activity is associated with better sleep quality, continuity and depth in midlife women: The SWAN sleep study. Sleep, 36(9), pp. 1279–88. Available at https://academic.oup.com/sleep/article/36/9/1279/2453863?login=true.

[72] Villaverde Gutierrez, C., Torres Luque, G., Abalos Medina, G. M., Argente del Castillo, M. J., Guisado, I. M., Guisado Barrilao, R. and Ramirez Rodrigo, J., 2012. Influence of exercise on mood in postmenopausal women. Journal of Clinical Nursing, 21(7–8), pp. 923–8. Available at https://onlinelibrary.wiley.com/doi/full/10.1111/j.1365-2702.2011.03972.x?casa_token=skeP0DOPJ9AAAAAA%3Ae2B_fzFXn2gY6psPKfUzyHfnPiqqqPi3TPXTA8780Lad3qXTzHxXY7nvBSLVzbmjdpePKfeDXZCG4ZNr; Elavsky, S. and McAuley, E., 2007. *Physical activity and mental health outcomes during menopause: A randomized controlled trial*. Annals of Behavioral Medicine, 33(2), pp. 132–42. Available at https://academic.oup.com/abm/

article/33/2/132/4569352.

[73] Wu, Y., Zhang, D. and Kang, S., 2013. Physical activity and risk of breast cancer: A meta-analysis of prospective studies. Breast Cancer Research and Treatment, 137(3), pp. 869–82. Available at https://link.springer.com/article/10.1007/s10549-012-2396-7; Monninkhof, E. M., Elias, S. G., Vlems, F. A., van der Tweel, I., Schuit, A. J., Voskuil, D. W. and van Leeuwen, F. E., 2007. Physical activity and breast cancer: A systematic review. Epidemiology, 18(1), pp. 137–57. Available at https://www.jstor.org/stable/20486329; McTiernan, A., Friedenreich, C. M., Katzmarzyk, P. T., Powell, K. E., Macko, R., Buchner, D., Pescatello, L. S., Bloodgood, B., Tennant, B., Vaux-Bjerke, A. and George, S. M., 2019. Physical activity in cancer prevention and survival: A systematic review. Medicine and Science in Sports and Exercise, 51(6), pp. 1252–61. Available at https://www.ncbi.nlm.nih.gov/pmc/articles/PMC6527123/.

[74] Thomas, A. and Daley, A. J., 2020. Women's views about physical activity as a treatment for vasomotor menopausal symptoms: A qualitative study. BMC Women's Health, 20(1), pp. 1–11. Available at https://bmcwomenshealth.biomedcentral.com/articles/10.1186/s12905-020-01063-w.

[75] Department of Health and Social Care, 7 Sep. 2019. UK Chief Medical Officer's physical activity guidelines. Available at https://assets.publishing.service.gov.uk/government/uploads/system/uploads/attachment_data/file/832868/uk-chief-medical-officers-physical-activity-guidelines.pdf.

[76] https://assets.publishing.service.gov.uk/government/uploads/system/uploads/attachment_data/file/832868/uk-chief-medical-officers-physical-activity-guidelines.pdf.

[77] Royal Osteoporosis Society, n.d. Exercise for bones. Available at https://theros.org.uk/information-and-support/bone-health/exercise-for-bones/.

[78] British Heart Foundation, Mar. 2017. Physical activity and sedentary behaviour repot 2017. Available at https://www.bhf.org.uk/informationsupport/publications/statistics/physical-inactivity-report-2017.

CH 03 - Mood

[1] Anxiety UK, n.d. Key facts and figures. Available at https://www.anxietyuk.org.uk/wp-content/uploads/2019/08/Key-Facts-and-Figures-2019.pdf.

[2] Chu, B., Marwaha, K., Sanvictores, T. and Ayers, D., 2021. Physiology, stress reaction. StatPearls [Internet]. Available at https://www.ncbi.nlm.nih.gov/books/NBK541120/.

[3] Thau, L., Gandhi, J. and Sharma, S., 2021. Physiology, cortisol. StatPearls [Internet]. Available at https://www.ncbi.nlm.nih.gov/books/NBK538239/.

[4] Yerkes, R. M. and Dodson, J. D., 1908. The relation of strength of stimulus to rapidity of habit-formation. Journal of Comparative Neurology and Psychology, 18, 459–82. Available at http://psychclassics.yorku.ca/Yerkes/Law/.

[5] Hammen, C., Kim, E. Y., Eberhart, N. K. and Brennan, P. A., 2009. Chronic and acute stress and the prediction of major depression in women. Depression and Anxiety, 26(8), pp. 718–23. Available at https://www.ncbi.nlm.nih.gov/pmc/articles/PMC3380803/.

[6] Chu, B., Marwaha, K., Sanvictores, T. and Ayers, D., 2021. Physiology, stress reaction. StatPearls [Internet]. Available at https://www.ncbi.nlm.nih.gov/books/NBK541120/.

[7] Chaplin, T. M., Hong, K., Bergquist, K. and Sinha, R., 2008. Gender differences in response to emotional stress: An assessment across subjective, behavioral, and physiological domains and relations to alcohol craving. Alcoholism: Clinical and Experimental Research, 32(7), pp. 1242–50. Available at https://www.ncbi.nlm.nih.gov/pmc/articles/PMC2575018/.

[8] Sharma, N., Chakrabarti, S. and Grover, S., 2016. Gender differences in caregiving among family-caregivers of people with mental illnesses. World Journal of Psychiatry, 6(1), pp. 7–17. Available at https://www.ncbi.nlm.nih.gov/pmc/articles/PMC4804270/.

[9] Zuckerman, M., Li, C. and Hall, J. A., 2016. When men and women differ in self-esteem and when they don't: A meta-analysis. Journal of Research in Personality, 64, pp. 34–51. Available at https://www.sciencedirect.com/science/article/abs/pii/S0092656616300873.

[10] Hallers-Haalboom, E. T., Maas, J., Kunst, L. E. and Bekker, M. H., 2020. The role of sex and gender in anxiety disorders: Being scared 'like a girl'? In Handbook of Clinical Neurology, 175, pp. 359–68. Elsevier. Available at https://www.sciencedirect.com/science/article/abs/pii/B9780444641236000242#bb0350; McLean, C. P., Asnaani, A., Litz, B. T. and Hofmann, S. G., 2011. Gender differences in anxiety disorders: Prevalence, course of illness, comorbidity and burden of illness. Journal of Psychiatric Research, 45(8), pp. 1027–35. Available at https://www.sciencedirect.com/science/article/abs/pii/S0022395611000458.

[11] Ibid.

[12] Eliot, L., Ahmed, A., Khan, H. and Patel, J., 2021. Dump the 'dimorphism': Comprehensive synthesis of human brain studies reveals few male-female differences beyond size. Neuroscience & Biobehavioral Reviews, 125, pp. 667–97. Available at https://www.sciencedirect.com/science/article/pii/S0149763421000804?via%3Dihub.

[13] Noordam, R., Aarts, N., Verhamme, K. M., Sturkenboom, M. C., Stricker, B. H. and Visser, L. E., 2015. Prescription and indication trends of antidepressant drugs in the Netherlands between 1996 and 2012: A dynamic population-based study. European Journal of Clinical Pharmacology, 71(3), pp. 369–75. Available at https://pubmed.ncbi.nlm.nih.gov/25560052/; Bacigalupe, A. and Martín, U., 2021. Gender inequalities in depression/anxiety and the consumption of psychotropic drugs: Are we medicalising women's mental health? Scandinavian Journal of Public Health, 49(3), pp. 317–24. Available at https://journals.sagepub.com/doi/pdf/10.1177/1403494820944736.

[14] Potts, M. K., Burnam, M. A. and Wells, K. B., 1991. Gender differences in depression detection: A comparison of clinician diagnosis and standardized assessment. Psychological Assessment: A Journal of Consulting and Clinical Psychology, 3(4), pp. 609–15. Available at https://www.rand.org/pubs/external_publications/EP19911208.html; Floyd, B. J., 1997. Problems in accurate medical diagnosis of depression in female patients. Social Science & Medicine, 44(3), pp. 403–12. Available at https://www.sciencedirect.com/science/article/abs/pii/S027795369600159I?via%3Dihub.

[15] McGregor, A. J., 2020. Sex Matters: How male-centric medicine endangers women's health and what we can do about it. Hachette UK. Available at https://books.google.ae/books?id=H2e2DwAAQBAJ&printsec=frontcover&dq=Dr+Alyson+McGregor,+author+of+Sex+Matters,&hl=en&sa=X&ved=2ahUKEwjA38TIrvT1AhWBzYUKHbIVAp0Q6AF-6BAgKEAI#v=onepage&q=Dr%20Alyson%20McGregor%2C%20author%20of%20Sex%20Matters%2C&f=false.

[16] Tasca, C., Rapetti, M., Carta, M. G. and Fadda, B., 2012. Women and hysteria in the history of mental health. Clinical Practice and Epidemiology in Mental Health, 8, pp. 110–19. Available at https://www.ncbi.nlm.nih.gov/pmc/articles/PMC3480686/.

[17] Maines, Rachel P., 1999. The Technology of Orgasm: "Hysteria", the Vibrator, and Women's Sexual Satisfaction. Baltimore: The Johns Hopkins University Press. p. 23. ISBN 0-8018-6646-4

[18] Carnlöf, C., Iwarzon, M., Jensen-Urstad, M., Gadler, F. and Insulander, P., 2017. Women with PSVT are often misdiagnosed, referred later than men, and have more symptoms after ablation. Scandinavian Cardiovascular Journal, 51(6), pp. 299–307. Available at https://www.tandfonline.com/doi/full/10.1080/14017431.2017.1385837?needAccess=true; Hamberg, K., Risberg, G. and Johansson, E. E., 2004. Male and female physicians show different patterns of gender bias: A paper-case study of management of irritable bowel syndrome. Scandinavian Journal of Public Health, 32(2), pp. 144–52. Available at https://journals.sagepub.com/doi/pdf/10.1080/14034940310015401.

[19] Hamberg, K., Risberg, G. and Johansson, E. E., 2004. Male and female physicians show different patterns of gender bias: A paper-case study of management of irritable bowel syndrome. Scandinavian Journal of Public Health, 32(2), pp. 144–52. Available at https://journals.sagepub.com/doi/pdf/10.1080/14034940310015401.

[20] Lichtman, J. H., Leifheit, E. C., Safdar, B., Bao, H., Krumholz, H. M., Lorenze, N. P., Daneshvar, M., Spertus, J. A. and D'Onofrio, G., 2018. Sex differences in the presentation

and perception of symptoms among young patients with myocardial infarction: Evidence from the VIRGO study (variation in recovery: role of gender on outcomes of young AMI patients). Circulation, 137(8), pp. 781–90. Available at https://www.ahajournals.org/doi/10.1161/CIRCULATIONAHA.117.031650; Carnlöf, C., Iwarzon, M., Jensen-Urstad, M., Gadler, F. and Insulander, P., 2017. Women with PSVT are often misdiagnosed, referred later than men, and have more symptoms after ablation. Scandinavian Cardiovascular Journal, 51(6), pp. 299–307. Available at https://www.tandfonline.com/doi/full/10.1080/14017431.2017.1385837?needAccess=true.

[21] BHF, 2017.

[22] Wilkinson, C., Bebb, O., Dondo, T. B., Munyombwe, T., Casadei, B., Clarke, S., Schiele, F., Timmis, A., Hall, M. and Gale, C. P., 2019. Sex differences in quality indicator attainment for myocardial infarction: A nationwide cohort study. Heart, 105(7), pp. 516–23. Available at https://pubmed.ncbi.nlm.nih.gov/30470725/.

[23] Nguyen, H. L., Saczynski, J. S., Gore, J. M. and Goldberg, R. J., 2010. Age and sex differences in duration of prehospital delay in patients with acute myocardial infarction: A systematic review. Circulation: Cardiovascular Quality and Outcomes, 3(1), pp. 82–92. Available at https://pubmed.ncbi.nlm.nih.gov/20123674/.

[24] Lichtman, J. H., Leifheit-Limson, E. C., Watanabe, E., Allen, N. B., Garavalia, B., Garavalia, L. S., Spertus, J. A., Krumholz, H. M. and Curry, L. A., 2015. Symptom recognition and health-care experiences of young women with acute myocardial infarction. Circulation: Cardiovascular Quality and Outcomes, 8(2 suppl 1), pp. S31–8. Available at https://pubmed.ncbi.nlm.nih.gov/25714826/.

[25] van Oosterhout, R. E., de Boer, A. R., Maas, A. H., Rutten, F. H., Bots, M. L. and Peters, S. A., 2020. Sex differences in symptom presentation in acute coronary syndromes: A systematic review and meta-analysis. Journal of the American Heart Association, 9(9), p. e014733. Available at https://pubmed.ncbi.nlm.nih.gov/32363989/.

[26] Wu, J., Gale, C. P., Hall, M., Dondo, T. B., Metcalfe, E., Oliver, G., Batin, P. D., Hemingway, H., Timmis, A. and West, R. M., 2018. Editor's choice – Impact of initial hospital diagnosis on mortality for acute myocardial infarction: A national cohort study. European Heart Journal: Acute Cardiovascular Care, 7(2), pp. 139–48. Available at https://pubmed.ncbi.nlm.nih.gov/27574333/; British Heart Foundation, 30 Aug. 2016. Women are 50% more likely than men to be given incorrect diagnosis following a heart attack. Available at https://www.bhf.org.uk/what-we-do/news-from-the-bhf/news-archive/2016/august/women-are-50-per-cent-more-likely-than-men-to-be-given-incorrect-diagnosis-following-a-heart-attack.

[27] Wu, J., Gale, C. P., Hall, M., Dondo, T. B., Metcalfe, E., Oliver, G., Batin, P. D., Hemingway, H., Timmis, A. and West, R. M., 2018. Editor's choice – Impact of initial hospital diagnosis on mortality for acute myocardial infarction: A national cohort study. European Heart Journal: Acute Cardiovascular Care, 7(2), pp. 139–48. Available at https://pubmed.ncbi.nlm.nih.gov/27574333/.

[28] Wilkinson, C., Bebb, O., Dondo, T. B., Munyombwe, T., Casadei, B., Clarke, S., Schiele, F., Timmis, A., Hall, M. and Gale, C. P., 2019. Sex differences in quality indicator attainment for myocardial infarction: A nationwide cohort study. Heart, 105(7), pp. 516–23. Available at https://pubmed.ncbi.nlm.nih.gov/30470725/.

[29] Solmi, M., Fiedorowicz, J., Poddighe, L., Delogu, M., Miola, A., Høye, A., Heiberg, I. H., Stubbs, B., Smith, L., Larsson, H. and Attar, R., 2021. Disparities in screening and treatment of cardiovascular diseases in patients with mental disorders across the world: Systematic review and meta-analysis of 47 observational studies. American Journal of Psychiatry, 178(9), pp. 793–803. Available at https://ajp.psychiatryonline.org/doi/10.1176/appi.ajp.2021.21010031.

[30] Wilkinson, C., Bebb, O., Dondo, T. B., Munyombwe, T., Casadei, B., Clarke, S., Schiele, F., Timmis, A., Hall, M. and Gale, C. P., 2019. Sex differences in quality indicator attainment for myocardial infarction: A nationwide cohort study. Heart, 105(7), pp. 516–23. Available at https://pubmed.ncbi.nlm.nih.gov/30470725/.

[31] British Heart Foundation, 29 Nov. 2018. National audit of cardiac rehabilitation (NACR) quality and outcomes report 2018. Available at https://www.bhf.org.uk/informationsupport/publications/statistics/national-audit-of-cardiac-rehabilitation-quality-and-outcomes-report-2018.

[32] Millett, E. R., Peters, S. A. and Woodward, M., 2018. Sex differences in risk factors for myocardial infarction: Cohort study of UK Biobank participants. BMJ, 363. Available at https://www.bmj.com/content/363/bmj.k4247.

[33] Hallers-Haalboom, E. T., Maas, J., Kunst, L. E. and Bekker, M. H., 2020. The role of sex and gender in anxiety disorders: Being scared 'like a girl'? In Handbook of Clinical Neurology, 175, pp. 359–68. Elsevier. Available at https://www.sciencedirect.com/science/article/abs/pii/B9780444641236000242#bb0115.

[34] Keenan, K. and Shaw, D., 1997. Developmental and social influences on young girls' early problem behavior. Psychological Bulletin, 121(1), pp. 95–113. Available at https://psycnet.apa.org/record/1997-02112-005.

[35] Hallers-Haalboom, E. T., Maas, J., Kunst, L. E. and Bekker, M. H., 2020. The role of sex and gender in anxiety disorders: Being scared 'like a girl'? In Handbook of Clinical Neurology, 175, pp. 359–68. Elsevier. Available at https://www.sciencedirect.com/science/article/abs/pii/B9780444641236000242#bb0115.

[36] Samaritans, n.d. Latest suicide data. Available at https://www.samaritans.org/about-samaritans/research-policy/suicide-facts-and-figures/latest-suicide-data/.

[37] Zorn, J. V., Schür, R. R., Boks, M. P., Kahn, R. S., Joëls, M. and Vinkers, C. H., 2017. Cortisol stress reactivity across psychiatric disorders: A systematic review and meta-analysis. Psychoneuroendocrinology, 77, pp. 25–36. Available at https://www.sciencedirect.com/science/article/abs/pii/S0306453016304735?via%3Dihub; Kirschbaum, C., Kudielka, B. M., Gaab, J., Schommer, N. C. and Hellhammer, D. H., 1999. Impact of gender, menstrual cycle phase, and oral contraceptives on the activity of the hypothalamus-pituitary-adrenal axis. Psychosomatic Medicine, 61(2), pp. 154–62. Available at https://pubmed.ncbi.nlm.nih.gov/10204967/; Stephens, M. A. C., Mahon, P. B., McCaul, M. E. and Wand, G. S., 2016. Hypothalamic–pituitary–adrenal axis response to acute psychosocial stress: Effects of biological sex and circulating sex hormones. Psychoneuroendocrinology, 66, pp. 47–55. Available at https://www.ncbi.nlm.nih.gov/pmc/articles/PMC4788592/.

[38] Ibid.

[39] Taylor, S. E., Klein, L. C., Lewis, B. P., Gruenewald, T. L., Gurung, R. A. and Updegraff, J. A., 2000. Biobehavioral responses to stress in females: Tend-and-befriend, not fight-or-flight. Psychological Review, 107(3), pp. 411–29. Available at https://pubmed.ncbi.nlm.nih.gov/10941275/.

[40] Verma, R., Balhara, Y. P. S. and Gupta, C. S., 2011. Gender differences in stress response: Role of developmental and biological determinants. Industrial Psychiatry Journal, 20(1), pp. 4–10. Available at https://www.ncbi.nlm.nih.gov/pmc/articles/PMC3425245/.

[41] Taylor, S. E., Klein, L. C., Lewis, B. P., Gruenewald, T. L., Gurung, R. A. and Updegraff, J. A., 2000. Biobehavioral responses to stress in females: Tend-and-befriend, not fight-or-flight. Psychological Review, 107(3), pp. 411–29. Available at https://pubmed.ncbi.nlm.nih.gov/10941275/; Olff, M., Frijling, J. L., Kubzansky, L. D., Bradley, B., Ellenbogen, M. A., Cardoso, C., Bartz, J. A., Yee, J. R. and Van Zuiden, M., 2013. The role of oxytocin in social bonding, stress regulation and mental health: An update on the moderating effects of context and interindividual differences. Psychoneuroendocrinology, 38(9), pp. 1883–94. Available at https://www.sciencedirect.com/science/article/pii/S0306453013002369#bib0225.

[42] McLean, C. P. and Anderson, E. R., 2009. Brave men and timid women? A review of the gender differences in fear and anxiety. Clinical Psychology Review, 29(6), pp. 496–505. Available at https://www.sciencedirect.com/science/article/abs/pii/S0272735809000671; Zuckerman, M., Li, C. and Hall, J. A., 2016. When men and women differ in self-esteem and when they don't: A meta-analysis. Journal of Research in Personality, 64, pp. 34–51. Available at https://www.sciencedirect.com/science/article/abs/pii/S0092656616300873; Hallers-Haalboom, E. T., Maas, J., Kunst, L. E. and Bekker, M. H., 2020. The role of sex and gender in anxiety disorders: Being scared 'like a girl'? In Handbook of Clinical Neurology, 175, pp. 359–68. Elsevier. Available at https://www.sciencedirect.com/science/article/abs/pii/B9780444641236000242#bb0450.

[43] Women's Aid, n.d. Domestic abuse is a gendered crime. Available at https://www.womensaid.org.uk/information-support/what-is-domestic-abuse/domestic-abuse-is-a-gendered-crime/; Hallers-Haalboom, E. T., Maas, J., Kunst, L. E. and Bekker, M. H., 2020. The role of sex and gender in anxiety disorders: Being scared 'like a girl'? In Handbook of Clinical Neurology, 175, pp. 359–68. Elsevier. Available at https://www.sciencedirect.com/science/article/abs/pii/B9780444641236000242#bbb0175.

[44] Labad, J., Menchón, J. M., Alonso, P., Jiménez, S. and Vallejo, J., 2005. Female reproductive cycle and obsessive-compulsive disorder. Journal of Clinical Psychiatry, 66(4), pp. 428–35. Available at https://pubmed.ncbi.nlm.nih.gov/15816784/.

[45] Angold, A. and Worthman, C. W., 1993. Puberty onset of gender differences in rates of depression: A developmental, epidemiologic and neuroendocrine perspective. Journal of Affective Disorders, 29(2–3), pp. 145–58. Available at https://pubmed.ncbi.nlm.nih.gov/8300975/; Cyranowski, J. M., Frank, E., Young, E. and Shear, M. K., 2000. Adolescent onset of the gender differ-

ence in lifetime rates of major depression: A theoretical model. Archives of General Psychiatry, 57(1), pp. 21–7. Available at https://pubmed.ncbi.nlm.nih.gov/10632229/.

[46] Balzer, B. W., Duke, S. A., Hawke, C. I. and Steinbeck, K. S., 2015. The effects of estradiol on mood and behavior in human female adolescents: A systematic review. European Journal of Pediatrics, 174(3), pp. 289–98. Available at https://pubmed.ncbi.nlm.nih.gov/25567794/.

[47] Winer, S. A. and Rapkin, A. J., 2006. Premenstrual disorders: Prevalence, etiology and impact. Journal of Reproductive Medicine, 51(4 Suppl). pp. 339–47. Available at https://pubmed.ncbi.nlm.nih.gov/16734317/.

[48] Schoep, M. E., Nieboer, T. E., van der Zanden, M., Braat, D. D. and Nap, A. W., 2019. The impact of menstrual symptoms on everyday life: A survey among 42,879 women. American Journal of Obstetrics and Gynecology, 220(6), pp. 569e1–e7. Available at https://pubmed.ncbi.nlm.nih.gov/30885768/.

[49] Mishra, S., Elliott, H. and Marwaha, R., 2021. Premenstrual dysphoric disorder. StatPearls [Internet]. Available at https://www.ncbi.nlm.nih.gov/books/NBK532307/.

[50] Geta, T. G., Woldeamanuel, G. G. and Dassa, T. T., 2020. Prevalence and associated factors of premenstrual syndrome among women of the reproductive age group in Ethiopia: Systematic review and meta-analysis. PLoS One, 15(11), p. e0241702. Available at https://journals.plos.org/plosone/article?id=10.1371/journal.pone.0241702.

[51] Romans, S. E., Clarkson, R., Einstein, G., Petrovic, M. and Stewart, D. E., 2012. Mood and the menstrual cycle: A review of prospective data studies. Gender Medicine, 9(5), pp. 361–84. Available at https://pubmed.ncbi.nlm.nih.gov/23036262/.

[52] Romans, S. E., Kreindler, D., Asllani, E., Einstein, G., Laredo, S., Levitt, A., Morgan, K., Petrovic, M., Toner, B. and Stewart, D. E., 2013. Mood and the menstrual cycle. Psychotherapy and Psychosomatics, 82(1), pp. 53–60. Available at http://einsteinlab.ca/wp-content/uploads/2016/04/Mood-and-the-Menstrual-Cycle-Psychotherapy-and-Psychosomatics.pdf.

[53] Skovlund, C. W., Mørch, L. S., Kessing, L. V. and Lidegaard, Ø., 2016. Association of hormonal contraception with depression. JAMA Psychiatry, 73(11), pp. 1154–62. Available at https://jamanetwork.com/journals/jamapsychiatry/fullarticle/2552796.

[54] Ibid.

[55] Keyes, K. M., Cheslack-Postava, K., Westhoff, C., Heim, C. M., Haloossim, M., Walsh, K. and Koenen, K., 2013. Association of hormonal contraceptive use with reduced levels of depressive symptoms: A national study of sexually active women in the United States. American Journal of Epidemiology, 178(9), pp. 1378–88. Available at https://www.ncbi.nlm.nih.gov/pmc/articles/PMC3888252/.

[56] Zettermark, S., Perez Vicente, R. and Merlo, J., 2018. Hormonal contraception increases the risk of psychotropic drug use in adolescent girls but not in adults: A pharmacoepidemiological study on 800 000 Swedish women. PLoS One, 13(3), p. e0194773. Available at https://www.ncbi.nlm.nih.gov/pmc/articles/PMC5864056/.

[57] Toohey, J., 2012. Depression during pregnancy and postpartum. Clinical Obstetrics and Gynecology, 55(3), pp. 788–97. Available at https://pubmed.ncbi.nlm.nih.gov/22828111/; Lindahl, V., Pearson, J. L. and Colpe, L., 2005. Prevalence of suicidality during pregnancy and the postpartum. Archives of Women's Mental Health, 8(2), pp. 77–87. Available at https://pubmed.ncbi.nlm.nih.gov/15883651/.

[58] Goodman, J. H., Watson, G. R. and Stubbs, B., 2016. Anxiety disorders in postpartum women: A systematic review and meta-analysis. Journal of Affective Disorders, 203, pp. 292–331. Available at https://pubmed.ncbi.nlm.nih.gov/27317922/.

[59] Vigod, S. N., Wilson, C. A. and Howard, L. M., 2016. Depression in pregnancy. BMJ, 352. Available at https://www.bmj.com/content/352/bmj.i1547.full; Biaggi, A., Conroy, S., Pawlby, S. and Pariante, C.M., 2016. Identifying the women at risk of antenatal anxiety and depression: A systematic review. Journal of Affective Disorders, 191, pp. 62–77. Available at https://www.ncbi.nlm.nih.gov/pmc/articles/PMC4879174/#bib20.

[60] Vigod, S. N., Wilson, C. A. and Howard, L. M., 2016. Depression in pregnancy. BMJ, 352. Available at https://www.bmj.com/content/352/bmj.i1547.full.

[61] Glover, V., 2014. Maternal depression, anxiety and stress during pregnancy and child outcome; what needs to be done. Best Practice & Research Clinical Obstetrics & Gynaecology, 28(1), pp. 25–35. Available at https://pubmed.ncbi.nlm.nih.gov/24090740/; Li, X., Gao, R., Dai, X., Liu, H., Zhang, J., Liu, X., Si, D., Deng, T. and Xia, W., 2020. The association between symptoms of depression during pregnancy and low birth weight: A prospective study. BMC Pregnancy and Childbirth, 20(147), pp. 1–7. Available at https://bmcpregnancychildbirth.biomedcentral.com/articles/10.1186/s12884-020-2842-1.

[62] Biaggi, A., Conroy, S., Pawlby, S. and Pariante, C.M., 2016. Identifying the women at risk of antenatal anxiety and depression: A systematic review. Journal of Affective Disorders, 191, pp. 62–77. Available at https://www.ncbi.nlm.nih.gov/pmc/articles/PMC4879174/#bib20.

[63] Vink, A. S., Clur, S. A. B., Wilde, A. A. and Blom, N. A., 2018. Effect of age and gender on the QTc-interval in healthy individuals and patients with long-QT syndrome. Trends in Cardiovascular Medicine, 28(1), pp. 64–75. Available at https://www.researchgate.net/publication/318896767_Effect_of_age_and_gender_on_the_QTc-interval_in_healthy_individuals_and_patients_with_Long-QT_syndrome.

[64] Yim, I. S., Tanner Stapleton, L. R., Guardino, C. M., Hahn-Holbrook, J. and Dunkel Schetter, C., 2015. Biological and psychosocial predictors of postpartum depression: Systematic review and call for integration. Annual Review of Clinical Psychology, 11, pp. 99–137. Available at https://www.ncbi.nlm.nih.gov/pmc/articles/PMC5659274/#R18.

[65] Figueiredo, B., Canário, C. and Field, T., 2014. Breastfeeding is negatively affected by prenatal depression and reduces postpartum depression. Psychological Medicine, 44(5), pp. 927–36. Available at https://pubmed.ncbi.nlm.nih.gov/23822932/.

[66] Hamdan, A. and Tamim, H., 2012. The relationship between postpartum depression and breastfeeding. International Journal of Psychiatry in Medicine, 43(3), pp. 243–59. Available at https://pubmed.ncbi.nlm.nih.gov/22978082/.

[67] Kennedy, R. L., Malabu, U. H., Jarrod, G., Nigam, P., Kannan, K. and Rane, A., 2010. Thyroid function and pregnancy: Before, during and beyond. Journal of Obstetrics and Gynaecology, 30(8), pp. 774–83. Available at https://pubmed.ncbi.nlm.nih.gov/21126112/.

[68] Yim, I. S., Tanner Stapleton, L. R., Guardino, C. M., Hahn-Holbrook, J. and Dunkel Schetter, C., 2015. Biological and psychosocial predictors of postpartum depression: Systematic review and call for integration. Annual Review of Clinical Psychology, 11, pp. 99–137. Available at https://www.ncbi.nlm.nih.gov/pmc/articles/PMC5659274/#R120.

[69] Freeman, E. W., Sammel, M. D., Boorman, D. W. and Zhang, R., 2014. Longitudinal pattern of depressive symptoms around natural menopause. JAMA Psychiatry, 71(1), pp. 36–43. Available at https://www.ncbi.nlm.nih.gov/pmc/articles/PMC4576824/; Clayton, A. H. and Ninan, P. T., 2010. Depression or menopause? Presentation and management of major depressive disorder in perimenopausal and postmenopausal women. Primary Care Companion to the Journal of Clinical Psychiatry, 12(1). Available at https://www.ncbi.nlm.nih.gov/pmc/articles/PMC2882813/.

[70] Chidi-Ogbolu, N. and Baar, K., 2019. Effect of estrogen on musculoskeletal performance and injury risk. Frontiers in Physiology, 9, p. 1834. Available at https://www.frontiersin.org/articles/10.3389/fphys.2018.01834/full.

[71] Weber, M. T., Maki, P. M. and McDermott, M. P., 2014. Cognition and mood in perimenopause: A systematic review and meta-analysis. The Journal of Steroid Biochemistry and Molecular Biology, 142, pp. 90–8. Available at https://pubmed.ncbi.nlm.nih.gov/23770320/; Georgakis, M. K., Beskou-Kontou, T., Theodoridis, I., Skalkidou, A. and Petridou, E. T., 2019. Surgical menopause in association with cognitive function and risk of dementia: A systematic review and meta-analysis. Psychoneuroendocrinology, 106, pp. 9–19. Available at https://www.sciencedirect.com/science/article/abs/pii/S0306453018311478?via%3Dihub.

[72] Greendale, G. A., Huang, M. H., Wight, R. G., Seeman, T., Luetters, C., Avis, N. E., Johnston, J. and Karlamangla, A. S., 2009. Effects of the menopause transition and hormone use on cognitive performance in midlife women. Neurology, 72(21), pp. 1850–7. Available at https://pubmed.ncbi.nlm.nih.gov/19470968/; Weber, M. T., Rubin, L. H. and Maki, P. M., 2013. Cognition in perimenopause: The effect of transition stage. Menopause, 20(5), pp. 511–7. Available at https://www.ncbi.nlm.nih.gov/pmc/articles/PMC3620712/.

[73] Dementia Statistics Hub, 5 Jul. 2018. Prevalence by gender in the UK. Alzheimer's Research UK. Available at https://www.dementiastatistics.org/statistics/prevalence-by-gender-in-the-uk/.

[74] Harlow, B. L., Wise, L. A., Otto, M. W., Soares, C. N. and Cohen, L. S., 2003. Depression and its influence on reproductive endocrine and menstrual cycle markers associated with perimenopause: The Harvard Study of Moods and Cycles. *Archives of General Psychiatry*, 60(1), pp. 29–36. Available at https://pubmed.ncbi.nlm.nih.gov/12511170/.

[75] Whitcomb, B. W., Purdue-Smithe, A. C., Szegda, K. L., Boutot, M. E., Hankinson, S. E., Manson, J. E., Rosner, B., Willett, W. C., Eliassen, A. H. and Bertone-Johnson, E. R., 2018. Cigarette smoking and risk of early natural menopause. *American Journal of Epidemiology*, 187(4), pp. 696–704. Available at https://www.ncbi.nlm.nih.gov/pmc/articles/PMC5888979/.

[76] Dugan, S. A., Bromberger, J. T., Segawa, E., Avery, E. and Sternfeld, B., 2015. Association between physical activity and depressive symptoms: Midlife women in SWAN. *Medicine and Science in Sports and Exercise*, 47(2), pp. 335–42. Available at https://www.ncbi.nlm.nih.gov/pmc/articles/PMC4280341/.

[77] Van Uffelen, J. G., van Gellecum, Y. R., Burton, N. W., Peeters, G., Heesch, K. C. and Brown, W. J., 2013. Sitting-time, physical activity, and depressive symptoms in mid-aged women. *American Journal of Preventive Medicine*, 45(3), pp. 276–81. Available at https://pubmed.ncbi.nlm.nih.gov/23953353/.

[78] Joffe, H., Petrillo, L. F., Koukopoulos, A., Viguera, A. C., Hirschberg, A., Nonacs, R., Somley, B., Pasciullo, E., White, D. P., Hall, J. E. and Cohen, L. S., 2011. Increased estradiol and improved sleep, but not hot flashes, predict enhanced mood during the menopausal transition. *Journal of Clinical Endocrinology & Metabolism*, 96(7), pp. E1044–54. Available at https://www.ncbi.nlm.nih.gov/pmc/articles/PMC3135198/.

[79] National Institute for Health and Care Excellence, 5 Dec. 2019. Menopause: Diagnosis and management. Available at https://www.nice.org.uk/guidance/ng23/chapter/Recommendations#managing-short-term-menopausal-symptoms.

[80] Shafiei, F., Salari-Moghaddam, A., Larijani, B. and Esmaillzadeh, A., 2019. Adherence to the Mediterranean diet and risk of depression: A systematic review and updated meta-analysis of observational studies. *Nutrition Reviews*, 77(4), pp. 230–9. Available at https://pubmed.ncbi.nlm.nih.gov/30726966/; Firth, J., Solmi, M., Wootton, R. E., Vancampfort, D., Schuch, F. B., Hoare, E., Gilbody, S., Torous, J., Teasdale, S. B., Jackson, S. E. and Smith, L., 2020. A meta-review of 'lifestyle psychiatry': The role of exercise, smoking, diet and sleep in the prevention and treatment of mental disorders. *World Psychiatry*, 19(3), pp. 360–80. Available at https://pubmed.ncbi.nlm.nih.gov/32931092/; Jacka, F. N., O'Neil, A., Opie, R., Itsiopoulos, C., Cotton, S., Mohebbi, M., Castle, D., Dash, S., Mihalopoulos, C., Chatterton, M. L. and Brazionis, L., 2017. A randomised controlled trial of dietary improvement for adults with major depression (the 'SMILES' trial). *BMC Medicine*, 15(23), pp. 1–13. Available at https://bmcmedicine.biomedcentral.com/articles/10.1186/s12916-017-0791-y.

[81] Sinclair, A., Begg, D., Mathai, M. and Weisinger, R., 2007. Omega 3 fatty acids and the brain: Review of studies in depression. *Asia Pacific Journal of Clinical Nutrition*, 16(S1), pp. S391–7. Available at https://pubmed.ncbi.nlm.nih.gov/17392137/; Calder, P. C., 2006. n− 3 Polyunsaturated fatty acids, inflammation, and inflammatory diseases. *American Journal of Clinical Nutrition*, 83(6), pp. 1505S–19S. Available at https://pubmed.ncbi.nlm.nih.gov/16841861/.

[82] Ciesielski, T. H. and Williams, S. M., 2020. Low Omega-3 intake is associated with high rates of depression and preterm birth on the country level. *Scientific Reports*, 10(19749), pp. 1–13. Available at https://www.nature.com/articles/s41598-020-76552-x; Zhang, M. M., Zou, Y., Li, S. M., Wang, L., Sun, Y. H., Shi, L., Lu, L., Bao, Y. P. and Li, S. X., 2020. The efficacy and safety of omega-3 fatty acids on depressive symptoms in perinatal women: A meta-analysis of randomized placebo-controlled trials. *Translational Psychiatry*, 10(193), pp. 1–9. Available at https://www.nature.com/articles/s41398-020-00886-3.

[83] Gerster, H., 1998. Can adults adequately convert a-linolenic acid (18: 3n-3) to eicosapentaenoic acid (20: 5n-3) and docosahexaenoic acid (22: 6n-3)? *International Journal for Vitamin and Nutrition Research*, 68(3), pp. 159–73. Available at https://pubmed.ncbi.nlm.nih.gov/9637947/.

[84] Pérez-Jiménez, J., Neveu, V., Vos, F. and Scalbert, A., 2010. Identification of the 100 richest dietary sources of polyphenols: An application of the Phenol-Explorer database. *European Journal of Clinical Nutrition*, 64(3), pp. S112–20. Available at https://www.nature.com/articles/ejcn2010221.pdf?origin=ppub.

[85] McDonald, D., Hyde, E., Debelius, J. W., Morton, J. T., Gonzalez, A., Ackermann, G., Aksenov, A. A., Behsaz, B., Brennan, C., Chen, Y. and DeRight Goldasich, L., 2018. American Gut: An open platform for citizen science microbiome research. *mSystems*, 3(3), pp. e00031–18. Available at https://www.ncbi.nlm.nih.gov/pmc/articles/PMC5954204/.

[86] Almeida, O. P., Ford, A. H. and Flicker, L., 2015. Systematic review and meta-analysis of randomized placebo-controlled trials of folate and vitamin B12 for depression. *International Psychogeriatrics*, 27(5), pp. 727–37. Available at https://www.cambridge.org/core/journals/international-psychogeriatrics/article/abs/systematic-review-and-metaanalysis-of-randomized-placebocontrolled-trials-of-folate-and-vitamin-b12-for-depression/9DF1E65CA9BFE49370312D75C78BCEBF.

[87] Ibid.

[88] Hughes, C. F., Ward, M., Tracey, F., Hoey, L., Molloy, A. M., Pentieva, K. and McNulty, H., 2017. B-vitamin intake and biomarker status in relation to cognitive decline in healthy older adults in a 4-year follow-up study. *Nutrients*, 9(1), p. 53. Available at https://www.mdpi.com/2072-6643/9/1/53; Behrens, A., Graessel, E., Pendergrass, A. and Donath, C., 2020. Vitamin B – Can it prevent cognitive decline? A systematic review and meta-analysis. *Systematic Reviews*, 9(111), pp. 1–21. Available at https://systematicreviewsjournal.biomedcentral.com/articles/10.1186/s13643-020-01378-7.

[89] Silva, Y. P., Bernardi, A. and Frozza, R. L., 2020. The role of short-chain fatty acids from gut microbiota in gut-brain communication. *Frontiers in Endocrinology*, 11, p. 25. Available at https://www.ncbi.nlm.nih.gov/pmc/articles/PMC7005631/.

[90] Skonieczna-Żydecka, K., Grochans, E., Maciejewska, D., Szkup, M., Schneider-Matyka, D., Jurczak, A., Łoniewski, I., Kaczmarczyk, M., Marlicz, W., Czerwińska-Rogowska, M. and Pełka-Wysiecka, J., 2018. Faecal short chain fatty acids profile is changed in Polish depressive women. *Nutrients*, 10(12), p. 1939. Available at https://www.mdpi.com/2072-6643/10/12/1939; Zheng, P., Zeng, B., Zhou, C., Liu, M., Fang, Z., Xu, X., Zeng, L., Chen, J., Fan, S., Du, X. and Zhang, X., 2016. Gut microbiome remodeling induces depressive-like behaviors through a pathway mediated by the host's metabolism. *Molecular Psychiatry*, 21(6), pp. 786–96. Available at https://pubmed.ncbi.nlm.nih.gov/27067014/.

[91] Knowles, S. R., Nelson, E. A. and Palombo, E. A., 2008. Investigating the role of perceived stress on bacterial flora activity and salivary cortisol secretion: A possible mechanism underlying susceptibility to illness. *Biological Psychology*, 77(2), pp. 132–7. Available at https://researchbank.swinburne.edu.au/file/ef1fc8d1-ee61-402a-b150-eabe280e0648/1/PDF%20%28Accepted%20manuscript%29.pdf.

[92] Noonan, S., Zaveri, M., Macaninch, E. and Martyn, K., 2020. Food & mood: A review of supplementary prebiotic and probiotic interventions in the treatment of anxiety and depression in adults. *BMJ Nutrition, Prevention & Health*, 3, p. e000053. Available at https://nutrition.bmj.com/content/bmjnph/3/2/351.full.pdf.

[93] Sanders, L. M. and Zeisel, S. H., 2007. Choline: Dietary requirements and role in brain development. *Nutrition Today*, 42(4), pp. 181–6. Available at https://www.ncbi.nlm.nih.gov/pmc/articles/PMC2518394/.

[94] Choi, K. W., Stein, M. B., Nishimi, K. M., Ge, T., Coleman, J. R., Chen, C. Y., Ratanatharathorn, A., Zheutlin, A. B., Dunn, E. C., 23andMe Research Team and Major Depressive Disorder Working Group of the Psychiatric Genomics Consortium, 2020. An exposure-wide and Mendelian randomization approach to identifying modifiable factors for the prevention of depression. *American Journal of Psychiatry*, 177(10), pp. 944–54. Available at https://ajp.psychiatryonline.org/doi/10.1176/appi.ajp.2020.19111158.

[95] Mental Health Foundation, 9 Mar. 2021. Smoking and mental health. Available at https://www.mentalhealth.org.uk/a-to-z/s/smoking-and-mental-health.

[96] Firth, J., Solmi, M., Wootton, R. E., Vancampfort, D., Schuch, F. B., Hoare, E., Gilbody, S., Torous, J., Teasdale, S. B., Jackson, S. E. and Smith, L., 2020. A meta-review of 'lifestyle psychiatry': The role of exercise, smoking, diet and sleep in the prevention and treatment of mental disorders. *World Psychiatry*, 19(3), pp. 360–80. Available at https://pubmed.ncbi.nlm.nih.gov/32931092/; Wootton, R. E., Richmond, R. C., Stuijfzand, B. G., Lawn, R. B., Sallis, H. M., Taylor, G. M., Hemani, G., Jones, H. J., Zammit, S., Smith, G. D. and Munafò, M. R., 2020. Evidence for causal effects of lifetime smoking on risk for depression and schizophrenia: A Mendelian randomisation study. *Psychological Medicine*, 50(14), pp. 2435–43. Available at https://pubmed.ncbi.nlm.nih.gov/31689377/.

[97] Peltier, M. R., Flores, J. M., Smith, P. H., Roberts, W., Verplaetse, T. L., Moore, K. E., Hacker, R., Oberleitner, L. M. and McKee, S. A., 2020. Smoking across the menopausal transition in a 10-year longitudinal sample: The role of sex hormones and depressive symptoms. *Nicotine and Tobacco Research*, 22(6), pp. 872–7. Available at https://pubmed.ncbi.nlm.nih.gov/31058288/; Chen, H. L., Cai, J. Y., Zha, M. L. and Shen, W. Q., 2019. Prenatal smoking and postpartum depression: A meta-analysis. *Journal of Psychosomatic Obstetrics & Gynecology*, 40(2), pp. 97–105. Available at https://www.researchgate.net/profile/Hong-Lin-Chen/publication/323642207_Prenatal_smoking_and_postpartum_depression_a_meta-analysis/links/5dc37557299bf1a47b1c03bf/Prenatal-smoking-and-postpartum-depression-a-meta-analysis.pdf.

[98] Wilsnack, S. C., Wilsnack, R. W. and Kantor, L. W., 2013. Focus on: Women and the costs of alcohol use. *Alcohol Research*, 35(2), pp. 219–28. Available at https://www.ncbi.nlm.nih.gov/pmc/articles/PMC3908713/#b73-arcr-35-2-219.

[99] Sharma, A., 2006. Exercise for mental health. The Primary Care Companion for CNS Disorders, 8(2), p. 106. Available at https://www.ncbi.nlm.nih.gov/pmc/articles/PMC1470658/.

[100] Kołomańska-Bogucka, D. and Mazur-Bialy, A. I., 2019. Physical activity and the occurrence of postnatal depression – a systematic review. *Medicina*, 55(9), p. 560. Available at https://pubmed.ncbi.nlm.nih.gov/31480778/; Kołomańska, D., Zarawski, M. and Mazur-Bialy, A., 2019. Physical activity and depressive disorders in pregnant women – a systematic review. *Medicina*, 55(5), p. 212. Available at https://pubmed.ncbi.nlm.nih.gov/31130705/; Carter, T., Bastounis, A., Guo, B. and Morrell, C. J., 2019. The effectiveness of exercise-based interventions for preventing or treating postpartum depression: A systematic review and meta-analysis. *Archives of Women's Mental Health*, 22(1), pp. 37–53. Available at https://pubmed.ncbi.nlm.nih.gov/29882074/.

[101] Kołomańska, D., Zarawski, M. and Mazur-Bialy, A., 2019. Physical activity and depressive disorders in pregnant women – a systematic review. *Medicina*, 55(5), p. 212. Available at https://pubmed.ncbi.nlm.nih.gov/31130705/.

[102] Nelson, D. B., Sammel, M. D., Freeman, E. W., Lin, H., Gracia, C. R. and Schmitz, K. H., 2008. Effect of physical activity on menopausal symptoms among urban women. *Medicine and Science in Sports and Exercise*, 40(1), pp. 50–8. Available at https://pubmed.ncbi.nlm.nih.gov/18091021/; Mansikkamäki, K., Raitanen, J., Malila, N., Sarkeala, T., Männistö, S., Fredman, J., Heinävaara, S. and Luoto, R., 2015. Physical activity and menopause-related quality of life – a population-based cross-sectional study. Maturitas, 80(1), pp. 69–74. Available at https://pubmed.ncbi.nlm.nih.gov/25449820/.

[103] Firth, J., Solmi, M., Wootton, R. E., Vancampfort, D., Schuch, F. B., Hoare, E., Gilbody, S., Torous, J., Teasdale, S. B., Jackson, S. E. and Smith, L., 2020. A meta-review of 'lifestyle psychiatry': The role of exercise, smoking, diet and sleep in the prevention and treatment of mental disorders. *World Psychiatry*, 19(3), pp. 360–80. Available at https://www.ncbi.nlm.nih.gov/pmc/articles/PMC7491615/.

[104] Sharma, A., Barrett, M. S., Cucchiara, A. J., Gooneratne, N. S. and Thase, M. E., 2017. A breathing-based meditation intervention for patients with major depressive disorder following inadequate response to antidepressants: A randomized pilot study. *Journal of Clinical Psychiatry*, 78(1), p. 493. Available at https://www.psychiatrist.com/jcp/depression/adjunctive-yoga-for-mdd/.

CH 04 Sleep

[1] Institute of Medicine (US) Committee on Sleep Medicine and Research, Colten H. R., Altevogt B. M. [eds], 2006. Extent and health consequences of chronic sleep loss and sleep disorders. In *Sleep Disorders and Sleep Deprivation: An Unmet Public Health Problem*. National Academies Press. Available at https://www.ncbi.nlm.nih.gov/books/NBK19961.

[2] Cohen, S., Doyle, W. J., Alper, C. M., Janicki-Deverts, D. and Turner, R. B., 2009. Sleep habits and susceptibility to the common cold. *Archives of Internal Medicine*, 169(1), pp. 62–7. Available at https://jamanetwork.com/journals/jamainternalmedicine/fullarticle/414701; Kalmbach, D. A., Arnedt, J. T., Pillai, V. and Ciesla, J. A., 2015. The impact of sleep on female sexual response and behavior: A pilot study. *The Journal of Sexual Medicine*, 12(5), pp. 1221–32. Available at https://pubmed.ncbi.nlm.nih.gov/25772315/.

[3] Burgard, S. A. and Ailshire, J. A., 2013. Gender and time for sleep among US adults. *American Sociological Review*, 78(1), pp. 51–69. Available at https://www.ncbi.nlm.nih.gov/pmc/articles/PMC4164903/.

[4] Meers, J., Stout-Aguilar, J. and Nowakowski, S., 2019. Sex differences in sleep health. *Sleep and Health*, pp. 21–9. Available at https://www.sciencedirect.com/science/article/pii/B9780128153734000034?via%3Dihub.

[5] Reynolds, W. S., Fowke, J. and Dmochowski, R., 2016. The burden of overactive bladder on US public health. *Current Bladder Dysfunction Reports*, 11(1), pp. 8–13. Available at https://www.ncbi.nlm.nih.gov/pmc/articles/PMC4821440/; Weiss, J. P., 2012. Nocturia: Focus on etiology and consequences. *Reviews in Urology*, 14(3–4), pp. 48–55. Available at https://pubmed.ncbi.nlm.nih.gov/23526404/.

[6] Kim, Y. S., Kim, N. and Kim, G. H., 2016. Sex and gender differences in gastroesophageal reflux disease. *Journal of Neurogastroenterology and Motility*, 22(4), pp. 575–88. Available at https://www.ncbi.nlm.nih.gov/pmc/articles/PMC5056567/.

[7] Shahrbabaki, S. S., Linz, D., Hartmann, S., Redline, S. and Baumert, M., 2021. Sleep arousal burden is associated with long-term all-cause and cardiovascular mortality in 8001 community-dwelling older men and women. *European Heart Journal*, 42(21), pp. 2088–99. Available at https://academic.oup.com/eurheartj/article/42/21/2088/6239256.

[8] Meers, J., Stout-Aguilar, J. and Nowakowski, S., 2019. Sex differences in sleep health. *Sleep and Health*, pp. 21–9. Available at https://www.sciencedirect.com/science/article/pii/B9780128153734000034?via%3Dihub.

[9] Greenblatt, D. J., Harmatz, J. S. and Roth, T., 2019. Zolpidem and gender: Are women really at risk? *Journal of Clinical Psychopharmacology*, 39(3), pp. 189–99. Available at https://pubmed.ncbi.nlm.nih.gov/30939589/.

[10] Mong, J. A. and Cusmano, D. M., 2016. Sex differences in sleep: Impact of biological sex and sex steroids. *Philosophical Transactions of the Royal Society B: Biological Sciences*, 371(1688), p. 20150110. Available at https://royalsocietypublishing.org/doi/10.1098/rstb.2015.0110.

[11] Nolen-Hoeksema, S., Larson, J. and Grayson, C., 1999. Explaining the gender difference in depressive symptoms. *Journal of Personality and Social Psychology*, 77(5), pp. 1061–72. Available at https://doi.apa.org/doiLanding?doi=10.1037%2F0022-3514.77.5.1061.

[12] Burgard, S. A. and Ailshire, J. A., 2013. Gender and time for sleep among US adults. *American Sociological Review*, 78(1), pp. 51–69. Available at https://www.ncbi.nlm.nih.gov/pmc/articles/PMC4164903/.

[13] Kuljis, D. A., Loh, D. H., Truong, D., Vosko, A. M., Ong, M. L., McClusky, R., Arnold, A. P. and Colwell, C. S., 2013. Gonadal-and sex-chromosome-dependent sex differences in the circadian system. *Endocrinology*, 154(4), pp. 1501–12. Available at https://pubmed.ncbi.nlm.nih.gov/23439698/.

[14] Institute of Medicine (US) Committee on Sleep Medicine and Research, Colten H. R., Altevogt B. M. [eds], 2006. Sleep physiology. In *Sleep Disorders and Sleep Deprivation: An Unmet Public Health Problem*. National Academies Press. Available at https://www.ncbi.nlm.nih.gov/books/NBK19956/.

[15] Roth, T., 2009. Slow wave sleep: Does it matter?. *Journal of Clinical Sleep Medicine*, 5(2 suppl), pp. S4–5. Available at https://www.ncbi.nlm.nih.gov/pmc/articles/PMC2824210/.

[16] Walker, M. P. and van Der Helm, E., 2009. Overnight therapy? The role of sleep in emotional brain processing. *Psychological Bulletin*, 135(5), pp. 731–48. Available at https://www.ncbi.nlm.nih.gov/pmc/articles/PMC2890316/; Institute of Medicine (US) Committee on Sleep Medicine and Research, Colten H. R., Altevogt B. M. [eds], 2006. Sleep physiology. In *Sleep Disorders and Sleep Deprivation: An Unmet Public Health Problem*. National Academies Press. Available at https://www.ncbi.nlm.nih.gov/books/NBK19956/.

[17] Goldstein, A. N. and Walker, M. P., 2014. The role of sleep in emotional brain function. *Annual Review of Clinical Psychology*, 10, pp. 679–708. Available at https://www.ncbi.nlm.nih.gov/pmc/articles/PMC4286245/.

[18] Kirsch, D., Benca, R. and Eichler, A., 2015. Stages and architecture of normal sleep. UpToDate. Available at https://www.uptodate.com/contents/stages-and-architecture-of-normal-sleep.

[19] Lee, J., Han, Y., Cho, H. H. and Kim, M. R., 2019. Sleep disorders and menopause. *Journal of Menopausal Medicine*, 25(2), pp. 83–7. Available at https://www.ncbi.nlm.nih.gov/pmc/articles/PMC6718648/.

[20] Ibid.

[21] Johnson, E. O., Roth, T., Schultz, L. and Breslau, N., 2006. Epidemiology of DSM-IV insomnia in adolescence: Lifetime prevalence, chronicity, and an emergent gender difference. *Pediatrics*, 117(2), pp. e247–56. Available at https://publications.aap.org/pediatrics/article-abstract/117/2/e247/68471/Epidemiology-of-DSM-IV-Insomnia-in-Adolescence?redirectedFrom=fulltext.

[22] Ibid

[23] Baker, F. C. and Lee, K. A., 2018. Menstrual cycle effects on sleep. *Sleep Medicine Clinics*, 13(3), pp. 283–94. Available at https://pubmed.ncbi.nlm.nih.gov/30098748/#:~:text=Subjective%20and%20objective%20sleep%20changes,luteal%20phase%2C%20potentially%20progesterone%20related.

[24] Van Reen, E. and Kiesner, J., 2016. Individual differences in self-reported difficulty sleeping across the menstrual cycle. *Archives of Women's Mental Health*, 19(4), pp. 599–608. Available at https://pubmed.ncbi.nlm.nih.gov/26973332/.

[25] Driver, H. S., Werth, E., Dijk, D. J. and Borbély, A. A., 2008. The menstrual cycle effects on sleep. *Sleep Medicine Clinics*, 3(1), pp. 1–11. Available at https://www.sciencedirect.com/science/article/abs/pii/S1556407X07001142; Dorsey, A., De Lecea, L. and Jennings, K. J., 2021. Neurobiological and hormonal mechanisms regulating women's sleep. *Frontiers in Neuroscience*, p. 1446. Available at https://www.frontiersin.org/articles/10.3389/fnins.2020.625397/full#B17.

[26] Baker, F. C., Mitchell, D. and Driver, H. S., 2001. Oral contraceptives alter sleep and raise body temperature in young women. *Pflügers Archiv*, 442(5), pp. 729–37. Available at https://pubmed.ncbi.nlm.nih.gov/11512029/.

[27] Baker, F. C. and Lee, K. A., 2018. Menstrual cycle effects on sleep. *Sleep Medicine Clinics*, 13(3), pp. 283–94. Available at https://pubmed.ncbi.nlm.nih.gov/30098748/#:~:text=Subjective%20and%20objective%20sleep%20changes,luteal%20phase%2C%20potentially%20progesterone%20related.

[28] Sedov, I. D., Cameron, E. E., Madigan, S. and Tomfohr-Madsen, L. M., 2018. Sleep quality during pregnancy: A meta-analysis. *Sleep Medicine Reviews*, 38, pp. 168–76. Available at https://pubmed.ncbi.nlm.nih.gov/28866020/.

[29] Dorsey, A., De Lecea, L. and Jennings, K. J., 2021. Neurobiological and hormonal mechanisms regulating women's sleep. *Frontiers in Neuroscience*, p. 1446. Available at https://www.frontiersin.org/articles/10.3389/fnins.2020.625397/full#B16; Lara-Carrasco, J., Simard, V., Saint-Onge, K., Lamoureux-Tremblay, V. and Nielsen, T., 2014. Disturbed dreaming during the third trimester of pregnancy. *Sleep Medicine*, 15(6), pp. 694–700. Available at https://pubmed.ncbi.nlm.nih.gov/24780135/.

[30] Hertz, G., Fast, A., Feinsilver, S. H., Albertario, C. L., Schulman, H. and Fein, A. M., 1992. Sleep in normal late pregnancy. *Sleep*, 15(3), pp. 246–51. Available at https://academic.oup.com/sleep/article/15/3/246/2749272?login=true.

[31] Ibid.

[32] Tsai, S. Y., Lee, C. N., Wu, W. W. and Landis, C. A., 2016. Sleep hygiene and sleep quality of third-trimester pregnant women. *Research in Nursing & Health*, 39(1), pp. 57–65. Available at https://pubmed.ncbi.nlm.nih.gov/26650922/.

[33] Hertz, G., Fast, A., Feinsilver, S. H., Albertario, C. L., Schulman, H. and Fein, A. M., 1992. Sleep in normal late pregnancy. *Sleep*, 15(3), pp. 246–51. Available at https://academic.oup.com/sleep/article/15/3/246/2749272?login=true.

[34] Moszeik, E. N., von Oertzen, T. and Renner, K. H., 2020. Effectiveness of a short Yoga Nidra meditation on stress, sleep, and well-being in a large and diverse sample. *Current Psychology*, pp. 1–15. Available at https://link.springer.com/article/10.1007/s12144-020-01042-2.

[35] Lee, J., Han, Y., Cho, H. H. and Kim, M. R., 2019. Sleep disorders and menopause. *Journal of Menopausal Medicine*, 25(2), pp. 83–7. Available at https://www.ncbi.nlm.nih.gov/pmc/articles/PMC6718648/#B7.

[36] Dorsey, A., De Lecea, L. and Jennings, K. J., 2021. Neurobiological and hormonal mechanisms regulating women's sleep. *Frontiers in Neuroscience*, p. 1446. Available at https://www.frontiersin.org/articles/10.3389/fnins.2020.625397/full.

[37] Baker, F. C., Lampio, L., Saaresranta, T. and Polo-Kantola, P., 2018. Sleep and sleep disorders in the menopausal transition. *Sleep Medicine Clinics*, 13(3), pp. 443–56. Available at https://www.ncbi.nlm.nih.gov/pmc/articles/PMC6092036/.

[38] Polo-Kantola, P., Erkkola, R., Irjala, K., Pullinen, S., Virtanen, I. and Polo, O., 1999. Effect of short-term transdermal estrogen replacement therapy on sleep: A randomized, double-blind crossover trial in postmenopausal women. *Fertility and Sterility*, 71(5), pp. 873–80. Available at https://www.sciencedirect.com/science/article/abs/pii/S001502829900062X.

[39] Guthrie, K. A., Larson, J. C., Ensrud, K. E., Anderson, G. L., Carpenter, J. S., Freeman, E. W., Joffe, H., LaCroix, A. Z., Manson, J. E., Morin, C. M. and Newton, K. M., 2018. Effects of pharmacologic and nonpharmacologic interventions on insomnia symptoms and self-reported sleep quality in women with hot flashes: A pooled analysis of individual participant data from four MsFLASH trials. *Sleep*, 41(1), p. zsx190. Available at https://pubmed.ncbi.nlm.nih.gov/29165623/.

[40] Conley, S., Knies, A., Batten, J., Ash, G., Miner, B., Hwang, Y., Jeon, S. and Redeker, N. S., 2019. Agreement between actigraphic and polysomnographic measures of sleep in adults with and without chronic conditions: A systematic review and meta-analysis. *Sleep Medicine Reviews*, 46, pp. 151–60. Available at https://pubmed.ncbi.nlm.nih.gov/31154154/; Gavriloff, D., Sheaves, B., Juss, A., Espie, C. A., Miller, C. B. and Kyle, S. D., 2018. Sham sleep feedback delivered via actigraphy biases daytime symptom reports in people with insomnia: Implications for insomnia disorder and wearable devices. *Journal of Sleep Research*, 27(6), p. e12726. Available at https://pubmed.ncbi.nlm.nih.gov/29989248/.

[41] Blume, C., Garbazza, C. and Spitschan, M., 2019. Effects of light on human circadian rhythms, sleep and mood. *Somnologie*, 23(3), pp. 147–56. Available at https://www.ncbi.nlm.nih.gov/pmc/articles/PMC6751071/.

[42] Ibid. Available at https://www.ncbi.nlm.nih.gov/pmc/articles/PMC6751071/#:~:text=Roughly%20speaking%2C%20the%20effect%20of,phase%20%5B43%2C%2066%5D.

[43] Terman, J. S., Terman, M., Lo, E. S. and Cooper, T. B., 2001. Circadian time of morning light administration and therapeutic response in winter depression. *Archives of General Psychiatry*, 58(1), pp. 69–75. Available at https://jamanetwork.com/journals/jamapsychiatry/fullarticle/481701.

[44] NHS, 30 Jul. 2018. Treatment – seasonal affective disorder (SAD). Available at https://www.nhs.uk/mental-health/conditions/seasonal-affective-disorder-sad/treatment/.

[45] Teran, E., Yee-Rendon, C. M., Ortega-Salazar, J., De Gracia, P., Garcia-Romo, E. and Woods, R. L., 2020. Evaluation of two strategies for alleviating the impact on the circadian cycle of smartphone screens. *Optometry and Vision Science*, 97(3), pp. 207–17. Available at https://pubmed.ncbi.nlm.nih.gov/32168244/; Lawrenson, J. G., Hull, C. C. and Downie, L. E., 2017. The effect of blue-light blocking spectacle lenses on visual performance, macular health and the sleep-wake cycle: A systematic review of the literature. *Ophthalmic and Physiological Optics*, 37(6), pp. 644–54. Available at https://pubmed.ncbi.nlm.nih.gov/29044670/.

[46] Jackson, S. B., 2020. Rolling my third eye: The third eye and pineal gland connection. *DU Quark*, 5(1), pp. 6–13. Available at https://dsc.duq.edu/cgi/viewcontent.cgi?article=1075&context=duquark.

[47] Grivas, T. B. and Savvidou, O. D., 2007. Melatonin the 'light of night' in human biology and adolescent idiopathic scoliosis. *Scoliosis*, 2(1), pp. 1–14. Available at https://www.ncbi.nlm.nih.gov/pmc/articles/PMC1855314/#B11.

[48] Greendale, G. A., Witt-Enderby, P., Karlamangla, A. S., Munmun, F., Crawford, S., Huang, M. and Santoro, N., 2020. Melatonin patterns and levels during the human menstrual cycle and after menopause. *Journal of the Endocrine Society*, 4(11), p. bvaa115. Available at https://academic.oup.com/jes/article/4/11/bvaa115/5898237.

[49] Herxheimer, A. and Petrie, K. J., 2002. Melatonin for the prevention and treatment of jet lag. *Cochrane Database of Systematic Reviews*, (2). Available at https://pubmed.ncbi.nlm.nih.

gov/12076414/; Ferracioli-Oda, E., Qawasmi, A. and Bloch, M. H., 2013. Meta-analysis: Melatonin for the treatment of primary sleep disorders. *PloS One*, 8(5), p. e63773. Available at https://pubmed.ncbi.nlm.nih.gov/23691095/.

50 Amstrup, A. K., Sikjaer, T., Mosekilde, L. and Rejnmark, L., 2015. The effect of melatonin treatment on postural stability, muscle strength, and quality of life and sleep in postmenopausal women: A randomized controlled trial. *Nutrition Journal*, 14(102), pp. 1–8. Available at https://pubmed.ncbi.nlm.nih.gov/26424587/.

51 Costello, R. B., Lentino, C. V., Boyd, C. C., O'Connell, M. L., Crawford, C. C., Sprengel, M. L. and Deuster, P. A., 2014. The effectiveness of melatonin for promoting healthy sleep: A rapid evidence assessment of the literature. *Nutrition Journal*, 13(1), p. 106. Available at https://www.ncbi.nlm.nih.gov/pmc/articles/PMC4273450/.

52 Pro, L. P. F. and Con, L. M., 2019. Should melatonin be used as a sleeping aid for elderly people? *Canadian Journal of Hospital Pharmacy*, 72(4), pp. 327–9. Available at https://www.ncbi.nlm.nih.gov/pmc/articles/PMC6699865/.

53 Erland, L. A. and Saxena, P. K., 2017. Melatonin natural health products and supplements: Presence of serotonin and significant variability of melatonin content. *Journal of Clinical Sleep Medicine*, 13(2), pp. 275–81. Available at https://jcsm.aasm.org/doi/10.5664/jcsm.6462.

54 Erland, L. A. and Saxena, P. K., 2017. Melatonin natural health products and supplements: Presence of serotonin and significant variability of melatonin content. *Journal of Clinical Sleep Medicine*, 13(2), pp. 275–81. Available at https://jcsm.aasm.org/doi/10.5664/jcsm.6462.

55 Wang, F., Lee, O. E. K., Feng, F., Vitiello, M. V., Wang, W., Benson, H., Fricchione, G. L. and Denninger, J. W., 2016. The effect of meditative movement on sleep quality: A systematic review. *Sleep Medicine Reviews*, 30, pp. 43–52. Available at https://pubmed.ncbi.nlm.nih.gov/26802824/; Reid, K. J., Baron, K. G., Lu, B., Naylor, E., Wolfe, L. and Zee, P. C., 2010. Aerobic exercise improves self-reported sleep and quality of life in older adults with insomnia. *Sleep Medicine*, 11(9), pp. 934–40. Available at https://pubmed.ncbi.nlm.nih.gov/20813580/; Kovacevic, A., Mavros, Y., Heisz, J. J. and Singh, M. A. F., 2018. The effect of resistance exercise on sleep: A systematic review of randomized controlled trials. *Sleep Medicine Reviews*, 39, pp. 52–68. Available at https://pubmed.ncbi.nlm.nih.gov/28919335/.

56 Stutz, J., Eiholzer, R. and Spengler, C. M., 2019. Effects of evening exercise on sleep in healthy participants: A systematic review and meta-analysis. *Sports Medicine*, 49(2), pp. 269–87. Available at https://pubmed.ncbi.nlm.nih.gov/30374942/.

57 Ibid.

58 Savoie, M. B., Lee, K. A., Subak, L. L., Hernandez, C., Schembri, M., Fung, C. H., Grady, D. and Huang, A. J., 2020. Beyond the bladder: poor sleep in women with overactive bladder syndrome. *American Journal of Obstetrics and Gynecology*, 222(6), pp. 600e1–e13. Available at https://www.ncbi.nlm.nih.gov/pmc/articles/PMC7263944/.

59 Crosby, P., Hamnett, R., Putker, M., Hoyle, N. P., Reed, M., Karam, C. J., Maywood, E. S., Stangherlin, A., Chesham, J. E., Hayter, E. A. and Rosenbrier-Ribeiro, L., 2019. Insulin/IGF-1 drives PERIOD synthesis to entrain circadian rhythms with feeding time. *Cell*, 177(4), pp. 896–909. Available at https://linkinghub.elsevier.com/retrieve/pii/S0092867419301667.

60 Al Khatib, H. K., Harding, S. V., Darzi, J. and Pot, G. K., 2017. The effects of partial sleep deprivation on energy balance: A systematic review and meta-analysis. *European Journal of Clinical Nutrition*, 71(5), pp. 614–24. Available at https://www.nature.com/articles/ejcn2016201.

61 Kitano, N., Tsunoda, K., Tsuji, T., Osuka, Y., Jindo, T., Tanaka, K. and Okura, T., 2014. Association between difficulty initiating sleep in older adults and the combination of leisure-time physical activity and consumption of milk and milk products: A cross-sectional study. *BMC Geriatrics*, 14(118), pp. 1–7. Available at https://pubmed.ncbi.nlm.nih.gov/25407520/; Fakhr-Movahedi, A., Mirmohammadkhani, M. and Ramezani, H., 2018. Effect of milk-honey mixture on the sleep quality of coronary patients: A clinical trial study. Clinical Nutrition ESPEN, 28, pp. 132–5. Available at https://pubmed.ncbi.nlm.nih.gov/30390870/; Komada, Y., Okajima, I. and Kuwata, T., 2020. The effects of milk and dairy products on sleep: A systematic review. *International Journal of Environmental Research and Public Health*, 17(24), p. 9440. Available at https://pubmed.ncbi.nlm.nih.gov/33339284/.

62 Wurtman, R. J. and Wurtman, J. J., 1986. Carbohydrate craving, obesity and brain serotonin. *Appetite*, 7, pp. 99–103. Available at https://www.sciencedirect.com/science/article/abs/pii/S0195666386800551.

63 Institute of Medicine (US) Committee on Military Nutrition Research, 2001. Pharmacology of caffeine. In *Caffeine for the Sustainment of Mental Task Performance: Formulations for Military Operations*. National Academies Press. Available at https://www.ncbi.nlm.nih.gov/books/NBK223808/#:~:text=The%20mean%20half%2Dlife%20of,et%20al.%2C%201989).

64 Ibid

65 Stein, M. D. and Friedmann, P. D., 2006. Disturbed sleep and its relationship to alcohol use. *Substance Abuse*, 26(1), pp. 1–13. Available at https://www.ncbi.nlm.nih.gov/pmc/articles/PMC2775419/.

66 Pacheco, D., 29 Nov. 2021. Alcohol and sleep. Sleep Foundation. Available at https://www.sleepfoundation.org/nutrition/alcohol-and-sleep.

67 Chaput, J. P., Dutil, C., Featherstone, R., Ross, R., Giangregorio, L., Saunders, T. J., Janssen, I., Poitras, V. J., Kho, M. E., Ross-White, A. and Zankar, S., 2020. Sleep timing, sleep consistency, and health in adults: A systematic review. *Applied Physiology, Nutrition, and Metabolism*, 45(10), pp. S232–47. Available at https://pubmed.ncbi.nlm.nih.gov/33054339/; Okano, K., Kaczmarzyk, J. R., Dave, N., Gabrieli, J. D. and Grossman, J. C., 2019. Sleep quality, duration, and consistency are associated with better academic performance in college students. *NPJ Science of Learning*, 4(16), pp. 1–5. Available at https://www.nature.com/articles/s41539-019-0055-z.

68 Mindell, J. A., Telofski, L. S., Wiegand, B. and Kurtz, E. S., 2009. A nightly bedtime routine: Impact on sleep in young children and maternal mood. *Sleep*, 32(5), pp. 599–606. Available at https://pubmed.ncbi.nlm.nih.gov/19480226/.

69 Johnson, D. P. and Whisman, M. A., 2013. Gender differences in rumination: A meta-analysis. *Personality and Individual Differences*, 55(4), pp. 367–74. Available at https://www.ncbi.nlm.nih.gov/pmc/articles/PMC3786159/.

70 Scullin, M. K., Krueger, M. L., Ballard, H. K., Pruett, N. and Bliwise, D. L., 2018. The effects of bedtime writing on difficulty falling asleep: A polysomnographic study comparing to-do lists and completed activity lists. *Journal of Experimental Psychology: General*, 147(1), pp. 139–46. Available at https://www.ncbi.nlm.nih.gov/pmc/articles/PMC5758411/.

71 Boggiss, A. L., Consedine, N. S., Brenton-Peters, J. M., Hofman, P. L. and Serlachius, A. S., 2020. A systematic review of gratitude interventions: Effects on physical health and health behaviors. *Journal of Psychosomatic Research*, 135, p. 110165. Available at https://www.sciencedirect.com/science/article/abs/pii/S0022399920301847.

72 Lastella, M., O'Mullan, C., Paterson, J. L. and Reynolds, A. C., 2019. Sex and sleep: Perceptions of sex as a sleep promoting behavior in the general adult population. *Frontiers in Public Health*, 7, p. 33. Available at https://www.ncbi.nlm.nih.gov/pmc/articles/PMC6409294/.

73 Ibid.

74 Ibid.

75 Kalmbach, D. A., Arnedt, J. T., Pillai, V. and Ciesla, J. A., 2015. The impact of sleep on female sexual response and behavior: A pilot study. *The Journal of Sexual Medicine*, 12(5), pp. 1221–32. Available at https://pubmed.ncbi.nlm.nih.gov/25772315/.

76 Lateef, O. M. and Akintubosun, M. O., 2020. Sleep and reproductive health. *Journal of Circadian Rhythms*, 18, p. 1. Available at https://www.ncbi.nlm.nih.gov/pmc/articles/PMC7101004/.

77 Leproult, R. and Van Cauter, E., 2011. Effect of 1 week of sleep restriction on testosterone levels in young healthy men. *JAMA*, 305(21), pp. 2173–4. Available at https://jamanetwork.com/journals/jama/article-abstract/1029127.

78 Frederick, D. A., John, H. K. S., Garcia, J. R. and Lloyd, E. A., 2018. Differences in orgasm frequency among gay, lesbian, bisexual, and heterosexual men and women in a US national sample. *Archives of Sexual Behavior*, 47(1), pp. 273–88. Available at https://link.springer.com/article/10.1007/s10508-017-0939-z.

79 Frederick, D. A., John, H. K. S., Garcia, J. R. and Lloyd, E. A., 2018. Differences in orgasm frequency among gay, lesbian, bisexual, and heterosexual men and women in a US national

sample. *Archives of Sexual Behavior*, 47(1), pp. 273–88. Available at https://link.springer.com/article/10.1007/s10508-017-0939-z.

[80] Garcia, J. R., Lloyd, E. A., Wallen, K. and Fisher, H. E., 2014. Variation in orgasm occurrence by sexual orientation in a sample of US singles. *The Journal Of Sexual Medicine*, 11(11), pp. 2645–52. Available at https://www.jsm.jsexmed.org/article/S1743-6095(15)30602-0/fulltext; Mahar, E. A., Mintz, L. B. and Akers, B. M., 2020. Orgasm equality: Scientific findings and societal implications. *Current Sexual Health Reports*, 12(1), pp. 24–32. Available at https://link.springer.com/article/10.1007/s11930-020-00237-9.

[81] Mahar, E. A., Mintz. L. B. and Akers, B. M., 2020. Orgasm equality: Scientific findings and societal implications. *Current Sexual Health Reports*, 12(1), pp. 24–32. Available at https://link.springer.com/article/10.1007/s11930-020-00237-9.

[82] Muehlenhard, C. L. and Shippee, S. K., 2010. Men's and women's reports of pretending orgasm. *Journal of Sex Research*, 47(6). pp. 552–67. Available at https://www.tandfonline.com/doi/abs/10.1080/00224490903171794.

[83] Mahar, E. A., Mintz, L. B. and Akers, B. M., 2020. Orgasm equality: Scientific findings and societal implications. *Current Sexual Health Reports*, 12(1), pp. 24–32. Available at https://link.springer.com/article/10.1007/s11930-020-00237-9.

[84] Guitelman, J., Mahar, E. A., Mintz, L. B. and Dodd, H. E., 2019. Effectiveness of a bibliotherapy intervention for young adult women's sexual functioning. *Sexual and Relationship Therapy*, 36(2–3), pp. 198–218. Available at https://www.tandfonline.com/doi/full/10.1080/14681994.2019.1660761;

[85] Mahar, E. A., Mintz, L. B. and Akers, B. M., 2020. Orgasm equality: Scientific findings and societal implications. *Current Sexual Health Reports*, 12(1), pp. 24–32. Available at https://link.springer.com/article/10.1007/s11930-020-00237-9; Mintz, L. B., 2018. *Becoming Cliterate: Why orgasm equality matters – and how to get it*. HarperOne. Available at https://books.google.ae/books?id=2mRitAEACAAJ&dq=becoming+cliterate&hl=en&sa=X&ved=2ahUKEwjH88Lc2Pf1AhUIz4UKHb5wBmwQ6AF6BAgEEAI.

[86] Rivera, A. S., Akanbi, M., O'Dwyer, L. C. and McHugh, M., 2020. Shift work and long work hours and their association with chronic health conditions: A systematic review of systematic reviews with meta-analyses. *PloS One*, 15(4), p. e0231037. Available at https://journals.plos.org/plosone/article?id=10.1371/journal.pone.0231037.

Appendix 1: Polycystic ovary syndrome And Endometriosis

[1] Nardo, L. G., Patchava, S. and Laing, I., 2008. Polycystic ovary syndrome: Pathophysiology, molecular aspects and clinical implications. *Panminerva Medica*, 50(4), pp. 267–78. Available at https://pubmed.ncbi.nlm.nih.gov/19078868/.

[2] Eshre, R. and ASRM-Sponsored PCOS Consensus Workshop Group, 2004. Revised 2003 consensus on diagnostic criteria and long-term health risks related to polycystic ovary syndrome (PCOS). *Human Reproduction*, 19(1), pp. 41–7. Available at https://pubmed.ncbi.nlm.nih.gov/14688154/.

[3] Moran, L. J., Ko, H., Misso, M., Marsh, K., Noakes, M., Talbot, M., Frearson, M., Thondan, M., Stepto, N. and Teede, H. J., 2013. Dietary composition in the treatment of polycystic ovary syndrome: A systematic review to inform evidence-based guidelines. *Journal of the Academy of Nutrition and Dietetics*, 113(4), pp. 520–45. Available at https://pubmed.ncbi.nlm.nih.gov/23420000/; Mehrabani, H. H., Salehpour, S., Amiri, Z., Farahani, S. J., Meyer, B.J. and Tahbaz, F., 2012. Beneficial effects of a high-protein, low-glycemic-load hypocaloric diet in overweight and obese women with polycystic ovary syndrome: A randomized controlled intervention study. *Journal of the American College of Nutrition*, 31(2), pp. 117–25. Available at https://pubmed.ncbi.nlm.nih.gov/22855917/.

[4] Yang, K., Zeng, L., Bao, T. and Ge, J., 2018. Effectiveness of omega-3 fatty acid for polycystic ovary syndrome: A systematic review and meta-analysis. *Reproductive Biology and Endocrinology*, 16(1), p. 27. Available at https://www.ncbi.nlm.nih.gov/pmc/articles/PMC5870911/; Parker, D. R., Weiss, S. T., Troisi, R., Cassano, P. A., Vokonas, P. S. and Landsberg, L., 1993. Relationship of dietary saturated fatty acids and body habitus to serum insulin concentrations: The Normative Aging Study. *American Journal of Clinical Nutrition*, 58(2), pp. 129–36. Available at https://academic.oup.com/ajcn/article-abstract/58/2/129/4715905.

[5] Haidari, F., Banaei-Jahromi, N., Zakerkish, M. and Ahmadi, K., 2020. The effects of flaxseed supplementation on metabolic status in women with polycystic ovary syndrome: A randomized open-labeled controlled clinical trial. *Nutrition Journal*, 19(8). Available at https://nutritionj.biomedcentral.com/articles/10.1186/s12937-020-0524-5; Nowak, D. A., Snyder, D. C., Brown, A. J. and Demark-Wahnefried, W., 2007. The effect of flaxseed supplementation on hormonal levels associated with polycystic ovary syndrome: A case study. *Current Topics in Nutraceutical Research*, 5(4), pp. 177–81. Available at https://pubmed.ncbi.nlm.nih.gov/19789727/.

[6] Sørensen, L. B., Søe, M., Halkier, K. H., Stigsby, B. and Astrup, A., 2012. Effects of increased dietary protein-to-carbohydrate ratios in women with polycystic ovary syndrome. *The American Journal of Clinical Nutrition*, 95(1), pp. 39–48. Available at https://pubmed.ncbi.nlm.nih.gov/22158730/; Kasim-Karakas, S. E., Cunningham, W. M. and Tsodikov, A., 2007. Relation of nutrients and hormones in polycystic ovary syndrome. *American Journal of Clinical Nutrition*, 85(3), pp. 688–94. Available at https://pubmed.ncbi.nlm.nih.gov/17344488/.

[7] Leidy, H. J., Clifton, P. M., Astrup, A., Wycherley, T. P., Westerterp-Plantenga, M. S., Luscombe-Marsh, N. D., Woods, S. C. and Mattes, R. D., 2015. The role of protein in weight loss and maintenance. *American Journal of Clinical Nutrition*, 101(6), pp. 1320S–9S. Available at https://pubmed.ncbi.nlm.nih.gov/25926512/.

[8] Krul-Poel, Y. H. M., Koenders, P. P., Steegers-Theunissen, R. P., Ten Boekel, E., Wee, M. T., Louwers, Y., Lips, P., Laven, J. S. E. and Simsek, S., 2018. Vitamin D and metabolic disturbances in polycystic ovary syndrome (PCOS): A cross-sectional study. *PloS One*, 13(12), p. e0204748. Available at https://www.ncbi.nlm.nih.gov/pmc/articles/PMC6279035/.

[9] Thys-Jacobs, S., Donovan, D., Papadopoulos, A., Sarrel, P. and Bilezikian, J. P., 1999. Vitamin D and calcium dysregulation in the polycystic ovary syndrome. *Steroids*, 64(6), pp. 430–5. Available at https://pubmed.ncbi.nlm.nih.gov/10433180/.

[10] Amooee, S., Parsanezhad, M. E., Shirazi, M. R., Alborzi, S. and Samsami, A., 2013. Metformin versus chromium picolinate in clomiphene citrate-resistant patients with PCOs: A double-blind randomized clinical trial. *Iranian Journal of Reproductive Medicine*, 11(8), pp. 611–8. Available at https://pubmed.ncbi.nlm.nih.gov/24639797/.

[11] Izadi, A., Ebrahimi, S., Shirazi, S., Taghizadeh, S., Parizad, M., Farzadi, L. and Gargari, B. P., 2019. Hormonal and metabolic effects of coenzyme Q10 and/or vitamin E in patients with polycystic ovary syndrome. *Journal of Clinical Endocrinology & Metabolism*, 104(2), pp. 319–27. Available at https://pubmed.ncbi.nlm.nih.gov/30202998/; Izadi, A., Shirazi, S., Taghizadeh, S. and Gargari, B. P., 2019. Independent and additive effects of coenzyme Q10 and vitamin E on cardiometabolic outcomes and visceral adiposity in women with polycystic ovary syndrome., 50(2), pp. 1–10. Available at https://pubmed.ncbi.nlm.nih.gov/31349945/.

[12] Hajimonfarednejad, M., Nimrouzi, M., Heydari, M., Zarshenas, M. M., Raee, M. J. and Jahromi, B. N., 2018. Insulin resistance improvement by cinnamon powder in polycystic ovary syndrome: A randomized double-blind placebo controlled clinical trial. *Phytotherapy Research*, 32(2), pp. 276–83. Available at https://pubmed.ncbi.nlm.nih.gov/29250843/.

[13] All Party Parliamentary Group on Endometriosis, 2020. Endometriosis in the UK: Time for change. Available at https://www.endometriosis-uk.org/sites/endometriosis-uk.org/files/files/Endometriosis%20APPG%20Report%20Oct%202020.pdf; Husby, G. K., Haugen, R. S. and Moen, M. H., 2003. Diagnostic delay in women with pain and endometriosis. *Acta Obstetricia et Gynecologica Scandinavica*, 82(7), pp. 649–53. Available at https://pubmed.ncbi.nlm.nih.gov/12790847/.

[14] Royal College of Obstetricians & Gynaecologists, 29 Jun. 2018. *Endometriosis*. Available at https://www.rcog.org.uk/en/patients/patient-leaflets/endometriosis/.

[15] Missmer, S. A., Chavarro, J. E., Malspeis, S., Bertone-Johnson, E. R., Hornstein, M. D., Spiegelman, D., Barbieri, R. L., Willett, W. C. and Hankinson, S. E., 2010. A prospective study of dietary fat consumption and endometriosis risk. *Human Reproduction*, 25(6), pp. 1528–35. Available at https://academic.oup.com/humrep/article/25/6/1528/2915756?login=true; Hopeman, M. M., Riley, J. K., Frolova, A. I., Jiang, H. and Jungheim, E. S., 2015. Serum polyunsaturated fatty acids and endometriosis. *Reproductive Sciences*, 22(9), pp. 1083–7. Available at https://pubmed.ncbi.nlm.nih.gov/25539770/.

[16] Missmer, S. A., Chavarro, J. E., Malspeis, S., Bertone-Johnson, E. R., Hornstein, M. D., Spiegelman, D., Barbieri, R. L., Willett, W. C. and Hankinson, S. E., 2010. A prospective study of dietary fat consumption and endometriosis risk. Human Reproduction, 25(6), pp. 1528–35. Available at https://academic.oup.com/humrep/article/25/6/1528/2915756?login=true.

[17] Yamamoto, A., Harris, H. R., Vitonis, A. F., Chavarro, J. E. and Missmer, S. A., 2018. A prospective cohort study of meat and fish consumption and endometriosis risk. *American Journal Of Obstetrics And Gynecology*, 219(2), pp. 178e1–e10. Available at https://www.ajog.org/article/S0002-9378(18)30444-7/fulltext; Parazzini, F., Chiaffarino, F., Surace, M., Chatenoud, L., Cipriani, S., Chiantera, V., Benzi, G. and Fedele, L., 2004. Selected food intake and risk of endometriosis. *Human Reproduction*, 19(8), pp. 1755–9. Available at https://academic.oup.com/humrep/article/19/8/1755/2356458?login=true.

[18] Gołąbek, A., Kowalska, K. and Olejnik, A., 2021. Polyphenols as a diet therapy concept for endometriosis – current opinion and future perspectives. *Nutrients*, 13(4), p. 1347. Available at https://pubmed.ncbi.nlm.nih.gov/33919512/; Afrin, S., AlAshqar, A., El Sabeh, M., Miyashita-Ishiwata, M., Reschke, L., Brennan, J. T., Fader, A. and Borahay, M. A., 2021. Diet and nutrition in gynecological disorders: A focus on clinical studies. *Nutrients*, 13(6), p. 1747. Available at https://www.mdpi.com/2072-6643/13/6/1747.

[19] Qi, X., Zhang, W., Ge, M., Sun, Q., Peng, L., Cheng, W. and Li, X., 2021. Relationship between dairy products intake and risk of endometriosis: A systematic review and dose-response meta-analysis. *Frontiers in Nutrition*, 8, p. 449. Available at https://www.ncbi.nlm.nih.gov/pmc/articles/PMC8339299/.

[20] Marziali, M., Venza, M., Lazzaro, S., Lazzaro, A., Micossi, C. and Stolfi, V. M., 2012. Gluten-free diet: A new strategy for management of painful endometriosis related symptoms. *Minerva Chir*, 67(6), pp. 499–504. Available at https://pubmed.ncbi.nlm.nih.gov/23334113/.

Appendix 2 - Glossary Of Nutrients

[1] Jäger, R., Kerksick, C. M., Campbell, B. I., Cribb, P. J., Wells, S. D., Skwiat, T. M., Purpura, M., Ziegenfuss, T. N., Ferrando, A. A., Arent, S. M. and Smith-Ryan, A. E., 2017. International Society of Sports Nutrition position stand: Protein and exercise. *Journal of the International Society of Sports Nutrition*, 14(20). Available at https://pubmed.ncbi.nlm.nih.gov/28642676/.

[2] Public Health England, 11 Dec. 2020. NDNS: Results from years 9 to 11 (combined) – statistical summary. Available at https://www.gov.uk/government/statistics/ndns-results-from-years-9-to-11-2016-to-2017-and-2018-to-2019/ndns-results-from-years-9-to-11-combined-statistical-summary.

[3] Scientific Advisory Committee on Nutrition, Jul. 2017. Update on folic acid. Available at https://assets.publishing.service.gov.uk/government/uploads/system/uploads/attachment_data/file/637111/SACN_Update_on_folic_acid.pdf.

[4] NHS, 3 Aug. 2020. Vitamin E. Available at https://www.nhs.uk/conditions/vitamins-and-minerals/vitamin-e/.

[5] The British Dietetic Association, 8 Jun. 2021. Calcium: Food fact sheet. Available at https://www.bda.uk.com/resource/calcium.html.

[6] Anderson, J. J., Kruszka, B., Delaney, J. A., He, K., Burke, G. L., Alonso, A., Bild, D. E., Budoff, M. and Michos, E. D., 2016. Calcium intake from diet and supplements and the risk of coronary artery calcification and its progression among older adults: 10-year follow-up of the Multi-Ethnic Study of Atherosclerosis (MESA). *Journal of the American Heart Association*, 5(10), p. e003815. Available at https://www.ahajournals.org/doi/10.1161/JAHA.116.003815.

[7] Public Health England, 25 Mar. 2020. National diet and nutrition survey: Assessment of salt intake from urinary sodium in adults (aged 19 to 64 years) in England, 2018 to 2019. Available at https://www.gov.uk/government/statistics/national-diet-and-nutrition-survey-assessment-of-salt-intake-from-urinary-sodium-in-adults-aged-19-to-64-years-in-england-2018-to-2019

[8] COMA, 1991. Dietary reference values for food energy and nutrients for the United Kingdom – report of the Committee on Medical Aspects of Food Policy (COMA). TSO; Scientific Advisory Committee on Nutrition, 2015. Carbohydrates and health. Available at https://assets.publishing.service.gov.uk/government/uploads/system/uploads/attachment_data/file/445503/SACN_Carbohydrates_and_Health.pdf; Scientific Advisory Committee on Nutrition, 2019. Saturated fats and health. Available at https://assets.publishing.service.gov.uk/government/uploads/system/uploads/attachment_data/file/814995/SACN_report_on_saturated_fat_and_health.pdf; Scientific Advisory Committee on Nutrition, 2016. Vitamin D and health. Available at https://assets.publishing.service.gov.uk/government/uploads/system/uploads/attachment_data/file/537616/SACN_Vitamin_D_and_Health_report.pdf; Scientific Advisory Committee on Nutrition, Jul. 2017. Update on folic acid. Available at https://assets.publishing.service.gov.uk/government/uploads/system/uploads/attachment_data/file/637111/SACN_Update_on_folic_acid.pdf; Institute of Medicine. Food and Nutrition Board, 1998. Dietary Reference Intakes: Thiamin, riboflavin, niacin, vitamin B6, folate, vitamin B12, pantothenic acid, biotin, and choline. National Academy Press.

Acknowledgments

This book was the most challenging piece of written work I've ever done, but the most rewarding. However, I could not have done it without the incredible people around me.

Firstly, to start with my inspiration for the book – all of the female patients I've had the pleasure to look after. I've learned more about the female body and mind from you than I could ever learn from the pages of a textbook.

To my family – my mum and my sisters. The strongest women I've ever known and, I'm sure, will ever know. To DB, for being my hype man.

To Carly Cook, my book agent – 6 years later we have three books together, many shared bottles of wine, and a very strong friendship. Not forgetting Nora Millar, the embodiment of Girl Boss and my right hand (wo)man. Thank you for always believing in me – regardless of how wild my ideas sometimes are. I am eternally grateful to you.

My Yellow Kite family – Liz Gough, Issy Gonzalez-Prendergast, and Becca Mundy – thank you for taking a leap of faith with me on this book and bringing my vision to life. A big thank you to Elaine O'Neill and Julia Kellaway who helped soften my science chat and inject some fun back into the book.

Margaux Carpentier, thank you for your beautiful illustrations, and thank you Abi Hartshorne for designing the most gorgeous book that I am so proud to call my own. To the book shoot team – Lizzie Mayson, Jordan Bourke, and Louie Waller – you were a joy to work with (and eat with!) and did such a beautiful job with the recipes.

A special thank you to all the incredible researchers, academics and practitioners who contributed to the book – Dr Sarah McKay, Dr Brendon Stubbs, Alan Flanagan, Dr Sophie Bostock, Dr Marlize De Vivo, Emma Brockwell, Kelly McNulty, and Maeve Hanan, Reene McGregor and Dr Philippa Kaye. Your expertise and insight was invaluable in shaping this book. I feel very fortunate to call many of you colleagues and also friends now.

Finally – to you, my reader. Thank you for purchasing this book and supporting my work. But don't stop here – continue the conversation with other women, and men, in your life. The power for change is greater if we do it together.

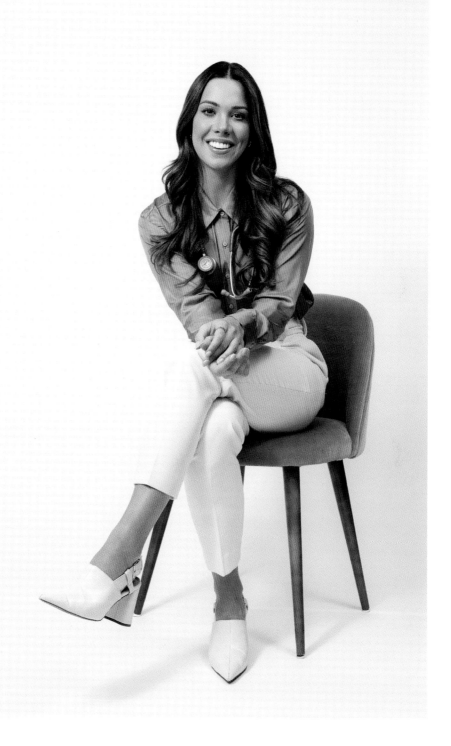

First published in Great Britain in 2022 by Yellow Kite Books
An Imprint of Hodder & Stoughton
An Hachette UK company

2

Executive Publisher: Liz Gough
Project Editor: Isabel Gonzalez-Prendergast
Copyeditor: Julia Kellaway
Designer: Hart Studio
Photographer: Lizzie Mayson
Food Stylist: Jordan Bourke
Prop Stylist: Louie Waller
Illustrator: Margaux Carpentier
Production Controller: Matthew Everett

A CIP catalogue record for this title is available from the British Library

Hardback ISBN 978 1 529 38286 0
eBook ISBN 978 1 529 38435 2

Colour origination by Alta London
Printed and bound in Germany by Mohn Media GmbH

Hodder & Stoughton policy is to use papers that are natural, renewable and recyclable products and made from wood grown in sustainable forests. The logging and manufacturing processes are expected to conform to the environmental regulations of the country of origin.

Yellow Kite
Hodder & Stoughton Ltd
Carmelite House
50 Victoria Embankment
London EC4Y 0DZ

www.yellowkitebooks.co.uk
www.hodder.co.uk